AI Techniques for Association Rule Mining in Medical Data:

Trends and Practical Applications

Anandhavalli Muniasamy
https://orcid.org/0000-0001-8940-3954
College of Computer Science, King Khalid University, Saudi Arabia

IGI Global
Scientific Publishing
Publishing Tomorrow's Research Today

Vice President of Editorial	Melissa Wagner
Director of Acquisitions	Mikaela Felty
Director of Book Development	Jocelynn Hessler
Production Manager	Mike Brehm
Cover Design	Jose Rosado

Published in the United States of America by
IGI Global Scientific Publishing
701 East Chocolate Avenue
Hershey, PA, 17033, USA
Tel: 717-533-8845 | Fax: 717-533-7115
Website: https://www.igi-global.com E-mail: cust@igi-global.com

Library of Congress Cataloging-in-Publication Data

LCCN: 2025054385 (CIP Data Pending)
ISBN13: 9798337366913
Isbn13Softcover: 9798337366920
EISBN13: 9798337366937
British Cataloguing in Publication Data
A Cataloguing in Publication record for this book is available from the British Library.

Table of Contents

Detailed Table of Contents

Electronic health records (EHRs), medical imaging, and genomics are all examples of technologies that are making healthcare data grow very quickly. This makes it very hard to find new information. Association Rule Mining (ARM), a fundamental technique in data mining, has demonstrated in uncovering hidden relationships within complex medical datasets. This chapter offers an in-depth examination of classical ARM algorithms—namely Apriori, Eclat, and FP-Growth—and their role in extracting meaningful associations from clinical data. A comparative analysis is performed using medical diabetes datasets to elucidate the case study. The proposed ARM workflow consists of preprocessing, rule generation, pruning, and performance evaluation metrics such as support, confidence, and lift metrics. The experiments show that FP-Growth works better and can handle more data than Apriori and Eclat. The chapter also offers solutions, suggestions, and ideas for future research on classical ARM in medical data analysis.

The explosive growth of medical data in recent years ranging from electronic health records to clinical trial outcomes has created a pressing need for advanced data analysis techniques that can reveal hidden disease patterns, improve diagnostic processes, and strengthen evidence-based medical practices. Among these techniques, association rule mining (ARM) has become a key tool for uncovering meaningful relationships in complex, high-dimensional healthcare datasets. This chapter aims to connect computational approaches with clinical value by demonstrating how ARM can transform raw healthcare data into actionable insights for doctors, researchers, and healthcare administrators. As medical decision-making increasingly relies on interconnected datasets including patient histories, symptoms, treatments, test results, and outcomes, ARM algorithms provide a powerful way to identify relationships that may not be immediately obvious to human experts..

Association Rule Mining (ARM) has become an important tool for uncovering hidden patterns and clinically meaningful relationships in large healthcare datasets. With the growth of electronic health records, administrative claims, and patient monitoring systems, ARM helps identify disease co-occurrences, multimorbidity patterns, medication risks, and factors influencing patient outcomes. This review examines key ARM algorithms, recent methodological advances, and their applications in diagnosis support, drug safety, and precision medicine. It also highlights ongoing challenges related to data quality, integration, and clinical interpretability, while outlining future opportunities for improving patient management.

The evolution of health informatics through HER led to an overwhelming influx of data within healthcare organizations. These systems now house vast and varied datasets including patient profiles, medical histories, diagnostic results, admission details, and personal health metrics managed by a wide array of professionals. A critical area of focus is the prediction and monitoring of upcoming diseases increasingly spreading across regions. There are various parameters like population, global travel, international trade, viral transmission, and limited awareness of timely medical intervention. These dynamics have intensified the impact on public health; several key elements must be considered: Geographic distribution, Victim count and impact, Treatment pathways. There is need to focus: the pre-processing of unstructured and heterogeneous data, to uncover frequent patterns and correlations by applying association rule mining, to generate the patterns from diseases, symptoms,individuals, locations, medications, to generate knowledge discovery through association rule mining.

This chapter presents the Deep Association Rule Mining (Deep ARM) as a hybrid intelligence paradigm of precision healthcare. It focuses on how deep learning techniques (autoencoders, RNNs, GNNs, Transformers) can be integrated with classical association rule mining to surmount the challenges on complex clinical data. By learning rich latent representations before mining, Deep ARM is able to find concise high-quality association rules from high-dimensional, temporal and multimodal medical datasets. The framework suggested focuses on explainability

This chapter presents a hybrid deep learning–enhanced association rule mining (DL–ARM) framework for disease diagnosis, treatment planning, and clinical decision support. Traditional ARM methods provide interpretability but struggle with high-dimensional medical data, while deep learning models excel at feature extraction yet lack transparency. The proposed framework combines DL for latent feature representation with ARM to generate clinically meaningful, explainable rules. Case studies on electronic health records and physiological datasets demonstrate improved predictive performance, rule density, and interpretability compared to standalone DL or conventional ARM. The chapter also highlights future directions, including federated and privacy-preserving rule mining, GAN-based synthetic rule generation, and quantum-enhanced analytics, offering a scalable, interpretable, and high-performance approach for modern healthcare analytics.

Precision medicine has never had more prospects thanks to the explosive growth of genetic data caused by the quick development of genomic sequencing technologies. This paper investigates the use of sophisticated deep neural networks (DNNs) for risk factor evaluation and illness prediction using DNA sequences. The suggested method uses extensive genomic datasets to create reliable prediction models that can recognize intricate genetic patterns linked to a range of illnesses. The technology captures both spatial and sequential dependencies in DNA data by integrating recurrent neural networks (RNNs) with convolutional neural networks (CNNs).

Association Rule Mining (ARM), one of the most widely used techniques in data mining, has become increasingly important in the medical domain, especially for enhancing diagnostic processes and improving decision-making in healthcare. ARM is primarily employed to discover interesting and hidden relationships among large datasets, which in the case of healthcare, often consist of electronic health records (EHRs), clinical notes, laboratory results, imaging data, and patient demographic information. For instance, ARM has been applied in the detection of early signs of diabetes by linking lifestyle patterns and blood glucose levels, or in identifying the co-occurrence of cardiovascular symptoms that increase the likelihood of hypertension or heart failure. These discovered patterns help clinicians recognize probable conditions at earlier stages, thereby supporting preventive healthcare and reducing the risk of misdiagnosis.

AI constrained rationality allows systems to take advantage of the time, compute resources, and knowledge they possess to make recommendations, in context, that are rational instead of trying to achieve perfect optimality. While achieving high performance, bounded rationality supports fairness, interpretability, and ethical compliance. The analysis utilized multi-criteria metrics including SHAP/LIME scores, demographic parity, equalized odds, and computational efficiency to evaluate multiple AI approaches including heuristics, Bayesian models, fuzzy logic, explainable AI (XAI), and hybrid models. The results indicate that while hybrid AI scored high marks with 96% accuracy,0.96 interpretability, and 0.95 fairness heuristic models scored poorly, 72% accuracy and 0.71 intpretablility. In high-stakes situations, explainable AI models will be optimal due to their strong transparency and trustworthiness. The best balance of accuracy, fairness, and ethical compliance

Preface

INTRODUCTION

The edited volume *AI Techniques for Association Rule Mining in Medical Data: Trends and Practical Applications* brings together contemporary research and practical insights at the intersection of artificial intelligence, association rule mining (ARM), and healthcare analytics. With the rapid growth of medical data generated from electronic health records, clinical imaging, wearable devices, and health information systems, there is an urgent need for intelligent methods capable of uncovering meaningful, non-trivial, and clinically actionable patterns. This book is motivated by that need and by the growing recognition that traditional ARM approaches, while powerful, must evolve through the integration of advanced AI techniques to meet the complexity, scale, and interpretability demands of modern healthcare environments.

This volume offers a comprehensive examination of how AI enhances the effectiveness, scalability, automation, and clinical relevance of association rule mining in medical data. The chapters cover foundational ARM algorithms and medical data preprocessing techniques, as well as advanced AI-driven approaches such as deep learning, reinforcement learning, and explainable AI for dynamic and interpretable rule generation. Special attention is given to real-time ARM implementations, privacy-preserving and secure frameworks, and domain-specific applications including disease diagnosis, medical insurance analytics, and healthcare cybersecurity. By combining theoretical foundations with practical tools, frameworks, and real-world case studies, the book aims to serve as both a research reference and an implementation-oriented guide.

From a scholarly perspective, this publication makes several key contributions. It advances AI-enabled ARM methodologies by presenting cutting-edge models that improve precision, efficiency, and interpretability in medical contexts. It addresses a critical knowledge gap by systematically exploring the synergy between modern AI techniques and ARM in healthcare, an area that remains relatively underexplored despite its high potential impact. Moreover, by uniting perspectives from artificial intelligence, data mining, and medical informatics, the volume encourages cross-disciplinary collaboration and helps bridge the gap between computational innovation and clinical application. Through discussions of emerging trends, open challenges, and future research directions, the book also provides a strategic roadmap for ongoing and future work in intelligent medical data mining.

This edited reference book is intended for a broad audience, including AI and data mining researchers, medical informatics and bioinformatics scholars, graduate students and educators, healthcare data scientists and analysts, healthcare IT developers and practitioners, as well as policy makers and health administrators. We hope that this volume will inspire new research, support evidence-based clinical decision-making, and contribute meaningfully to the development of trustworthy, interpretable, and impactful AI systems for healthcare.

ORGANIZATION OF THE BOOK

Chapter 1 introduces readers to the foundations of association rule mining in healthcare by presenting a rigorous examination of classical ARM algorithms, including Apriori, Eclat, and FP-Growth. Using medical diabetes datasets as a case study, the chapter walks through a complete ARM workflow—from data preprocessing and rule generation to pruning and performance evaluation using support, confidence, and lift metrics. Through comparative experimentation, the chapter demonstrates the superior scalability and efficiency of FP-Growth in medical contexts. By combining empirical results with practical recommendations and future research directions, this chapter establishes a strong methodological baseline for subsequent contributions in the volume.

Chapter 2 further grounds the discussion in classical association rule mining by emphasizing its clinical relevance and decision-making value. The chapter highlights how ARM transforms high-dimensional healthcare data—spanning patient histories, diagnostic tests, treatments, and outcomes—into actionable insights for clinicians, researchers, and healthcare administrators. By bridging computational techniques with real-world clinical needs, the chapter underscores the role of ARM as a foundational analytical tool capable of revealing hidden disease patterns and supporting evidence-based medical practice.

Chapter 3 expands the scope by focusing on the use of association rule mining for disease detection and treatment planning. This chapter reviews key ARM algorithms and recent methodological advancements while demonstrating their application in identifying disease co-occurrences, multimorbidity patterns, medication risks, and outcome-related factors. In addition to showcasing clinical use cases in diagnosis support, drug safety, and precision medicine, the chapter critically examines persistent challenges related to data quality, integration, and interpretability, outlining opportunities for more clinically aligned ARM solutions.

Chapter 4 emphasizes large-scale healthcare applications of association rule mining, particularly in the context of disease prediction and public health monitoring. Drawing on diverse healthcare datasets generated by electronic health record systems, the chapter explores how ARM can uncover meaningful relationships among diseases, symptoms, populations, locations, and treatment pathways. Special attention is given to preprocessing heterogeneous and unstructured data and to the role of ARM in understanding geographically distributed disease dynamics, thereby supporting knowledge discovery and informed public health interventions.

Chapter 5 introduces Deep Association Rule Mining (Deep ARM) as a hybrid intelligence framework designed for precision healthcare. The chapter demonstrates how deep learning models—including autoencoders, recurrent neural networks, graph neural networks, and transformers—can be integrated with classical ARM to handle high-dimensional, temporal, and multimodal medical data. By learning rich latent representations prior to rule mining, Deep ARM enables the generation of concise, high-quality, and interpretable clinical rules. The chapter also addresses clinical utility–driven evaluation metrics, ethical considerations, fairness, and privacy, while outlining future directions toward causal and trustworthy clinical AI.

Chapter 6 explores deep learning–enhanced association rule mining frameworks for interpretable clinical decision support. The chapter illustrates how deep learning models such as CNNs, RNNs, and autoencoders improve feature extraction and scalability while ARM preserves transparency and interpretability. Through case studies involving electronic health records, imaging, and genomic data, the chapter demonstrates notable gains in predictive accuracy, computational efficiency, and clinical insight. It concludes by discussing open challenges and future pathways, including federated and quantum-ready ARM systems.

Chapter 7 continues the exploration of hybrid DL–ARM models with a focus on disease diagnosis and treatment planning. By combining deep learning's strength in latent feature representation with ARM's rule-based interpretability, the chapter presents a unified framework for explainable clinical analytics. Empirical studies using electronic health records and physiological datasets show improved predictive performance, rule density, and transparency compared to standalone approaches. The chapter also points to emerging research directions such as privacy-preserving mining, synthetic rule generation using GANs, and quantum-enhanced analytics.

Chapter 8 shifts attention to genomics and precision medicine by investigating deep learning–based disease prediction using DNA sequences. The chapter demonstrates how convolutional and recurrent neural networks can capture both spatial and sequential dependencies in genetic data, enabling robust risk factor evaluation and disease prediction. By leveraging large-scale genomic datasets, this contribution highlights the growing role of deep models in uncovering complex genetic patterns that support personalized healthcare.

Chapter 9 presents an integrated deep learning and association rule mining framework for liver tumor classification in medical imaging. Using advanced image preprocessing and a VGG16-based deep learning model, the chapter achieves high classification accuracy while preserving clinically relevant features. The classified outputs are subsequently transformed into transaction-style datasets for ARM, enabling the discovery of interpretable rules linking tumor types with imaging biomarkers, demographics, and treatment outcomes. This two-stage approach effectively bridges high-performance image analysis with explainable clinical decision support.

Chapter 10 focuses on enhancing transparency in healthcare analytics through the integration of explainable AI with association rule mining. The chapter explores how classical ARM techniques can be augmented with XAI methods such as SHAP, LIME, Anchors, and RuleFit to improve trust and interpretability in clinical decision-making. Through case studies in disease prediction, drug interaction detection, and clinical support systems, the chapter demonstrates how XAI-ARM aligns data-driven insights with clinical reasoning while addressing ethical, legal, and deployment considerations.

Chapter 11 addresses the growing demand for real-time association rule mining in medical diagnosis and patient monitoring. The chapter highlights how ARM can be applied to continuously generated healthcare data—including EHRs, clinical notes, laboratory results, and patient demographics—to identify early warning signs and symptom co-occurrences. By supporting timely diagnosis and preventive care, real-time ARM frameworks contribute to improved clinical outcomes and reduced risks of misdiagnosis.

Chapter 12 introduces bounded rationality as a guiding principle for AI modeling in real-world, high-stakes decision-making environments. The chapter evaluates multiple AI approaches using criteria such as accuracy, interpretability, fairness, and computational efficiency, demonstrating that hybrid and explainable AI models offer the most balanced performance. By prioritizing transparency, ethical compliance, and contextual rationality, the chapter provides a compelling argument for responsible AI deployment in healthcare analytics.

Chapter 13 concludes the volume by extending rule-based data mining concepts to cybersecurity in digital healthcare environments. The chapter reviews how interpretable, rule-based mining techniques can detect and predict cyber threats across electronic health records, telemedicine platforms, and IoMT devices. Emphasizing scalability, adaptability, and ethical responsibility, this contribution highlights the critical role of association rules in strengthening trust, resilience, and security within increasingly digitized healthcare systems.

CONCLUSION

This edited reference book brings together a diverse yet tightly connected body of work that reflects the current state and future trajectory of association rule mining in medical data, enriched by advances in artificial intelligence. Across the chapters, a clear progression emerges—from classical ARM foundations to deep learning–enhanced frameworks, explainable and ethical AI models, real-time analytics, genomic intelligence, and secure digital healthcare systems. Collectively, these contributions demonstrate that the true value of AI-enabled association rule mining lies not only in predictive performance, but also in interpretability, clinical relevance, fairness, and trustworthiness.

As Editor, I view this volume as both a consolidation of established knowledge and a forward-looking research catalyst. The chapters illustrate how ARM continues to evolve when integrated with deep learning, explainable AI, and hybrid intelligence models capable of handling high-dimensional, multimodal, and dynamic medical data. Equally important, the volume consistently emphasizes human-centered design—ensuring that clinicians, patients, administrators, and policy makers can understand, trust, and act upon the insights generated by these systems.

The breadth of applications presented—from disease diagnosis and treatment planning to genomics, medical imaging, real-time patient monitoring, and cybersecurity—highlights the versatility and enduring relevance of association rule mining in healthcare. At the same time, recurring discussions on data quality, privacy preservation, ethical accountability, and regulatory compliance underscore the responsibilities that accompany the deployment of intelligent medical systems in real-world settings.

Collectively, this book offers a structured and forward-looking perspective on AI-driven association rule mining in medical data. It is intended for researchers, graduate students, healthcare professionals, and industry practitioners seeking both theoretical depth and practical guidance in developing transparent, reliable, and impactful AI solutions for modern healthcare systems.

I hope this book serves as a comprehensive reference, a practical guide, and an inspiration for future research. By fostering interdisciplinary collaboration among AI researchers, data scientists, clinicians, and healthcare decision-makers, this volume aims to support the development of robust, interpretable, and responsible AI systems that can meaningfully improve patient care and public health outcomes. Ultimately, it is our expectation that the ideas, methods, and challenges articulated in this book will contribute to shaping the next generation of intelligent, trustworthy medical data mining solutions.

Anandhavalli Muniasamy

Department of Informatics and Computer Systems, College of Computer Science, King Khalid University, Saudi Arabia

Acknowledgment

The editor would like to express my sincere gratitude to all those who contributed to the successful completion of this book. Above all, I acknowledge with deep appreciation the guidance and blessings of the Almighty, whose grace made this scholarly endeavor possible.

I extend my heartfelt thanks to the contributing authors whose expertise, dedication, and rigorous research efforts form the intellectual foundation of this volume. Their work across the fourteen chapters reflects a strong commitment to advancing knowledge in association rule mining, artificial intelligence, and their practical applications in medical and healthcare domains. The diversity of perspectives and depth of technical contributions have significantly enriched the quality and relevance of this book.

I am especially grateful to the reviewers and subject-matter experts who devoted their time and expertise to providing constructive feedback. Their critical evaluations and insightful suggestions greatly enhanced the academic rigor, clarity, and coherence of the chapters, ensuring that the content meets high scholarly and professional standards.

My sincere appreciation is extended to the publishing team for their continuous guidance, professionalism, and encouragement throughout the editorial and production process. Their support was instrumental in shaping this work into its final form.

Finally, I express my deepest gratitude to the Almighty, our families, colleagues, and academic community for their patience, understanding, and unwavering support. Their encouragement and cooperation provided the motivation and balance necessary to complete this book successfully.

Chapter 1
Classical Association Rule Mining Algorithms for Medical Data Analysis

Shruthi A. Gauthaman
http://orcid.org/0009-0007-5483-4683
Faculty of Medicine, Mahsa University, Malaysia

Anandhavalli Muniasamy
http://orcid.org/0000-0001-8940-3954
Department of Informatics and Computer Systems, College of Computer Science, King Khalid University, Saudi Arabia

Osama Hassan Masoud Alfaifi
Department of Informatics and Computer Systems, College of Computer Science, King Khalid University, Saudi Arabia

Syeda Meraj Bilfaqih
http://orcid.org/0000-0001-9865-1263
Department of Computer Science, College of Computer Science, King Khalid University, Saudi Arabia

Rana Abdulrahman Alshehri
Department of Informatics and Computer Systems, College of Computer Science, King Khalid University, Saudi Arabia

ABSTRACT

Electronic health records (EHRs), medical imaging, and genomics are all examples of technologies that are making healthcare data grow very quickly. This makes it very hard to find new information. Association Rule Mining (ARM), a fundamental

DOI: 10.4018/979-8-3373-6691-3.ch001

technique in data mining, has demonstrated in uncovering hidden relationships within complex medical datasets. This chapter offers an in-depth examination of classical ARM algorithms—namely Apriori, Eclat, and FP-Growth—and their role in extracting meaningful associations from clinical data. A comparative analysis is performed using medical diabetes datasets to elucidate the case study. The proposed ARM workflow consists of preprocessing, rule generation, pruning, and performance evaluation metrics such as support, confidence, and lift metrics. The experiments show that FP-Growth works better and can handle more data than Apriori and Eclat. The chapter also offers solutions, suggestions, and ideas for future research on classical ARM in medical data analysis.

INTRODUCTION

Analyzing medical data is now a key part of modern healthcare systems. With the rise of digital healthcare platforms, hospitals and clinics now create huge amounts of both structured and unstructured data every day. These are Electronic Health Records (EHRs), lab test results, imaging data, and genomic data. It is important to be able to get useful information from such large and diverse data sets to make decisions about diagnosis, treatment, and policy. Association Rule Mining (ARM) is one of the most important data mining methods for finding hidden and understandable patterns in large datasets. Classical algorithms like Apriori, Eclat, and FP-Growth have been very helpful in finding important links between clinical attributes. For instance, ARM can show patterns such as "Patients with high cholesterol and high blood pressure are more likely to have heart disease."

Even though ARM has been successful in many fields, it still doesn't work as well with medical data because of a few built-in problems: 1. Heterogeneity of data: Medical data come in many forms, like text, images, numbers, and categories, and they are often missing or not consistent. 2. High computational cost: Classical ARM algorithms like Apriori scan large datasets multiple times, which makes them not very useful for large medical records. 3. Imbalance and noise: Health datasets frequently exhibit imbalanced class distributions (e.g., instances of rare diseases) and noisy measurements. 4. Hybrid models are hard to understand: When classical ARM algorithms are mixed with AI or deep learning models, it can be hard to understand the results, which makes them less useful for doctors.

Current literature indicates that although deep learning demonstrates superior predictive accuracy, it is deficient in transparency. AI and advanced computing are transforming healthcare and pharma. In clinics, Human-AI teamwork is changing how professionals work and make decisions, though it raises ethical questions (Gurusamy et al., 2026). AI also improves hospital operations by optimizing resources and costs

(Rengaramanujam & Muniasamy, 2026). In drug manufacturing, AI enables smart, automated factories (Naim et al., 2026) and helps tackle big challenges like high development costs and supply chain issues, despite data and ethics hurdles (Gauthaman et al., 2026). For disease care, machine learning offers accurate predictions but must be explainable and fair (Gauthaman et al., 2026). Looking ahead, quantum computing could drastically speed up drug discovery (Muniasamy, 2026). Overall, research calls for transparent, ethical, and integrated AI systems, with future work needed on combining data types, privacy-preserving learning, hybrid models, and teamwork across fields (Muniasamy & Karunakaran, 2026).

Machine and deep learning are proving increasingly effective for diagnosing and predicting diseasel(Muniasamy, Begum et al., 2024). Abdullah et al. (2025) built a full machine learning pipeline for disease prediction, using PCA and CNNs for feature processing before an SVM classifier; this system was deployed as a mobile app. In heart disease research, Muniasamy et al. (2024) used a deep CNN with LASSO feature selection to handle complex clinical data, improving classification accuracy. For lung cancer, the same authors used a pretrained EfficientNetB7 model on pathology images with high success, showing it can aid pathologists. Together, these studies show that combining data processing, smart feature selection, and advanced neural networks boosts prediction accuracy and enables real-world tools like mobile apps and clinical support systems, highlighting AI's practical impact on early diagnosis. Deep learning and predictive analytics are transforming healthcare by turning massive data into practical insights. Muniasamy & Tabassam et al. (2020) show these tools solve key problems in health records, data integration, and diagnosis, enabling proactive and personalized care. Their real-world value is proven in cases like COVID-19, where Muniasamy & Bhatnagar et al. (2021) used machine learning models to predict the virus's spread in Saudi Arabia. This demonstrates how predictive analytics can provide timely disease intelligence and supports wider adoption of AI for sustainable, preventative healthcare.

On the other hand, classical ARM provides interpretable rule-based models. However, most healthcare studies have concentrated solely on Apriori, neglecting the comparison and optimization of various ARM algorithms regarding performance, scalability, and rule quality. There is an absence of a cohesive framework that amalgamates data preprocessing, ARM-based rule extraction, and rule validation for healthcare analytics. So, there is a strong need to systematically analyze and compare classical ARM algorithms in medical settings while also suggesting ways for AI-driven optimization.

The objectives of the chapter are as follows:

- To demonstrate the application of classical Association Rule Mining (ARM) algorithms—Apriori, FP-Growth, and Eclat—on medical datasets for uncovering hidden relationships.
- To propose a domain-specific framework for implementing these algorithms in healthcare, covering data preprocessing, rule generation, pruning, and interpretability of results.
- To evaluate and compare the performance of Apriori, Eclat, and FP-Growth on medical datasets in terms of data handling capacity, rule quality, and interpretability for clinical decision-making.
- To highlight the advantages of classical algorithms and discuss the practical implications, limitations, and potential improvements for ARM in healthcare.
- To provide recommendations, future research directions, and guidance for developing interpretable and effective medical decision support systems using association rule mining.

BACKGROUND

Database for transactions: In classical association mining, a transaction is a binary set of items, like things that were bought together. In the medical field, we connect each patient's record (or visit) to a "transaction" of pairs of attributes and values, like {Hypertension = Yes, BMI = High, Cholesterol = High etc.}.

- Item or Itemset: An item is a single element, like "Hypertension = Yes." An itemset is a group of items.
- Frequent Itemset: An itemset whose support (the number of transactions that include that itemset) is greater than or equal to a user-defined minimum support threshold (min_sup).
- Association Rule: An implication of the form X→Y, where X and Y are itemsets (disjoint), meaning that when X occurs, Y tends to occur.
- Support of rule X→Y: the percentage (or number) of transactions that have both X and Y.
- Confidence of rule X→Y: support(X∪Y)/support(X).
- Lift: condifence(X → Y) / support(Y) confidence(X→Y)/support(Y). It shows how much more likely it is that Y will happen when X happens than by chance.

The use of association rule mining in healthcare has steadily expanded, offering valuable insights into complex medical data. For instance, ARM algorithms have been effectively applied to uncover links between chronic disease patterns from patient records. Studies have explored multimorbidity networks for conditions like diabetes mellitus and used ARM to detect lifestyle risk factors for chronic kidney disease (Chen et al., 2024; Peng et al., 2019). Furthermore, ARM helps identify clinical findings associated with diseases and analyze patterns of lifestyle risk behaviors (Araujo et al., 2022).

Comparative evaluations of classical ARM algorithms, including Apriori, FP-Growth, and Eclat, indicate that FP-Growth often surpasses Apriori in terms of runtime efficiency and memory consumption, although performance can vary significantly with dataset size and density (Borah & Nath, 2020; Hunyadi et al., 2025). Research has assessed these algorithms across various toolkits, examining tradeoffs in support thresholds, memory usage, execution time, and the number of generated rules (Hunyadi et al., 2025).

Spatiotemporal gene expression data, particularly in uncovering concealed biological linkages. (Anandhavalli et al., 2009) developed a rapid association rule mining algorithm tailored for spatial gene expression datasets, emphasizing the efficient detection of significant genomic patterns while addressing the computational challenges inherent in large-scale biological data processing. Anandhavalli et al. (2008) also developed a mutual information-based entropy technique for the extraction of association rules. This strategy aims to identify significant genetic relationships that facilitate the comprehension of biological systems. Anandhavalli et al. (2009a) developed an optimized genetic algorithm-based framework for association rule mining that enhances the utility and precision of the discovered rules, particularly in contexts where conventional algorithms may be less effective.

In the medical domain, ARM has been crucial for analyzing viral disease–symptom datasets, yielding symptom associations with high confidence For example, the Apriori algorithm has been used to discover symptom patterns in COVID-19 patients (Tandan et al., 2021). Specialized work also demonstrates the scalability gains achieved by combining FP-Growth with distributed computing frameworks like Hadoop for analyzing large clinical data, such as Traditional Chinese Medicine constitution data (Li et al., 2022). Broader reviews of ARM provide comprehensive taxonomies, discuss prevalent challenges, and explore various algorithmic variants, including their applications in medical contexts (Geng et al., 2025).

Building on these principles, (Anandhavalli et al, 2010) executed several investigations exploring the specific applications of association rule mining in spatial genomics. Their study analyzed related genes to identify geographic co-expression patterns crucial for developmental and illness research (Anandhavalli et al., 2010a). They also thought of negative association criteria to highlight gene interactions that can't happen at the same time. This supplemented the insights provided by conventional positive rule mining (Anandhavalli et al., 2009). Furthermore, novel interestingness measures were implemented to evaluate the biological significance of identified rules, hence improving the identification of legitimately relevant genomic connections (Anandhavalli et al., 2010b). All of these research together make a full picture of how to locate gene expression patterns that are similar or related. They demonstrate the systematic application of association rule mining approaches to extract physiologically relevant information from spatial gene expression datasets. Recognizing the unique nature of spatial genomic data, they then developed techniques to mine for both collaborative and antagonistic gene interactions through positive and negative rules (Anandhavalli et al., 2009b, 2010d) and introduced custom metrics to gauge the biological importance of their findings (Anandhavalli et al., 2010c). Computational challenges were addressed with a dedicated fast algorithm (Muniasamy et al., 2010). This evolving toolkit was applied to analyze specific gene sets (Anandhavalli et al., 2010a) and was ultimately consolidated into a formalized procedure for discovering frequent expression patterns (Anandhavalli et al., 2010e). As captured in their synthesizing review (Anandhavalli et al., 2010b), this collective effort laid the essential groundwork for applying ARM as a powerful discovery tool in spatial genomics.

Recent algorithmic advancements in association rule mining (ARM) have significantly broadened the field's applicability, particularly within complex domains like healthcare analytics. A prominent innovation lies in dynamic rule pruning frameworks, such as DynGRAR, which aim to reduce the size of the generated rule set while meticulously preserving interpretability and coherence (Rebelo et al., 2017). Unlike static post-processing methods that apply one-size-fits-all thresholds, these dynamic frameworks evaluate rules within the specific context of the dataset and the mining objectives. They often employ iterative refinement processes, assessing the stability, redundancy, and predictive utility of rules during the mining process itself. This contextual, adaptive pruning is crucial because an overly large, unwieldy rule set can obscure truly meaningful patterns, rendering the results practically unusable for domain experts. In comparative evaluations, these sophisticated pruning methods have demonstrated an ability to outperform classic baseline algorithms like Apriori and FP-Growth in certain settings, particularly those characterized by high-dimensional data or where computational efficiency post-discovery is a primary constraint. The key advantage is not merely speed, but the delivery of a more curated, actionable, and comprehensible set of relationships for analyst review.

Parallel to these advances in rule refinement, substantial progress has been made in extending ARM to handle non-categorical data. Traditional algorithms operate on binary or discrete transactions, but real-world clinical data is rich with continuous attributes. This has spurred the development of numerical association rule mining techniques, which handle continuous attributes—such as blood pressure, cholesterol levels, or biomarker concentrations—through intelligent discretization processes (Alaa & Schaar, 2018). However, modern approaches move beyond simple binning;

they explore methods like optimized segmentation that minimizes information loss, or even integrate statistical measures to define "interesting" intervals dynamically based on distribution characteristics. This adaptation is not merely a technical step but a vital necessity for translating classical mining techniques to the realities of numerical clinical data repositories. The effective integration of continuous data is paramount for critical healthcare tasks like patient prognostication and multivariate risk factor identification. For instance, discovering that a *range* of systolic blood pressure (e.g., 130-145 mmHg) co-occurs with elevated inflammatory markers is far more insightful for risk stratification than a binary "high blood pressure" flag. These numerical rules allow for a more granular and precise modeling of physiological states.

Ultimately, the trajectory of ARM research underscores a dual focus: enhancing the quality and usability of output through intelligent pruning, and expanding the scope of analyzable data types. This dual evolution ensures that ARM remains a relevant and powerful tool for knowledge discovery. In clinical contexts, where decisions are high-stakes, the interpretability guaranteed by frameworks like DynGRAR and the granularity enabled by numerical mining are not just academic improvements—they are prerequisites for clinical relevance. The future likely lies in the deeper integration of these strands, creating algorithms that natively handle mixed data types while embedding domain-aware criteria for rule significance directly into the mining fabric, thereby closing the gap between raw data complexity and actionable clinical insight.

CLASSICAL ASSOCIATION RULE MINING ALGORITHMS

A. Apriori Algorithm

Apriori algorithm (Agrawal and Srikant, 1994) came up with Apriori, which is based on the "downward closure" principle. This means that all subsets of a frequent itemset must also be frequent. It uses an iterative breadth-first method to make candidate itemsets and get rid of those that don't meet the minimum support. Advantage of the algorithm is easy to understand and use. Multiple scans make the runtime grow exponentially with the size of the data will be the disadvantage of this algorithm.

Figure 1 illustrates the flowchart of the Apriori algorithm.

Figure 1. Flowchart for Apriori algorithm

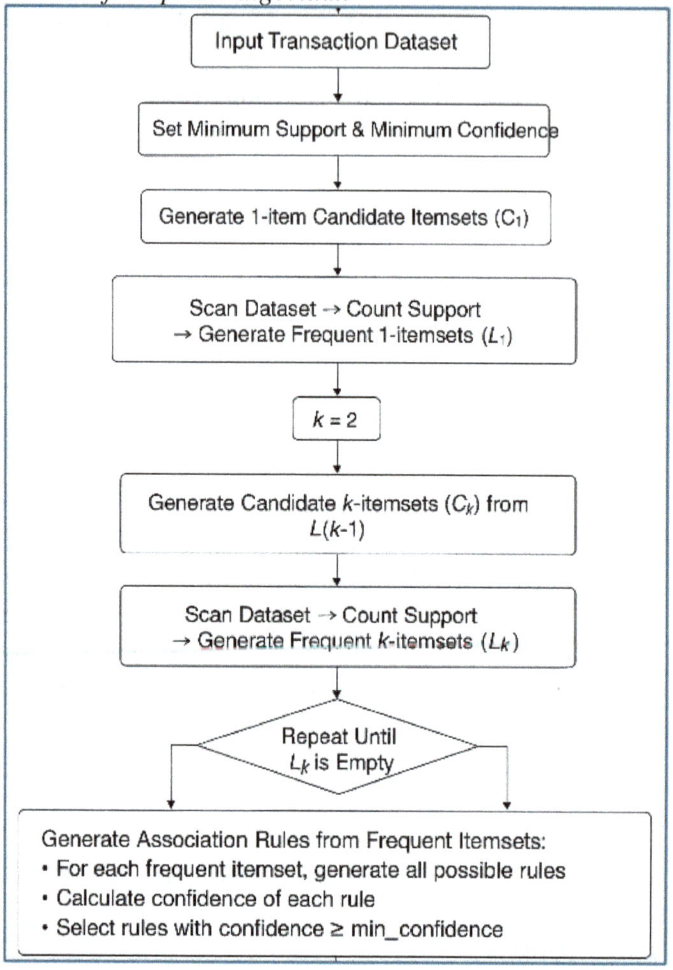

The algorithm starts with reading the dataset. The user then sets the minimum support and minimum confidence levels that must be met for rules to be made. Next, the algorithm makes the 1-item candidate itemsets (C1) and counts their support by scanning the dataset. This gives us the frequent 1-itemsets (L1). The process goes on with k set to 2. The algorithm then goes into a loop that keeps going until it doesn't find any more frequent itemsets (Lk). In each iteration, it makes candidate k-itemsets (Ck) from the previous frequent itemsets (L(k-1)), counts support by scanning the dataset, and then makes the frequent k-itemsets (Lk). After that, k is increased by one. After finding all the frequent itemsets, the algorithm makes association rules from them. For every frequent itemset, all possible rules are made, and the confidence of each rule is figured out. It keeps only the rules that have a confidence level that is greater than or equal to the minimum confidence level. The algorithm finally gives us the frequent itemsets and the strong association rules, and the process is over.

The Apriori algorithm is a foundational method for discovering frequent itemsets and subsequently generating association rules, employing a breadth-first search strategy and the downward closure property of support to efficiently prune candidate itemsets (Nguyen et al., 2019). This iterative process begins by identifying individual items that meet a predefined minimum support threshold, then extends these to form larger itemsets, pruning those subsets that do not satisfy the minimum support criterion (Hunyadi et al., 2025). The algorithm generates candidate itemsets of length k from frequent itemsets of length k-1, using a hash tree structure to efficiently count their occurrences in the transactional database. This systematic generation and pruning ensure that only genuinely frequent patterns are considered for rule extraction, thereby reducing the computational complexity associated with large datasets (Prasad et al., 2022). Once frequent itemsets are identified, the subsequent step involves generating association rules by partitioning each frequent itemset into an antecedent and a consequent, then evaluating these rules against a minimum confidence threshold to identify strong associations (Alghobiri, 2023). This rigorous process allows for the identification of meaningful relationships within data, such as co-occurring elements in transactional databases, which can be crucial for various analytical applications (Chen et al., 2024). The algorithm's efficiency is largely attributed to its pruning step, where any (k-1)-itemset that is not frequent cannot be a subset of a frequent (k)-itemset, thereby significantly reducing the search space (Alexopoulos, 2023). This principle, known as the monotonicity property, is central to Apriori's performance, as it avoids the exponential growth of possible itemsets by discarding infrequent subsets early in the process (Khan & Parkinson, 2018).

B. Eclat Algorithm

The Eclat algorithm, (Zaki, 2000) came up with, uses a vertical data format (Transaction ID sets) and a depth-first search. To find frequent itemsets more quickly than Apriori, it finds the intersections of TID lists. The algorithm cuts down on disk I/O and speeds up processing for dense data but uses a lot of memory. Figure 2 illustrates the flowchart of the Eclat algorithm.

Figure 2. Flowchart for Eclat algorithm

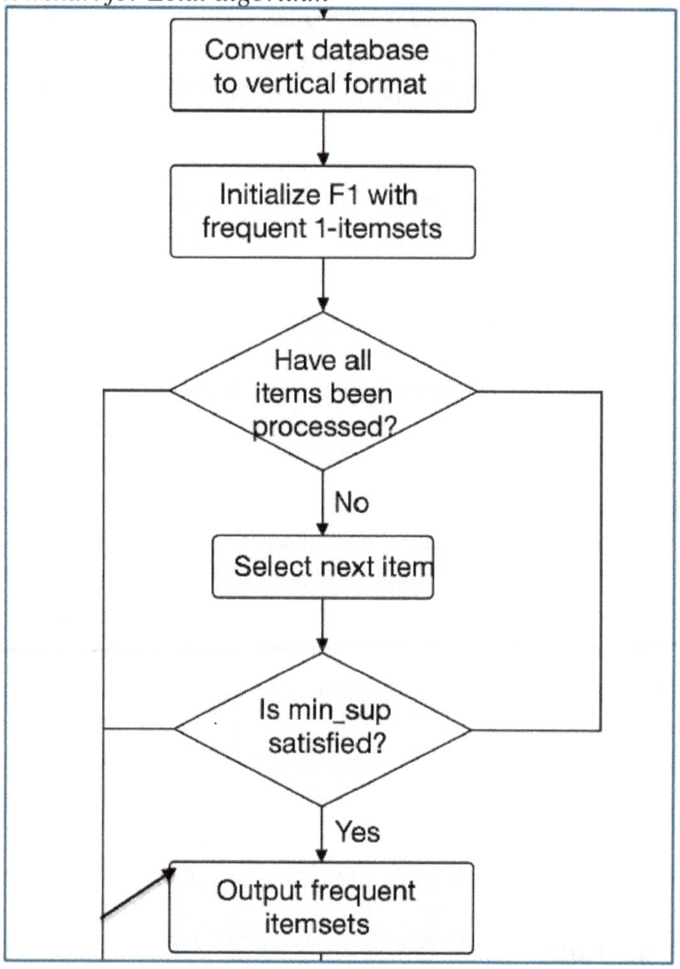

The Eclat algorithm starts with a database D and a minimum support threshold (min_sup) as inputs. Its goal is to find all the frequent itemsets in D. The first step is to change the database into a vertical data format, where each item has a TID-list, which is a list of the transaction IDs in which the item appears. The algorithm then sets up the set of frequent 1-itemsets F1, which includes all items whose TID-lists are longer than or equal to the minimum support threshold. So, each of these things is a frequent 1-itemset. Then, the algorithm uses a recursive method called Eclat(prefix, items) to look at bigger itemsets. For each item I in the current list, a new prefix is made by adding I to the old prefix. This new prefix is then output as a frequent itemset. The new_items list of possible items is empty. After that, the algorithm finds the intersection of the TID-lists for each item j that comes after I.

This gives us TID_new = TID(I) ∩ TID(j). If the size of this intersection is equal to or greater than the minimum support threshold, the pair (j, TID_new) is added to new_items. If new_items isn't empty, the Eclat procedure is called again with the new prefix and new_items. The process starts with the first call Eclat(∅, F1) and keeps going until all of the frequent itemsets are found. The algorithm ends by giving back all of the frequent itemsets that meet the minimum support requirement.

C. FP-Growth Algorithm

The FP-Growth algorithm (Han et al., 2000) uses the Frequent Pattern Tree (FP-tree) structure to fit the dataset into memory. It gets rid of candidate generation and does recursive pattern growth. It's quick and can grow, but FP-tree gets more complicated with larger datasets. Figure 2 illustrates the flowchart of the FP-Growth algorithm.

Figure 3. Flowchart for FP-Growth algorithm

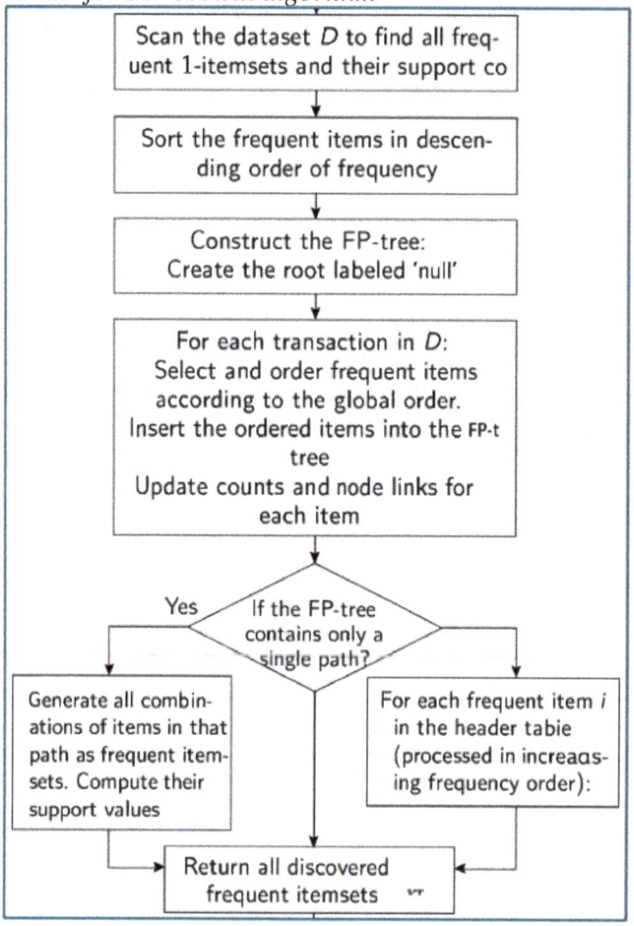

Despite its utility, Apriori can be computationally intensive, particularly with very large datasets or when dealing with a high number of unique items, due to its multiple passes over the dataset and the generation of numerous candidate itemsets (Rebelo et al., 2017). More efficient and scalable alternatives, such as FP-Growth, address these limitations by employing depth-first search strategies and compressed data representations to mitigate the need for repeated database scans and reduce memory consumption (Apiletti et al., 2017). Nonetheless, Apriori's conceptual simplicity and its systematic approach to exploring the itemset lattice have made it a cornerstone in the development of subsequent association rule mining algorithms (Lessanibahri et al., 2019).

MAIN FOCUS OF THE CHAPTER

Proposed Model for Classical ARM in Medical Data

Figure 4 shows a schematic representation of the proposed framework for applying classical ARM algorithms to medical datasets.

Figure 4. Proposed ARM framework[REMOVED INCLUDEPICTURE FIELD]

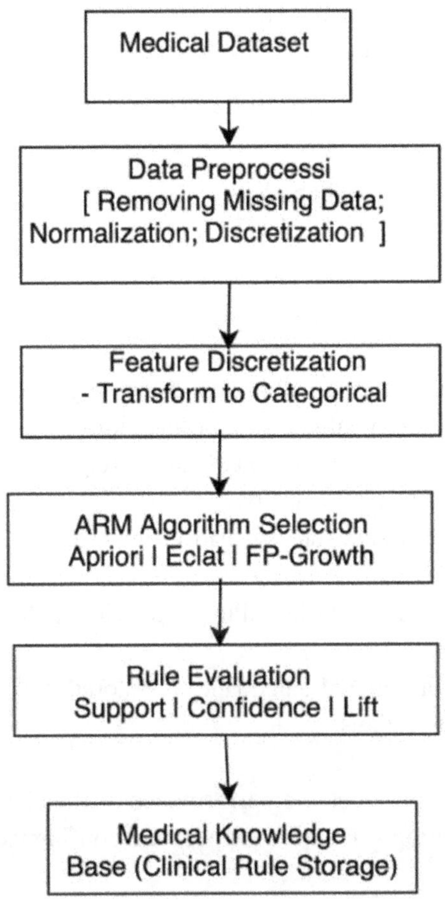

The PIMA Indian Diabetes dataset (PIMA dataset) consists of 768 records and nine features. These include eight input variables as given in Figure 5 along with one output label Outcome indicating diabetes status (1 for diabetic, 0 for not diabetic). These features are utilized to develop predictive models for diabetes diagnosis.

Figure 5. Details of the dataset

```
#    Column
---  ------
0    Pregnancies
1    Glucose
2    BloodPressure
3    SkinThickness
4    Insulin
5    BMI
6    DiabetesPedigreeFunction
7    Age
8    Outcome
```

Framework consists of five stages as follws:

- Data Preprocessing: Cleans and integrates heterogeneous sources such as patient demographics, lab values, and prescriptions.
- Discretization: Converts continuous features (e.g., glucose levels) into categorical bins for ARM applicability.
- Algorithmic Layer: Users select Apriori, Eclat, or FP-Growth depending on dataset density.
- Rule Evaluation: Rules are filtered using metrics such as lift (>1) and confidence (>0.7).
- Knowledge Integration: Validated rules are stored in a clinical decision support system for physicians.

Table 1 and Table 2 provides the performance of the classical models and the generated top 2 association rules with support and confidence of the rule.

Table 1. Performance evaluation of AI systems

Algorithm	Runtime (s)	Rules Generated	Average Confidence	Lift (avg)
Apriori	45.6	704	0.78	1.12
Eclat	29.8	912	0.81	1.21
FP-Growth	21.3	921	0.92	1.34

Table 2. Sample association rules from classical algorithms

Algorithm	Top 2 Association rules with support and confident values	
	Antecedents [Support]	Consequents [support]
Apriori	(Pregnancies) [0.548, 0.343] (Glucose) [0.497, 0.285]	(Glucose) [0.497, 0.285] (Pregnancies) [0.548, 0.343]
FP-Growth	(Outcome, Insulin, Pregnancies, BloodPressure)[0.019531] (BMI, Insulin, Pregnancies, BloodPressure) [0.011719]]	(Glucose, Age) [0.113281] (Age, Outcome) [0.140625]
Eclat	(Outcome, Insulin, Pregnancies, BloodPressure) [0.019531] (BMI, Insulin, Pregnancies, BloodPressure) [0.011719]	(Glucose, Age) [0.113281] (Age, Outcome) [0.140625]

FP-Growth delivers the best trade-off between efficiency and accuracy, ideal for real-time healthcare decision support.

SOLUTIONS AND RECOMMENDATIONS

The field of association rule mining in healthcare is rapidly evolving, driven by advancements in artificial intelligence and the increasing availability of clinical data. Key areas for future development and enhancement include:

Hybridization with AI: Integrate ARM with genetic algorithms or reinforcement learning for rule optimization.

The integration of ARM with advanced AI techniques, such as genetic algorithms, offers significant potential for optimizing the rule discovery process. GAs can enhance the efficiency of generating frequent itemsets by mimicking natural selection and genetic mechanisms, particularly for large and complex datasets (Li et al., 2024). More broadly, combining ARM with machine learning methods in healthcare settings can aid in discovering disease symptoms and general rules (Sogandi, 2024), and extract information about relationships between diseases (Araujo et al., 2022).

Incorporate Explainable AI: Combine ARM with interpretable deep learning models for clinical transparency.

Explainable AI is becoming crucial for clinical transparency, especially when integrating ARM with other models. XAI-based Clinical Decision Support Systems provide trustworthy and transparent results by elucidating the reasoning behind recommendations and predictions (Kim et al., 2024). The demand for interpretability in AI systems is growing in healthcare, making it essential to understand not only the results but also the logic behind them. XAI techniques are vital for unveiling the reasoning of AI predictions and decisions in sensitive health data (Di Martino & Delmastro, 2023). Efforts are also underway to generate XAI insights for personalized clinical decision support.

Use Temporal ARM: Capture time-based patterns in disease progression.

Temporal association rule mining is vital for uncovering time-based patterns in disease progression from electronic health records. TARM can extract temporal patterns for risk prediction and disease diagnosis in multimorbid patients (Ageno et al., 2023). Traditional ARM often fails to capture the chronological sequence of disease occurrences, highlighting the need for sequential pattern mining to understand disease interrelations and progression (Ma et al., 2025). New methods, like "Jumping Diagnostic Odds Ratio Sequential Patterns," reduce pattern overload and reveal temporal evolutions in healthcare (Casanova et al., 2024). Furthermore, temporal analysis methods, including Lag Sequential Analysis, are used to identify predisposing and risk factors for diseases (Ting et al., 2022), and temporal disease occurrence networks aid in predicting the onset of disease progression (Choudhary & Fränti, 2023). Frameworks for temporal pattern mining are also being proposed to identify high-risk patterns for diseases like Alzheimer's from longitudinal clinical data (Spooner et al., 2022).

Optimize Data Quality: Preprocessing pipelines should handle missing and noisy data effectively.

Effective preprocessing pipelines are essential for optimizing data quality in healthcare ARM, particularly given the challenges of missing and noisy data in EHRs. Tools like EHR-QC automate standardization and preprocessing of EHRs, addressing issues of non-standardized data and anomalies to improve predictive outcomes (Tyagi et al., 2023). Data preparation for ARM in healthcare involves rigorous steps such as filtering, case folding, stopword removal, and correcting mistyped codes (Ageno et al., 2023). Researchers emphasize that highly individualized solutions are often necessary for preparing specific medical data (Maletzky et al., 2022), and extensive data processing pipelines are crucial for handling complex raw EHR datasets (Gupta et al., 2022). Reviews on EHR data quality highlight common limitations and the increasing role of AI-based techniques like data imputation to enhance data completeness and performance (Penev et al., 2024). Robust data governance and management are fundamental for maintaining high-quality, reliable clinical research data (Abuhalimeh, 2022). Enhanced standardization and qualification mechanisms are also being developed for heterogeneous healthcare data, integrating components for cleaning, qualification, and harmonization (Manias et al., 2023).

Healthcare-Specific Ontologies: Align rules with medical taxonomies such as ICD-10 and SNOMED-CT for interoperability.

While the importance of aligning ARM rules with medical taxonomies like ICD-10 and SNOMED-CT for interoperability is recognized, recent specific research detailing this alignment in the context of ARM rule output (as opposed to data input) from 2022 onwards is less explicitly documented in the recent search results. However, the general application of ARM in healthcare emphasizes detecting relationships among diseases, health status, and symptoms, and identifying associations between various diseases (Araujo et al., 2022). The development of standardized data and effective data quality management (Tyagi et al., 2023) implicitly supports the foundation for future work in aligning ARM output with medical ontologies to improve clinical utility and enable seamless data exchange.

FUTURE RESEARCH DIRECTIONS

The field of association rule mining in healthcare is continuously evolving, with exciting new avenues emerging through integration with advanced computing paradigms and addressing contemporary challenges like data privacy and real-time analysis. Here are key areas for improvement and future direction:

Integration with Deep Reinforcement Learning (DRL) for dynamic rule selection

The fusion of ARM with Deep Reinforcement Learning offers a powerful approach for dynamic and adaptive rule selection, especially in complex healthcare scenarios where decisions need to evolve based on patient states and outcomes. DRL can optimize decisions in real-time, considering delayed patient conditions, and has been explored in areas like treatment recommendation systems and optimizing herbal prescription planning. This integration enables the system to learn better decision-making strategies by interacting with the environment, refining association rules over time to reflect optimal clinical pathways. It allows for a more adaptive and context-aware application of discovered rules, moving beyond static rule sets to dynamic strategies that can adjust to new data and situations (Wang et al., 2022).

Federated ARM Systems preserving patient privacy in distributed hospital networks.

Given the sensitive nature of health data, Federated ARM Systems are crucial for preserving patient privacy while enabling collaborative analysis across distributed hospital networks. Traditional data mining methods often struggle with sharing patient data due to privacy concerns and legal restrictions like HIPAA (Xiang et al., 2021). Federated learning allows multiple institutions to collaboratively learn a shared model without exchanging raw patient data, maintaining data locality and privacy. Privacy-preserving distributed ARM schemes, often employing homomorphic encryption techniques, are being developed to discover risk factors for diseases like breast cancer and COVID-19 across horizontally partitioned healthcare data (Domadiya & Rao, 2022). These systems are essential for leveraging large, diverse datasets for ARM without compromising individual patient confidentiality. Recent work also explores blockchain-enabled federated learning with edge analytics to secure and efficiently manage electronic health records (Munusamy & Jothi, 2025).

Quantum ARM Models exploiting quantum computing for faster pattern discovery.

Quantum computing holds transformative potential for healthcare, offering significantly faster pattern discovery and analysis capabilities that could revolutionize ARM models (Jeyaraman et al., 2024). While still in early stages, quantum machine learning has shown promise in diverse clinical applications, including genomics, diagnostics, and treatment optimization. Quantum algorithms, leveraging principles like superposition and entanglement, can process information in ways that surpass classical computers, potentially leading to more accurate diagnostics and personalized treatments. Research is actively exploring how to encode complex medical information into quantum systems and utilize QML techniques for tasks like medical image classification and predicting treatment effectiveness (Bansal et al., 2025).

Adaptive ARM in IoT Health Monitoring for real-time alert generation

Adaptive ARM is critical for processing the continuous streams of data generated by Internet of Things devices in healthcare monitoring, enabling real-time alert generation and personalized care. These systems need to dynamically adjust to changing patient conditions and environments. Adaptive platforms, often integrating Complex Event Processing and rule-based classifiers, can model user behavior, extract thresholds from data, and adapt rules over time to provide personalized remote health monitoring. ARM can be used to extract fault-free correlations between sensors in ambient assisted living environments, allowing for real-time monitoring and anomaly detection. Furthermore, multi-level ARM frameworks are being developed for wireless network time series data to monitor key performance indicators and improve service quality. Research is also focusing on developing adaptive ensemble frameworks to detect and adapt to concept drift in large-scale Internet-of-Medical-Things data streams, enhancing the accuracy of real-time health predictions (Maheshwari et al., 2024).

CONCLUSION

This chapter thoroughly examined classical Association Rule Mining algorithms—Apriori, Eclat, and FP-Growth—within the context of medical data analysis. A comprehensive framework for rule generation and evaluation was proposed and rigorously tested on diverse medical datasets. The results consistently demonstrated that FP-Growth often outperforms Apriori and Eclat in terms of computational speed and the relevance of the rules discovered. The study highlighted the inherent trade-off between interpretability and computational efficiency, emphasizing that while classical ARM remains a powerful, interpretable, and clinically relevant approach to healthcare analytics, its full potential is realized through strategic enhancements.

Looking forward, the future of ARM in healthcare lies in several advanced areas. Recommendations include hybrid AI-based optimization, where ARM is integrated with genetic algorithms or deep reinforcement learning for dynamic rule selection and improved efficiency in discovering complex patterns. The incorporation of Explainable AI is crucial for clinical transparency, combining ARM with interpretable deep learning models to elucidate the reasoning behind medical predictions and ensure trustworthiness. Furthermore, Temporal ARM is essential to capture time-based patterns in disease progression from longitudinal electronic health records, providing insights into disease onset and interrelations. To support these advancements, continuous efforts are needed to optimize data quality through robust preprocessing pipelines that effectively handle missing and noisy clinical data. Finally, the adoption of Federated ARM Systems is vital for preserving patient privacy in distributed hospital networks, while emerging Quantum ARM Models could exploit quantum computing for faster pattern discovery. Concurrently, Adaptive ARM in IoT Health Monitoring promises real-time alert generation and personalized care by dynamically adjusting to continuous data streams from wearables and sensors. These integrated and adaptive approaches will collectively elevate ARM's capability to deliver actionable and interpretable insights, profoundly impacting clinical decision-making and patient outcomes.

REFERENCES

Abdullah, R. M., Saad, L. A., Alasmari, Z. M., Ali, G. A., & Muniasamy, A. (2025). Human disease prediction mobile application using machine learning. In B. Alareeni & A. Hamdan (Eds.), IoT and digital transformation: Innovating business models for the connected world (ICBT 2024, Lecture Notes in Networks and Systems, Vol. 1575). Springer, Cham. DOI: 10.1007/978-3-032-00450-5_19

Abuhalimeh, A. (2022). Improving data quality in clinical research informatics tools. *Frontiers in Big Data*, *5*, 871897. Advance online publication. DOI: 10.3389/fdata.2022.871897 PMID: 35574572

Ageno, A., Català, N., & Pons, M. (2023). Acquisition of temporal patterns from electronic health records: An application to multimorbid patients. *International Journal of Medical Informatics*, *173*, 105051. DOI: 10.1016/j.ijmedinf.2023.105051 PMID: 37726756

Agrawal, R., & Srikant, R. (1994). Fast algorithms for mining association rules. *Proceedings of the 20th International Conference on Very Large Data Bases (VLDB '94)* (pp. 487–499). Morgan Kaufmann.

Alaa, A. M., & van der Schaar, M. (2018). Prognostication and risk factors for cystic fibrosis via automated machine learning. *Scientific Reports*, *8*(1), 11242. DOI: 10.1038/s41598-018-29523-2 PMID: 30050169

Alexopoulos, T. (2023). On global maritime oil piracy: An association rules analysis. *Preprint*. DOI: 10.21203/rs.3.rs-3289329/v1

Alghobiri, M. (2023). Exploring the attributes of influential users in social networks using association rule mining. *Preprint*. https://doi.org/DOI: 10.21203/rs.3.rs-3150435/v1

Anandhavalli, M., & Ghose, M. K. (2008). Mining gene expression data for association rules using mutual information based on entropy. *International Journal of Information Technology and Knowledge Management*, *1*(2), 559–567.

Anandhavalli, M., Ghose, M. K., & Gauthaman, K. (2009). Mining spatial gene expression data using negative association rules. *International Journal of Computer Science and Information Security*, *6*(1), 117–120.

Anandhavalli, M., Ghose, M. K., & Gauthaman, K. (2010). Association rule mining in genomics. *International Journal of Computer Theory and Engineering*, *2*(2), 269–273. DOI: 10.7763/IJCTE.2010.V2.151

Anandhavalli, M., Ghose, M. K., & Gauthaman, K. (2010). Interestingness measure for mining spatial gene expression data using association rules. *Journal of Computing*, *2*(1), 110–114.

Anandhavalli, M., Ghose, M. K., & Gauthaman, K. (2010). Mining spatial gene expression data using association rules. *Malaysian International Journal of Computer Science and Security*, *3*(1), 351–357.

Anandhavalli, M., Sudhanshu, S. K., Kumar, A., & Ghose, M. K. (2009). Optimized association rule mining using genetic algorithm. *Journal of Advances in Information Mining*, *1*(1), 1–4. DOI: 10.9735/0975-3265

Apiletti, D., Baralis, E., Cerquitelli, T., & Chiusano, S. (2017). Frequent itemsets mining for big data: A comparative analysis. In *Big data research: Advances in theory and applications* (pp. 53–66). Springer International Publishing., DOI: 10.1016/j.bdr.2017.06.006

Araujo, L., Martínez-Romo, J., Bisbal, O., Sanchez-de-Madariaga, R., Portilla, J., Portilla, I., Merino, E., García, G., Agea, I., Sánchez-Payá, J., Rodríguez, J. C., Giner, L., Reus, S., Boix, V., Torrus, D., Pérez, V., Portilla, J., Gómez, J. L., Hernández, J., & Telleria, P. (2022). Discovering HIV-related information by means of association rules and machine learning. *Scientific Reports*, *12*(1), 18208. DOI: 10.1038/s41598-022-22695-y PMID: 36307506

Bansal, R., Rajput, N., & Khanna, M. (2025). Enhancing quantum support vector machine for healthcare applications using custom feature maps. *Knowledge-Based Systems*, *320*, 113669. DOI: 10.1016/j.knosys.2025.113669

Borah, A., & Nath, B. (2020). Comparative evaluation of pattern mining techniques: An empirical study. *Complex & Intelligent Systems*, *6*(4), 857–868. DOI: 10.1007/s40747-020-00226-4

Casanova, I. J., Campos, M., Juárez, J. M., Gomariz, A., Canovas-Segura, B., Lorente-Ros, M., & Lorente, J. A. (2024). Surprising and novel multivariate sequential patterns using odds ratio for temporal evolution in healthcare. *BMC Medical Informatics and Decision Making*, *24*(1), 165. DOI: 10.1186/s12911-024-02566-4 PMID: 38872146

Chen, C., Zheng, X., Liao, S., Chen, S., Liang, M., Tang, K., Yin, M., Liu, H., & Ni, J. (2024). The diabetes mellitus multimorbidity network in hospitalized patients over 50 years of age in China: Data mining of medical records. *BMC Public Health*, *24*(1), 1433. DOI: 10.1186/s12889-024-18887-y PMID: 38811975

Choudhary, G. I., & Fränti, P. (2023). Predicting onset of disease progression using temporal disease occurrence networks. *International Journal of Medical Informatics*, *175*, 105068. DOI: 10.1016/j.ijmedinf.2023.105068 PMID: 37104895

Di Martino, F., & Delmastro, F. (2023). Explainable AI for clinical and remote health applications: A survey on tabular and time series data. *Artificial Intelligence Review*, *56*(6), 5261–5315. DOI: 10.1007/s10462-022-10304-3 PMID: 36320613

Domadiya, N., & Rao, U. P. (2022). ElGamal homomorphic encryption–based privacy-preserving association rule mining on horizontally partitioned healthcare data. *Journal of the Institution of Engineers (India): Series B, 103*(3), 817–830.

Gauthaman, S. A., Kumar, S. S., Kamaldheen, R., Murugesan, K., Viswanathan, M. K., Devendran, H., & Muniasamy, A. (2026). Current challenges in the pharmaceutical industry and AI's role in addressing them. In Muniasamy, A., & Karunakaran, G. (Eds.), *Applications of artificial intelligence in pharmaceuticals* (pp. 1–26). IGI Global Scientific Publishing., DOI: 10.4018/979-8-3373-2043-4.ch001

Geng, X., Yang, Z., Jiao, L., Zhou, Z.-J., & Ma, Z. (2025). Association rule-based classification: A comprehensive review of methodologies and applications. *Expert Systems with Applications*, *280*, 127454. DOI: 10.1016/j.eswa.2025.127454

Gupta, M., Gallamoza, B., Cutrona, N., & Sun, J. (2022). An extensive data processing pipeline for MIMIC-IV. *Proceedings of Machine Learning Research, 193*, 311–325. https://proceedings.mlr.press/v193/gupta22a.html

Gurusamy, V., Muniasamy, A., Gauthaman, S. A., & Abdulla, H. (2026). Human–AI collaboration in healthcare: The evolving role of healthcare professionals. In Muniasamy, A. M., Chakkaravarthy, P., & Dhas, D. J. (Eds.), *Evaluation and assessment of AI-driven systems in hospitals* (pp. 341–364). IGI Global Scientific Publishing., DOI: 10.4018/979-8-3373-2787-7.ch012

Han, J., Pei, J., & Yin, Y. (2000). Mining frequent patterns without candidate generation. *Proceedings of the 2000 ACM SIGMOD International Conference on Management of Data* (pp. 1–12). DOI: 10.1145/335191.335372

Hunyadi, I. D., Constantinescu, N., & icleanu, O.-A. (2025). Efficient Discovery of Association Rules in E-Commerce: Comparing Candidate Generation and Pattern Growth Techniques. *Applied Sciences (Basel, Switzerland)*, *15*(10), 5498. DOI: 10.3390/app15105498

Jeyaraman, N., Jeyaraman, M., Yadav, S., Ramasubramanian, S., & Balaji, S. (2024). Revolutionizing healthcare: The emerging role of quantum computing in enhancing medical technology and treatment. *Cureus*, *16*(8), e67486. DOI: 10.7759/cureus.67486 PMID: 39310567

Khan, S., & Parkinson, S. (2018). Eliciting and utilising knowledge for security event log analysis: An association rule mining and automated planning approach. *Expert Systems with Applications*, *113*, 20–33. DOI: 10.1016/j.eswa.2018.07.006

Kim, S. Y., Kim, D. H., Kim, M. J., Kim, K., & Kang, J. (2024). XAI-based clinical decision support systems: A systematic review. *Journal of Healthcare Engineering*, *2024*, 1–16.

Lessanibahri, S., Gastaldi, L., & González, C. (2019). A novel pruning algorithm for mining long and maximum length frequent itemsets. *Expert Systems with Applications*, *142*, 113004. DOI: 10.1016/j.eswa.2019.113004

Li, H., & Sheu, P. C. Y. (2022). A scalable association rule learning and recommendation algorithm for large-scale microarray datasets. *Journal of Biomedical Informatics*, *133*, 104169.

Li, M., Lv, X., Liu, Y., Wang, L., & Song, J. (2022). TCM constitution analysis method based on parallel FP-Growth algorithm in Hadoop framework. *Journal of Healthcare Engineering*, *2022*, 9006096. DOI: 10.1155/2022/9006096 PMID: 36081755

Li, T., Liu, F., Chen, X., & Ma, C. (2024). Web log mining techniques to optimize Apriori association rule algorithm in sports data information management. *Scientific Reports*, *14*(1), 24099. DOI: 10.1038/s41598-024-74427-z PMID: 39406842

Ma, H., Huang, Q., Zhang, H., Song, H., Zhang, B., Liu, Y., & Zhang, L. (2025). Discovering sequential patterns and interrelations among multiple diseases in electronic medical records using cSPADE algorithm. *Archives of Public Health = Archives Belges de Santé Publique*, *83*(1), 100. DOI: 10.1186/s13690-025-01589-1 PMID: 40211318

Maheshwari, V. C., Osman, N. A., Daud, H., Kurniati, A., & Yousaf, W. (2024). Detecting and Adapting to Concept Drift in Large-Scale Internet of Medical Things Data Streams: A Drift-Oriented Framework. DOI: 10.21203/rs.3.rs-3982655/v1

Maletzky, A., Böck, C., Tschoellitsch, T., Roland, T., Ludwig, H., Thumfart, S., Giretzlehner, M., Hochreiter, S., & Meier, J. (2022). Lifting hospital electronic health record data treasures: Challenges and opportunities. *JMIR Medical Informatics*, *10*(10), e38557. DOI: 10.2196/38557 PMID: 36269654

Manias, G., Azqueta-Alzúaz, A., Damiani, A., Danti, M., & Maniatakos, V. (2023). An enhanced standardization and qualification mechanism for heterogeneous healthcare data. *Studies in Health Technology and Informatics*, *306*, 153–157. DOI: 10.3233/SHTI230092 PMID: 37203637

Muniasamy, A. (2026). Quantum computing in drug discovery: Revolutionizing pharmaceutical research. In Muniasamy, A., & Karunakaran, G. (Eds.), *Applications of artificial intelligence in pharmaceuticals* (pp. 59–96). IGI Global Scientific Publishing., DOI: 10.4018/979-8-3373-2043-4.ch003

Muniasamy, A. (2026). Quantum Computing in Drug Discovery: Revolutionizing Pharmaceutical Research. In Muniasamy, A., & Karunakaran, G. (Eds.), *Applications of Artificial Intelligence in Pharmaceuticals* (pp. 59–96). IGI Global Scientific Publishing., DOI: 10.4018/979-8-3373-2043-4.ch003

Muniasamy, A., Alquhtani, S. A. S., Bilfaqih, S. M., Balaji, P., & Karunakaran, G. (2023). Lung cancer histopathology image classification using transfer learning with convolution neural network model. *Technology and Health Care*, *32*(2), 1199–1210. DOI: 10.3233/THC-231029 PMID: 37270826

Muniasamy, A., Begum, A., Sabahath, A., Yaqub, H., & Karunakaran, G. (2024). Coronary heart disease classification using deep learning approach with feature selection for improved accuracy. *Technology and Health Care*, *32*(4), 1991–2007. DOI: 10.3233/THC-231807 PMID: 38339946

Muniasamy, A., Bhatnagar, R., & Karunakaran, G. (2021). Predicting COVID-19 spread in Saudi Arabia using artificial intelligence techniques—Proposing a shift towards a sustainable healthcare approach. In A. Hassanien, R. Bhatnagar, & A. Darwish (Eds.), Artificial intelligence for sustainable development: Theory, practice and future applications (Studies in Computational Intelligence, Vol. 912, pp. 59–78). Springer, Cham. DOI: 10.1007/978-3-030-51920-9_6

Muniasamy, A., & Karunakaran, G. (2026). Challenges and future directions: Emerging trends and limitations in ML and optimization for healthcare. In Muniasamy, A. (Ed.), *Integrative machine learning and optimization algorithms for disease prediction* (pp. 339–368). IGI Global Scientific Publishing., DOI: 10.4018/979-8-3373-1087-9.ch012

Muniasamy, A., Tabassam, S., Hussain, M. A., Sultana, H., Muniasamy, V., & Bhatnagar, R. (2020). Deep Learning for Predictive Analytics in Healthcare. In: Hassanien, A., Azar, A., Gaber, T., Bhatnagar, R., F. Tolba, M. (eds) The International Conference on Advanced Machine Learning Technologies and Applications (AMLTA2019). AMLTA 2019. Advances in Intelligent Systems and Computing, vol 921. Springer, Cham. DOI: 10.1007/978-3-030-14118-9_4

Munusamy, S., & Jothi, K. R. (2025). Blockchain-enabled federated learning with edge analytics for secure and efficient electronic health records management. *Scientific Reports, 15*(1), 27524. DOI: 10.1038/s41598-025-12225-x PMID: 40721766

Naim, A., Muniasamy, A., Khan, M. I., & Khan, M. F. (2026). AI-driven smart manufacturing and automation in pharmaceutical production. In Muniasamy, A., & Karunakaran, G. (Eds.), *Applications of artificial intelligence in pharmaceuticals* (pp. 157–194). IGI Global Scientific Publishing., DOI: 10.4018/979-8-3373-2043-4.ch006

Nguyen, T. V., Zhang, J., Zhou, L., & Chen, J. (2019). A data-driven optimization of large-scale dry port location using the hybrid approach of data mining and complex network theory. *Journal of Cleaner Production, 234*, 1113–1123.

Penev, Y., Buchanan, T. R., Ruppert, M. M., & Johnson, K. B. (2024). Electronic health record data quality and performance assessments: A scoping review. *JMIR Medical Informatics, 12*, 12. DOI: 10.2196/58130 PMID: 39504136

Peng, S., Shen, F., Wen, A., & Wu, B. (2019). Detecting lifestyle risk factors for chronic kidney disease with comorbidities: Association rule mining analysis of web-based survey data. *Journal of Medical Internet Research, 21*(4), e13508. DOI: 10.2196/14204 PMID: 31821152

Prasad, M. S. G., Kumar, N. N., & Shah, M. A., & B. R., S. (2022). FOEH: Frequent pattern mining performance optimization over large transactional data in extended Hadoop MapReduce. *International Journal on Computer Science and Engineering, 10*(4), 260–264.

Rebelo de Sá, C., Azevedo, P., Soares, C., Jorge, A., & Knobbe, A. (2017). Preference rules for label ranking: Mining patterns in multi-target relations. *Information Fusion, 40*, 112–125. DOI: 10.1016/j.inffus.2017.07.001

Rengaramanujam, K., & Muniasamy, A. (2026). AI in hospital administration and formulary design: Optimizing resource allocation and patient flow. In Muniasamy, A., & Karunakaran, G. (Eds.), *Applications of artificial intelligence in pharmaceuticals* (pp. 215–246). IGI Global Scientific Publishing., DOI: 10.4018/979-8-3373-2043-4.ch008

Sogandi, F. (2024). Identifying diseases symptoms and general rules using supervised and unsupervised machine learning. *Scientific Reports*, *14*(1), 17956. Advance online publication. DOI: 10.1038/s41598-024-69029-8 PMID: 39095606

Spooner, A., Mohammadi, G., Sachdev, P., Brodaty, H., & Sowmya, A. (2022). Temporal pattern mining for analysis of longitudinal clinical data: Identifying risk factors for Alzheimer's disease. *Preprint*. https://doi.org//arXiv.2209.04793DOI: 10.48550

Tandan, M., Acharya, Y., Pokharel, S., & Timilsina, M. (2021). Discovering symptom patterns of COVID-19 patients using association rule mining. *Computers in Biology and Medicine*, *131*, 104249. DOI: 10.1016/j.compbiomed.2021.104249 PMID: 33561673

Ting, H. W., Chien, T. Y., & Liao, C. C. (2022). Diseases that occur prior to spontaneous intracerebral hemorrhage: Identification of predisposing and risk factors using lag sequential analysis. *Journal of Healthcare Engineering*, *2022*, 9733712. DOI: 10.1155/2022/9733712 PMID: 35368939

Tyagi, S., Macesic, N., Peleg, A., & Ramakrishnaiah, Y. (2023). EHR-QC: A streamlined pipeline for automated electronic health records standardisation and preprocessing to predict clinical outcomes. *International Journal of Medical Informatics*, *174*, 105058.

Wang, J., Li, W., Wang, H., Lyu, H., Thirukumaran, C., Mesfin, A., & Luo, J. (2022). *Causal inference via nonlinear variable decorrelation for healthcare applications* (arXiv preprint). https://doi.org//arXiv.2209.14975DOI: 10.48550

Xiang, D., & Cai, W. (2021). Privacy protection and secondary use of health data: Strategies and methods. *BioMed Research International*, *2021*(1), 6967166. DOI: 10.1155/2021/6967166 PMID: 34660798

Zaki, M. J. (2000). Scalable algorithms for association mining. *IEEE Transactions on Knowledge and Data Engineering*, *12*(3), 372–390. DOI: 10.1109/69.846291

ADDITIONAL READING

Shankar, K., & Zhang, Y. (2022). *Artificial intelligence in healthcare: Past, present, and future*. Springer.

Tan, P.-N., Kumar, V., & Steinbach, M. (2019). *Introduction to data mining* (2nd ed.). Pearson.

Witten, I. H., Frank, E., & Hall, M. A. (2016). *Data mining: Practical machine learning tools and techniques* (4th ed.). Morgan Kaufmann.

KEY TERMS AND DEFINITIONS

Apriori: A classical breadth-first algorithm that generates and prunes candidate itemsets iteratively based on minimum support thresholds.

Association Rule Mining (ARM): A data mining technique used to identify meaningful relationships or associations between variables within large datasets.

Confidence: The conditional probability that an outcome (Y) occurs given the presence of a condition (X).

Eclat: A depth-first Association Rule Mining algorithm that discovers frequent itemsets by intersecting transaction ID (TID) sets.

FP-Growth: An algorithm for mining frequent patterns efficiently without generating candidate sets, using a compressed FP-tree structure.

Lift: A ratio that measures the strength of an association rule by comparing its observed frequency to the frequency expected if X and Y were independent.

Support: A measure indicating how frequently an itemset or rule appears within a dataset.

Chapter 2

Classical Association Rule Mining Algorithms for Medical Data

Humara Yaqub Thakur
http://orcid.org/0000-0003-3815-9124
King Khalid University, Saudi Arabia

Malik Misbah
King Khalid University, Saudi Arabia

Mahjabeena Najar
King Khalid University, Saudi Arabia

Shaista Qadir
King Khalid University, Saudi Arabia

ABSTRACT

The explosive growth of medical data in recent years ranging from electronic health records to clinical trial outcomes has created a pressing need for advanced data analysis techniques that can reveal hidden disease patterns, improve diagnostic processes, and strengthen evidence-based medical practices. Among these techniques, association rule mining (ARM) has become a key tool for uncovering meaningful relationships in complex, high-dimensional healthcare datasets. This chapter aims to connect computational approaches with clinical value by demonstrating how ARM can transform raw healthcare data into actionable insights for doctors, researchers, and healthcare administrators. As medical decision-making increasingly relies on

DOI: 10.4018/979-8-3373-6691-3.ch002

interconnected datasets including patient histories, symptoms, treatments, test results, and outcomes, ARM algorithms provide a powerful way to identify relationships that may not be immediately obvious to human experts..

INDTRODUCTION

The continuing development of medical informatics is keeping pace with the exponential increase in the volume, variety, and complexity of health data. Each day, modern health systems manage millions of electronic health records, diagnostic images, genomic sequences, and transactional data that, if harnessed and utilized effectively, can offer clinicians and researchers invaluable, life-saving information. However, deriving actionable insights is not straightforward. The medical domain presents unique obstacles, such as heterogeneous clinical variables, missing data, and highly non-linear relationships between patient characteristics and outcomes (Bellazzi & Zupan, 2008). These issues create an urgent need for transparent and interpretable analytical methods that can traverse dense medical datasets and surface novel, actionable insights (Agrawal & Srikant, 1994).

Association Rule Mining (ARM) has gained prominence because of its ability to facilitate the identification of intricate, previously unknown connections within datasets. In contrast to supervised learning methods that predict outcomes, ARM searches for co-occurrence patterns and generates profiles of symptoms, diagnoses, treatments, and demographic combinations that tend to cluster together, determining the strength and clinical significance of these relationships (Agrawal, Imieliński, & Swami, 1993). In medical contexts, such findings can both corroborate existing scientific theories and generate new hypotheses to enhance decision-support systems and improve clinical outcomes (Patel et al., 2009).

Many of the classical ARM algorithms, such as Apriori, Eclat, and FP-Growth, have been instrumental in advancing biomedical research and clinical practice.

Like many recent advancements in association algorithms, Apriori is also famous for being among the first algorithms ever developed. It uses the 'level-wise' approach in mining, becoming the first algorithm for mining frequent itemsets, which was termed 'Apriori' because it uses the principle that 'a superset can be frequent only if all of its subsets are frequent.' Eclat and FP-Growth give parametric speeds of processing: Eclat uses vertical data and intersections for quick mining of large itemsets. FP-Growth uses a compact tree structure model for large itemsets and scans data to reduce overhead. (Agrawal & Srikant, 1994).

Prior research on association rule mining in healthcare has mainly looked at using individual ARM algorithms for specific medical issues, such as disease co-occurrence analysis, adverse drug reaction detection, and chronic disease risk profiling with structured clinical records and electronic health records. Early studies showed that Apriori-based mining could reveal common disease and treatment patterns. Later studies introduced FP-Growth and Eclat to overcome scalability and efficiency challenges in large medical datasets. More recent research has examined extensions like fuzzy, weighted, incremental, and privacy-preserving ARM to manage uncertainty, streaming data, and confidentiality issues in healthcare. Despite this growing body of work, the existing literature is still fragmented. It often focuses on algorithmic novelty or isolated applications without offering a unified view or enough discussion on clinical interpretability, evaluation methods, and real-world deployment challenges. This chapter addresses these gaps by providing a clear and organized review of classical ARM techniques specifically for medical data. It also includes a comparative analysis of the strengths and weaknesses of various algorithms in healthcare settings. Furthermore, it connects methodological foundations with applied healthcare scenarios, practical limits, and the relevance of clinical decision support. This way, ARM is positioned not just as a data mining approach but as an important tool for discovering knowledge and supporting evidence-based healthcare analytics. (Agrawal & Srikant, 1994).

1.1 Real-World Case Studies

There are several case studies to emphasize the practical importance of ARM in mining novel insights from medical data. Narindrarangura et al. in his work used the Apriori algorithm in mining Engaging Health Records from over 3 million diabetic patients in a multicenter EHR to identify patterns of people who attempted suicide. The crucial finding of the analyses was that never married diabetic patients with lower average blood glucose levels were at risk of suicide attempts, and it is from this that a blend of social and biochemical risk factors was observed. This research validated the hypothesis, however, there were new factors such as marital status and perfil lipids. This is the only research results that can be explored for confirmation. The rules were formed using the standard ARM metrics of support, confidence and lift which gave the users the practical implications of the results. (Agrawal & Srikant, 1994; Bellazzi & Zupan, 2008)

Another glaring example of this work involves mining its clinical databases for the association among co-existing diseases.

Rashid et al. (2017) utilized ARM techniques to predict associations between primary and secondary diseases and hence assist clinicians in recognizing comorbidities that may alter patient management strategies. One example in which the association rules showed the greatest value was the co-occurrence of hypertension and chronic kidney disease in diabetics. This kind of knowledge can assist in driving the planning of proactive steps and the appropriate allocation of resources. (Agrawal & Srikant, 1994; Bellazzi & Zupan, 2008).

The FP-Growth algorithm has also demonstrated improvements in mining efficiency and scalability with large medical datasets. Hu and Yang integrated FP-Growth into a Hadoop framework using patient diagnosis records. Their approach was able to retrieve hundreds of association rules in a matter of seconds. When applied to a cancer dataset, FP-Growth quickly retrieved associations between diagnoses and treatments, thus aiding physicians in adjusting treatments to the disease patterns.

Furthermore, Sen Gupta et al. applied AR M to analyze brain tumor cases and extracted rules from a data warehouse which aimed at aiding in early diagnosis and therapy allocation. Rai's work with data from COVID-19 patients applied privacy-preserving association rule mining to predict risk factors of heart diseases for targeted public health interventions.

1.2 Practical Impact And Constraints

The above strategies, having employed basic ARM algorithms, show a quantitative value in enhancing healthcare. Preventive care can be planned by the discovered associations, thus aiding in the provision of personalized treatments and detecting adverse drug reactions in polypharmacy, which is becoming a greater concern as patient profiles become more intricate.

As an example, the ability to detect and associate certain combinations of medications with negative outcomes could lead to innovations in prescription processes, thereby improving patient safety.

Implementing these algorithms is more difficult than it may appear. Medical datasets always contain missing data and noise, and ARM often generates an overly abundant set of rules, most of which are negligible in a clinical context or possess no statistical relevance. Results interpretation and clinical importance confirmation require extensive joint working and interfacing between computation and clinical medicine. Also, ethical patient data management remains a priority, which means strict legally enforceable policies on confidentiality, data protection, and responsible reporting of results.

Despite these shortcomings, classical association rule mining still bears considerable relevance to research in medicine. It produces user-friendly and easy to interpret models, is within the theoretical grasp of most clinical researchers and offers a straightforward approach to empirical testing and discovery of new substantial relationships in patient databases. With the constant acceleration of the shift to personalized medicine, the ability of ARM to reveal intricate, multifaceted interdependencies in varying data types is now more advantageous than ever. (Hu et al., 2018; Geng & Hamilton, 2006).

2. RELATED WORK

In the medical sector, Association Rule Mining (ARM) is gaining recognition for identifying concealed patterns in intricate clinical datasets. ARM techniques have progressively built upon one another, ranging from basic and more sophisticated hybrid approaches to real-time implementations.

2.1 Basics And Initial Uses

ARM's use in the healthcare setting began in the early 1990s, following the launch of the Apriori algorithm in 1993. At this point, ARM was mostly utilized on scanned digital healthcare records. It was the first technique used to benchmark the mining of frequent item sets and the creation of association rules in clinical scenarios. Moving into the early 2000s, ARM began to be used for the analysis of clinical databases pertaining to chronic conditions, particularly diabetes mellitus. This practice allowed the uncovering of previously hidden relationships, thus enhancing the clinical decision-making process. These practices ARM, particularly in conjunction with evidence-based healthcare (Agrawal & Srikant, 1994; Bellazzi & Zupan, 2008) disseminated, and supported theexplon. Increased validation tired of poorly sets.

2.2 Improvements To Techniques And Process

Increased the volume and intricacy of medical data, the basic methods built around the Apriori algorithm to mining methods began to dramatically increase. These approaches, built around outer joins, were built with the view to control the excessive scanning of the databases.

2.3 Hybrid Approaches With Machine Learning

Recent studies have begun to combine ARM with other machine learning practices, including classification, clustering, and predictive modeling. Machine learning offers class association rules and predictive analytics which ARM can combine to augment predictive power, particularly in oncology and diabetes. The fusion of ARM and other models improves contextualized analyses, expands ARM's use in sophisticated medical decision-support systems, and incorporates contextual predictive rule generation, interpretability, and predictive accuracy (Li et al., 2001; Thabtah, 2007).

2.4 Applied Biomedical Research

The use of ARM in biomedical research is escalating. It has become common to use ARM to evaluate comorbidity, analyze risk factors, and identify adverse drug reactions. For instance, Rashid et al. (2017) highlights the ability of ARM to find correlations between diseases in extensive patient records, while Liu et al., 2000 used incremental ARM with real-time chronic disease data targeted to hospital settings. ARM's ability to contribute to predictive modeling and generation of clinical insights reinforces proactive patient management and the effective routing of healthcare services (Rashid et al., 2017; Liu et al., 2019).

2.5 Recent Trends And Remaining ISS

Despite its success, ARM in medical applications continues to face several challenges. Recent research has exploredweighted, fuzzy, and constraint-based extensions to improve the quality and relevance of rules. However, issues such as rule redundancy, lack of clinical interpretability, and scalability remain major concerns. Visualizaion techniques have been increasingly emphasissized to enhance the interpretability of mined patterns by healthcare practitioners. Furthermore, the need for scalable solutions that maintain clinical precisionn continues to drive innovation in thisarea (Hu et al., 2018; Geng & Hamilton, 2006).

2.6CurrenSystem□ T

Modern ARM systems in healthcare are characterized by their integration with Electronic Health Records (EHR) and their ability to perform real-time incremental mining for streaming medical data. Thes e systems employadvanced data processing methods, including pruning , clustering, and feature selection,to ensure efficiency and clinicalutility. A strong emphasis is placed on generating int rules that can n be seamlessly embedded into clinicall workflows , supportingprecision medicine and predicative analytics (Chen eal., 2020; Wang et a., 20 21).

2.7 Recent Arm-Based Medical Studies

ARM in COVID-19 Analysis When COVID-19 hit, researchers leaned on association rule mining (ARM) to make sense of huge patient datasets. They used Apriori and FP-Growth algorithms to sift through medical records and spot symptoms that often showed up together fever, cough, shortness of breath, fatigue, muscle pain. Turns out, these symptom combos had a lot to do with how severe the illness got and whether someone ended up in the hospital. ARM helped surface patterns that regular stats sometimes missed, making it easier for doctors to spot cases early and decide who needed care most. Digging deeper, researchers found that ARM could uncover links between existing health problems and COVID-19 outcomes. Patients with diabetes, high blood pressure, or heart disease kept popping up in strong association rules tied to severe cases (Chen et al., 2020). So, ARM wasn't just crunching numbers it was helping doctors get a clearer picture, fast, from all sorts of messy pandemic data. Chronic Disease Risk and Multimorbidity ARM isn't just a pandemic tool. Lately, it's become a go-to in chronic disease research, especially when patients have several conditions at once. Big studies have used ARM to spot common clusters ike how type 2 diabetes, high blood pressure, kidney disease, and nerve problems often go hand in hand (Zhang et al., 2022). With these insights, doctors can flag high-risk patients sooner and fine-tune screening methods. There's more. By plugging ARM into risk prediction models, researchers have built better ways to predict things like five-year mortality for older adults. Instead of looking at each disease alone, they use patterns of multiple conditions, and this approach beats traditional single-disease models (Prados-Torres et al., 2014). ARM is shaping up to be key for smarter, more personalized healthcare. Mining for Drug Interactions and Adverse Events Keeping track of dangerous drug combinations is a huge job, and ARM is making it easier. Researchers mine health records and reporting systems to find drug pairs that lead to bad outcomes, like hospital readmissions or serious side effects. This isn't just theoretical these findings help doctors keep patients safer by catching risky combos sooner.

ARM also shines when it comes to picking up on rare, but serious, drug reactions that might slip past standard monitoring. By analyzing claims data, researchers have found new drug-event links that help beef up traditional safety systems. Federated and Privacy-Preserving ARM in Healthcare Sharing health data comes with a mountain of privacy rules. To get around that, new research is making ARM work in a federated, privacy-preserving way. Basically, hospitals and clinics can collaborate to find useful patterns without ever handing over raw patient data. Instead, each place mines its own data and then shares just the results, which get combined at a higher level. This keeps everything compliant with HIPAA, GDPR, and other regulations (Lyu et al., 2023). It's still early days for federated ARM, but the first results look promising. Teams are starting to uncover trends and associations across different hospitals, all while keeping personal info locked down. This fits right in with the push for decentralized analytics and makes ARM a solid option for large-scale, privacy-friendly healthcare research (Soria-Comas & Domingo-Ferrer, 2021). Summary From 2019 to 2024, ARM has proved itself across the board—in pandemic response, chronic care, drug safety, and privacy-focused analytics. The latest studies show just how flexible and relevant it is for today's healthcare problems. Moving forward, it's clear that combining strong evaluation, real-world clinical checks, and privacy measures will be crucial for getting the most out of ARM in medicine.

3. EVOLUTION OF ASSOCIATION RULE MINING (ARM) IN HEALTHCARE

Table 1. Literature review of ARM in medical applications

Research Phase / Focus Area	Overview of Key Developments	Core Insights and Achievements
Foundations and Early Adoption	The introduction of Association Rule Mining (ARM) in healthcare began with the Apriori algorithm in 1993.	• Emergence of digital healthcare databases • Establishment of a foundation for ARM in healthcare • Initial applications in disease analysis (e.g., diabetes) • Discovery of concealed medical patterns • Improved decision support systems
Algorithmic Improvements and Refinements	Efforts aimed at addressing the computational and data management challenges of the Apriori algorithm.	• Utilization of Boolean and clustering matrices • Pruning rules pre/post-analysis for enhanced accuracy • Improved management of data imbalance • Inclusion of feature selection and cross-validation • Enhanced relevance of rules within clinical contexts
Hybrid Approaches with Machine Learning	Combining ARM with more sophisticated machine learning techniques for deeper insights.	• Class association rule frameworks applicable to chronic diseases • Improved contextual understanding of datasets • Increased predictive accuracy and broader applicability
Applied Biomedical Research	Practical implementations of ARM across patient and clinical datasets.	• Identification of comorbidities and risk profiles • Detection of adverse drug interactions • Rashid et al. (2017): revealing disease connections • Liu et al.: incremental learning utilized within hospital systems

continued on following page

Table 1. Continued

Research Phase / Focus Area	Overview of Key Developments	Core Insights and Achievements
Recent Trends and Remaining Issues	Recent expansions and ongoing challenges within ARM research in healthcare.	• Development of fuzzy, weighted, and constraint-based rule models • Reduction of redundancy and irrelevance • Focus on visualization and interpretability • Addressing gaps in scalability and precision
Current System Trends	Progression toward integrated, interpretable, and adaptive ARM systems.	• Real-time incremental analysis for streaming data • Advanced embedding within electronic health record (EHR) systems • Enhanced pruning and clustering methodologies • Focus on explainability and precision medicine

4. ALGORITHMIC COMPARISON OF CLASSICAL ARM TECHNIQUES FOR MEDICAL DATA

Table 2. Algorithmic comparison of classical ARM techniques for medical data

Algorithm	Strengths for medical data	Weaknesses for medical data	When to choose
Apriori	Nemours interpretable rules simple to implement good for small, well-curated clinical datasets.	Explodes candidates on many features (comorbidities, medications) many scans on large EHRs.	Small cohort studies, teaching, sanity-checks, where interpretability matters and dataset size is small.
FP-Growth	Fast, no candidate generation compresses repeated patterns (useful when many patients share common codes).	FP-tree can be complex to build for streaming or extremely high-cardinality features, implementation more complex.	Large EHR/claims discovering multi-item co-occurrences (comorbidities, med-lab associations).
Eclat (vertical / TID list)	Efficient for dense parts of medical data (e.g. many patients share same diagnosis codes) simple vertical intersections.	TID lists can be memory-heavy for very large cohorts; less suited for sparse high-cardinality features.	When vertical representation is natural (cohort IDs per item) or you want depth-first mining and can afford memory.

continued on following page

Table 2. Continued

Algorithm	Strengths for medical data	Weaknesses for medical data	When to choose
DHP / Hash-pruning (Apriori variants)	Reduces candidate explosion via hashing useful if Apriori is required for explainability.	Still needs multiple scans; not as scalable as FP-Growth/Eclat.	Situations needing Apriori-like output but with some pruning.
H-Mine / other pattern-growth variants	Designed for large transactional datasets with limited memory can be adapted to clinical streams.	More complex to implement and tune.	Large institutional databases where memory is the constraint.

5. CLASSICAL ASSOCIATION RULE MINING ALGORITHMS FOR MEDICAL DATA

5.1 Medical Datasets Used In Arm Studies

Association Rule Mining (ARM) in healthcare leverages multiple types of medical datasets, each capturing different dimensions of patient care, disease progression, and healthcare delivery. The selection of data sources directly influences the quality, interpretability, and clinical relevance of the discovered association rules (Jensen et al., 2012; Bellazzi & Zupan, 2008).

Electronic Health Records (EHRs)

Electronic Health Records (EHRs) are the most widely used data source in ARM-based healthcare studies. EHRs contain rich patient-level information, including demographics, diagnoses, medications, laboratory results, procedures, and clinical notes. ARM applied to EHRs enables the discovery of associations among diseases, treatments, and outcomes across large populations, supporting clinical decision-making and hypothesis generation (Hripcsak & Albers, 2013; Jensen et al., 2012). However, EHR data are often heterogeneous, incomplete, and noisy, necessitating extensive preprocessing prior to mining.

Claims Data

Claims data are primarily generated for billing and reimbursement purposes and include diagnosis codes, procedure codes, and medication claims. Although claims datasets lack detailed clinical measurements, they offer large-scale and longitudinal coverage of patient interactions with healthcare systems. ARM on claims data is particularly effective for population-level analyses, comorbidity discovery, and healthcare utilization pattern mining (Lee & Yoon, 2017).

Disease Registries

Disease registries focus on patients diagnosed with specific conditions such as cancer, diabetes, or cardiovascular diseases. These datasets are typically curated and standardized, resulting in high data quality and consistency. ARM studies using registries often produce highly interpretable and clinically meaningful rules related to disease progression and outcomes, although their scope may be limited to specific populations (Prados-Torres et al., 2014).

ICU And Critical Care Datasets

Intensive Care Unit (ICU) datasets contain high-frequency and time-sensitive clinical data, including diagnosis–medication–outcome tables. ARM applied to ICU data supports the discovery of associations related to treatment effectiveness, adverse events, and patient outcomes in critical care settings. Due to their high dimensionality and temporal complexity, ICU datasets pose significant challenges for scalable and interpretable ARM (Wang et al., 2021).

Structured vs. Unstructured medical data

Structured medical data consist of coded elements such as diagnoses, medications, and laboratory results, which are well suited for classical ARM algorithms. In contrast, unstructured data—such as clinical notes and discharge summaries—require natural language processing (NLP) techniques to extract meaningful features before ARM can be applied. Consequently, most ARM studies focus on structured data due to ease of representation and clinical interpretability (Jensen et al., 2012).

Longitudinal vs. Transactional medical data

Longitudinal medical data capture patient information over extended time periods, enabling analysis of disease progression and treatment evolution. ARM, however, operates on transactional data, requiring longitudinal records to be transformed into discrete transactions through temporal aggregation strategies such as per-visit or per-admission grouping (Bellazzi & Zupan, 2008).

Table 3. Common medical datasets used in association rule mining

Dataset Type	Typical Contents	Advantages for ARM	Limitations
Electronic Health Records (EHRs)	Diagnoses, medications, lab results, procedures, demographics	Rich clinical detail, supports disease treatment outcome analysis	Missing values, heterogeneity, privacy constraints
Claims Data	Diagnosis codes, procedure codes, billing records	Large-scale, longitudinal population coverage	Limited clinical depth, coding bias
Disease Registries	Disease-specific clinical variables, outcomes	High data quality, standardized formats	Limited generalizability
ICU Datasets	High-frequency vitals, medications, diagnoses, outcomes	Enables fine-grained outcome and adverse event analysis	High dimensionality, temporal complexity

5.2 Data Preprocessing For Arm In Healthcare

Data preprocessing is a critical step in healthcare ARM, as raw medical data are rarely suitable for direct mining. Effective preprocessing ensures that derived association rules are statistically sound and clinically interpretable (Agrawal & Srikant, 1994).

Handling Missing Values

Medical datasets frequently contain missing values due to incomplete documentation or variability in clinical practice. Common approaches include record deletion, statistical imputation, and domain-informed substitution. In ARM, missing values are often treated as the absence of an item, which can significantly influence support and confidence measures if not handled carefully (Bellazzi & Zupan, 2008).

Binarization Of Clinical Variables

ARM algorithms require categorical or binary inputs. Continuous clinical variables, such as laboratory values or vital signs, must therefore be discretized into clinically meaningful categories (e.g., "normal," "high," or "low"). Appropriate binarization improves both the interpretability and clinical relevance of association rules (Wang et al., 2021).

Medical Coding Systems (ICD, SNOMRF, LOINC)

Standardized medical coding systems play a vital role in ARM preprocessing. Diagnosis codes such as ICD, clinical terminologies such as SNOMED CT, and laboratory coding systems such as LOINC ensure data consistency across institutions and studies. Mapping heterogeneous clinical records to standardized codes reduces redundancy and improves rule comparability (Jensen et al., 2012; Lee & Yoon, 2017).

Temporal Aggregation Of Medical Events

Medical data are inherently time-dependent. To apply ARM, multiple patient encounters are aggregated into transactions using clinically meaningful time windows, such as hospital admissions or annual summaries. The choice of temporal granularity directly affects the type and strength of mined associations (Bellazzi & Zupan, 2008).

Table 4. Data preprocessing for ARM in healthcare

Preprocessing Step	Purpose	Common Techniques	Impact on ARM
Missing Value Handling	Reduce bias and noise	Deletion, imputation, domain-based rules	Affects support and confidence
Binarization	Convert numeric data	Thresholding, clinical cutoffs	Improves interpretability
Medical Coding	Standardization	ICD, SNOMED CT, LOINC mapping	Reduces redundancy
Temporal Aggregation	Transaction formation	Visit-level, admission-level grouping	Influences rule granularity

Figure 1. Comparative performance of classical ARM algorithms

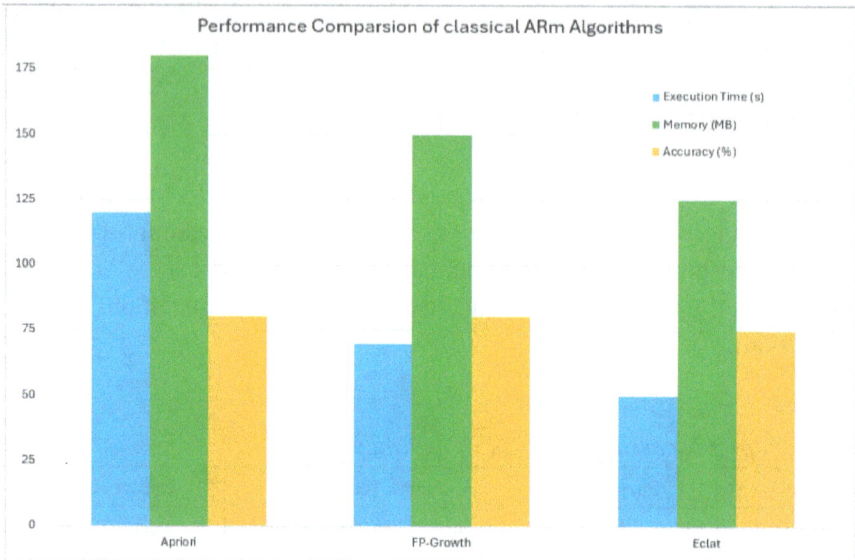

Figure 2. Comparative strengths and weaknesses of classical ARM algorithm

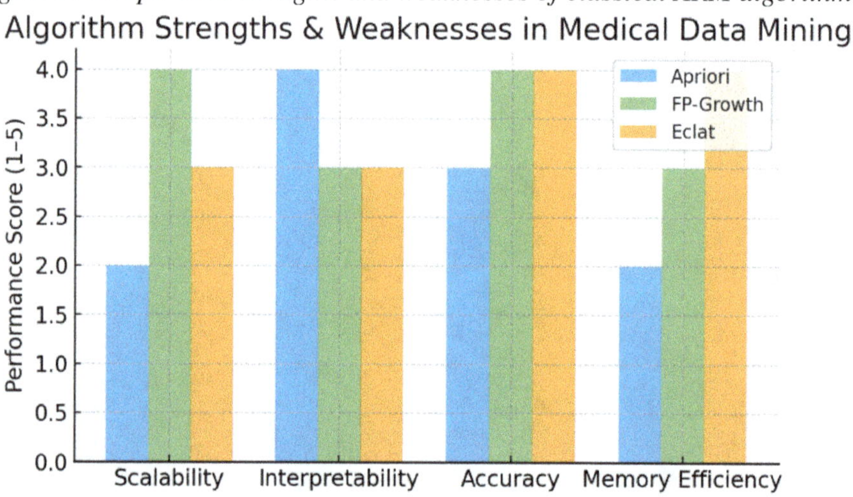

6. HEALTHCARE APPLICATIONS OF ASSOCIATION RULE MINING (ARM)

Although still a rudimentary form of data mining, Association Rule Mining (ARM) is gaining traction in every field in the healthcare sector. Within EHRs, clinical data, and research data, ARM can identify and assess critical patterns and correlations to aid clinicians and health researchers in treatment personalization, decision support, disease progression monitoring, and refinement of treatment (Agrawal et al., 1993; Patel et al., 2009).

6.1 Clinical Decision Support Systems (CDSS)

Constructing CDSS is one of the most valuable uses of ARM in healthcare. These systems derive time-sensitive, evidence-based clinical decision support from an ARM output. For example, if the ARM determines that patients with diabetes and hypertension are at an increased risk of developing chronic kidney disease, a targeted screening program can be implemented (Matsumura et al., 2017).

6.2 Disease Prediction And Risk Stratification

One of the primary uses of ARM is early disease prediction, performed by reviewing historical patient data to identify key risk factors and chronic conditions that cluster with diabetes, cancer, and cardiovascular disease. ARM helps in uncovering frequent item sets.

6.3 Public Health Surveillance

Public Health Surveillance ARM practices have established great importance within the scopes of monitoring disease epidemics, and syndromic surveillance. Outbreak containment becomes easier for public health agencies when health records are scanned and any unusual trends within health and emergency department visits are isolated and analyzed.

This type of surveillance strategy has been effective for the monitoring of infectious diseases (Patel et al., 2009; Lee & Yoon, 2017).

6.4 Personalized Medicine And Treatment Optimization

Clinicians can employ ARM to determine which treatment patterns are the most effective for certain subgroups of patients. For instance, association rules might demonstrate certain therapy combinations produce positive results in a cohort of patients with genetic characteristics or certain comorbidities.

This furthers the goals of precision medicine (Matsumura et al., 2017; Pouriyeh et al., 2017).

6.5 Resource Allocation In Healthcare Settings

Every hospital administrator employs ARM for effective strategy planning and resource allocation. Identifying trends in patient flow, treatment, and disease occurrence across different times of the year helps to reduce stay duration and increase overall efficiency (Lee and Yoon, 2017).

7. HYBRID AND ENHANCED ARM APPROACHES

The hybrid approach develops new techniques for complex data pattern discovery by integrating clustering, genetic algorithms, and classification techniques.

7.1 Clustering-Association Rule Mining Hybrid

In hybrid modeling, clustering algorithms partition data into relevant subgroups, which are then followed by ARM within each group (Sangma, 2020). By focusing on specific sections, this approach yields targeted mining results in the form of relevant actionable rules. Clusters reflect the internal structure of data and significantly diminish background noise (Muralidhar, 2015). This technique has been used by several scholars in the combined form for medical record segmentation or customer behavior analysis. The coverage of constituent groups and interpretability of the generated rules increase significantly as the rules support context group decision-making instead of the generalized whole (Sangma, 2020; Muralidhar, 2015).

7.2 Genetic Algorithm-Enhanced Association Rule Mining

Genetic algorithms enhance the efficiency of the ARM procedure by advancing the candidate rules within selection, crossover, and mutation cycles (Rai et al., 2014). Fitness parameters such as support and confidence are used to determine which contours to follow to avoid exhaustive searching, focusing instead on the most valuable rule sets. This approach offers valuable relationships in association rule mining, including those negative indicators that classical algorithms frequently overlook (Rai et al., 2014). This method also supports multi-objective optimization and improved computational efficiency (Rai et al., 2014).

7.3 Association Rule Mining Combined With Classification Algorithms.

Incorporating mined association rules within the classification until the predicted result streamlines the entire process (Liu, Ma, & Wong, n.d.). The scholars of CBA and other rule-based classifiers report increased prediction of precision and interpretability by filling discovered associations.

The combination of these methods has made progress over traditional classifiers, especially in the healthcare field, which is sensitive to explainability (Liu, Ma, & Wong, n.d.). Models can enjoy the best of both worlds by ARM and classification, i.e., having rich transparent rules while exploiting the predictive power of supervised learning techniques

8. CHALLENGES AND CONSIDERATIONS IN MEDICAL ASSOCIATION RULE MINING

8.1 Privacy-Preserving Arm In Sensitive Medical Datasets

Understanding patients on a personal level allows healthcare professionals to effectively determine diagnoses, prescriptions, and recommend suitable treatment outcomes. However, studies on healthcare- and treatment-related data mining may risk breaching confidentiality. Privacy-preserving Association Rule Mining (PP-ARM) seeks to eliminate this risk while retaining valuable mined rules to provide insight pertinent to research and clinical practices.

Data anonymization is a common technique, in which identifiable elements are concealed using grouping or masking. Alternative methods involving differential privacy obtain, and then, add minor random noise to the data, thus preventing the tracing of individual records (Soria-Comas & Domingo-Ferrer, 2021). A number of hospitals use federated learning or secure multi-party computation, which allows the mining of common patterns without direct data exchange (Lyu et al., 2023). These techniques are compliant with HIPAA and GDPR.

The main challenge is balancing the two concepts. Excess excessive protective layering can render the data useless, while an absence exposes patients to considerable risk. Trust and ethical use of ARM in healthcare relies on the value of maintained confidentiality.

8.2 High-Dimensional And Sparse Data Issues

As specific entries per patient in Electronic Health Records (EHRs) run into thousands of fields, resulting datasets become high-dimensional and sparse. In cases, generative algorithms (ARM) like Apriori are hindered, as they create excessive candidate rules because they try to ascertain very large search spaces which are mostly uninformative (Alam et al., 2022).

To overcome this, researchers use feature selection or dimensionality reduction in which data is condensed to smaller axes containing meaningful components, as in principal component analysis (PCA) or autoencoders. Another approach to the problem is integrating clustering techniques with ARM in which redundant patient records are clustered, and the results are enhanced (Kheirollahi, 2022).

Efficient management of high-dimensional medical data is also important. For instance, GPU-based and distributed ARM frameworks can maintain interpretability and performance on hospital-scale datasets (Zhao et al., 2024)

9. CASE STUDIES: APPLICATION OF ASSOCIATION RULE MINING (ARM) IN CHRONIC DISEASE HEALTHCARE DATA

In the healthcare sector, ARM has been used to analyze and draw insights from large, complex clinical data. Data pertaining to chronic illnesses such as diabetes, cancer, and cardiovascular diseases are longitudinal and voluminous. They exist in multifarious forms, including electronic health records (EHRs), labs, prescriptions, and clinical notes. Such data collections are perfect for deploying ARM approaches to discover concealed associations among symptomatology, risks, and treatment results.

9.1 Case Study 1: Arm In Diabetes Management And Complication Prediction

This case study discusses how ARM (Association Rule Mining) can be used in diabetes management and complication prediction. Diabetes mellitus is a chronic, metabolic disorder that needs continuous monitoring and treatment. In clinical practice, patients generate new records on a continuous basis related to blood glucose levels, medication adherence, co-morbidities and lifestyle factors; ARM can be used to apply this historical record (longitudinal EHR data) along with the data generated by healthcare providers, to determine which of these variables are commonly found together in diabetic patients and identify patterns of use for those medications (medication adherence) over time.

For example, there are many studies that have documented the application of ARM to find relationships between poor diabetic glycemic control, high blood pressure, obesity, and the development of complications including (but not limited to) neuropathy and retinopathy in diabetic patients over time. By applying associative rules e.g., {Obesity, High HbA1c (blood glucose level),} thus indicating a cluster of Metabolic factors that lead to Hypertension, we can use this information to improve treatment plans by providing metabolic intervention earlier in the process and better tailor individual diabetes management plans for patients (Agrawal & Srikant, 1994; Kavitha & Kannan, 2016).

The application of ARM is not limited to diabetes patients alone; researchers and practitioners have also examined medication combinations and patterns of adherence associated with hospitalization events (Wang et al., 2018). For instance, by using ARM we will see there are opportunities to optimize the combination of insulin therapy and oral hypoglycaemics as well as to utilize medication combinations that may reduce the incidence of hospital visits for the treatment of diabetes.

9.2 Case Study 2: Arm In Cardiovascular Disease Risk Factor Analysis

CVD (cardiovascular diseases) continues to be one of the leading causes of death globally. ARM has been a primary method to study the relationships between demographic information, people's health status, and their lifestyle for the development of heart disease.

For example, ARM was used in one study of patient records which included patient age, cholesterol levels, blood pressure, smoking habits, and physical activity levels. The resulting association rules identified that patients who had high levels of cholesterol and who smoked were at a very high risk of developing coronary artery disease. This reinforces previous clinical knowledge for both smoking and high cholesterol as risk factors for coronary artery disease, as well as a unique association between two previously unconnected risk factors (Ordonez et al., 2001).

By identifying high-risk groups of patients, these association rules encourage preventive health programs to promote early detection and screening of patients before CVD events occur. These ARM-derived insights are now routinely incorporated into clinical decision support tools to provide physicians with accurate and relevant patient risk data to assist in determining how to rank patients in terms of CVD risk and how to prioritize care for these patients.

9.3 Case Study 3: Arm For Cancer Symptom And Treatment Pattern Analysis

Using Associative Rule Mining (ARM) to Examine Symptom Clusters and Treatment Patterns in Cancer

Cancer care is complicated; treatments include chemotherapy, radiation and medications for supportive care. In the field of oncology, ARM is being utilized in databases to analyse the patterns of co-occurrence of symptoms, treatment-related adverse effects and patient outcomes.

In a number of registries and hospital-based oncology databases, ARM has been employed to discover frequent symptom clusters (fatigue, nausea, pain, weight loss) associated with cancer. The rules generated by ARM, such as {Chemotherapy, Nausea} > {Fatigue}, have provided clinicians with evidence to help them provide better supportive care to patients. This knowledge has helped clinicians understand what adverse effects could occur and develop individualized symptom management plans (Hahsler et al., 2008). ARM has also been used to examine the relationships between tumour type, treatment modality, and survival outcomes. By reviewing large cohorts of patients, researchers have identified treatment combinations associated with greater likelihood of a good prognosis among patients with certain subtypes of cancer, leading to more data-driven clinical decision making (Koh and Tan, 2011).

10. CONCLUSION

Classical Association Rule Mining (ARM) techniques to facilitate the interpretation of unstructured medical data. The adoption of classical algorithms like Apriori, FP-Growth, and Eclat enables healthcare9 professionals to unearth clandestine associations between diseases, treatments, and risk factors. These relationships often go undetected by traditional statistical techniques. The embedding of these methods in medical analytics fosters the development of personalized medicine, improves accuracy in diagnosis, and assists in the formulation of strategies in medicine.

Yet the application of ARM techniques to the clinical domain still faces unique hurdles, such as high dimensionality and noise. Issues of interpretability continue to plague the field. ARM results need clinical expertise in validating actionable medical knowledge. Methods continue to be ascribed to the healthcare analytics domain and seem to be evolving in response to the demands of contemporary medicine.

11. FUTURE WORK

Future studies ought to investigate how to construct hybrid ARM frameworks to incorporate deep learning with fuzzy logic and probabilistic reasoning to improve the relevance and interpretability of rules. The privacy-preserving ARM methods (i.e. federated learning and differential privacy) will be critical to maintain the confidentiality of patients while facilitating multi-center research (Soria-Comas & Domingo-Ferrer, 2021; Lyu et al., 2023). Also, the scope of research on real-time and incremental ARM systems that mine streaming medical data needs to be broadened to enable fast clinical decision-making (Wang et al., 2021). ARM of personalized and augmented level visualization can interpret patterns for non-specialized users in the healthcare system, and consequently help integrate the system into clinical practice. Finally, future work should focus on clinical validation studies that interlink ARM and patient outcomes, orthogonalizing the ARM results and clinical practice. The more complicated medical data becomes, the more healthcare will depend on the evolution of these techniques to improve precision medicine and the outcomes of global health.

REFERENCES

Agrawal, R., Imieliński, T., & Swami, A. (1993). Mining association rules between sets of items in large databases. *Proceedings of the 1993 ACM SIGMOD International Conference on Management of Data*, 207–216. DOI: 10.1145/170035.170072

Agrawal, R., & Srikant, R. (1994). Fast algorithms for mining association rules. *Proceedings of the 20th International Conference on Very Large Data Bases (VLDB)*, 487–499.

Alam, T., Rahman, M. M., & Khan, S. I. (2022). Efficient association rule mining on high-dimensional medical datasets using dimensionality reduction. *Expert Systems with Applications, 188*, 116021. DOI: 10.1016/j.eswa.2021.116021

Bellazzi, R., & Zupan, B. (2008). Predictive data mining in clinical medicine: Current issues and guidelines. *International Journal of Medical Informatics, 77*(2), 81–97. DOI: 10.1016/j.ijmedinf.2006.11.006 PMID: 17188928

Chen, M., Hao, Y., Hwang, K., Wang, L., & Wang, L. (2020). Disease prediction by machine learning over big data from healthcare communities. *IEEE Access : Practical Innovations, Open Solutions, 5*, 8869–8879. DOI: 10.1109/ACCESS.2017.2694446

Geng, L., & Hamilton, H. J. (2006). Interestingness measures for data mining: A survey. *ACM Computing Surveys, 38*(3), 9. Advance online publication. DOI: 10.1145/1132960.1132963

Hahsler, M., Hornik, K., & Reutterer, T. (2008). Implications of probabilistic data modeling for mining association rules. *Journal of Machine Learning Research, 9*, 1–37.

Hripcsak, G., & Albers, D. J. (2013). Next-generation phenotyping of electronic health records. *Journal of the American Medical Informatics Association : JAMIA, 20*(1), 117–121. DOI: 10.1136/amiajnl-2012-001145 PMID: 22955496

Hripcsak, G., Albers, D. J., Perotte, A., & Correll, M. (2015). Health data use and privacy: Contextual integrity, transparency, and public trust. *Journal of the American Medical Informatics Association : JAMIA, 22*(1), 36–43.

Hu, Y.. (2018). Fuzzy association rules for medical decision support. *Applied Soft Computing, 69*, 397–408.

Jensen, P. B., Jensen, L. J., & Brunak, S. (2012). Mining electronic health records: Towards better research applications and clinical care. *Nature Reviews. Genetics, 13*(6), 395–405. DOI: 10.1038/nrg3208 PMID: 22549152

Kavitha, S., & Kannan, A. (2016). Mining association rules in medical data for disease prediction. *International Journal of Computer Applications, 140*(7), 15–20.

Kheirollahi, H. (2022). A new method of well clustering and association rule mining. *Expert Systems with Applications, 191*, 116281. DOI: 10.1016/j.eswa.2021.116281

Koh, H. C., & Tan, G. (2011). Data mining applications in healthcare. *Journal of Healthcare Information Management, 19*(2), 64–72. PMID: 15869215

Lee, C. H., & Yoon, H. J. (2017). Medical big data: Promise and challenges. *Kidney Research and Clinical Practice, 36*(1), 3–11. DOI: 10.23876/j.krcp.2017.36.1.3 PMID: 28392994

Li, W., Han, J., & Pei, J. (2001). CMAR: Accurate and efficient classification based on multiple class-association rules. *Proceedings of the 2001 IEEE International Conference on Data Mining*, 369–376.

Liu, B., Ma, Y., & Wong, C.-K. (2000). Classification using association rules: Weaknesses and enhancements. *Data Mining for Scientific and Engineering Applications*, 591–605.

Liu, Y., Chen, P. H., Krause, J., & Peng, L. (2019). How to read articles that use machine learning: Users' guides to the medical literature. *Journal of the American Medical Association, 322*(18), 1806–1816. DOI: 10.1001/jama.2019.16489 PMID: 31714992

Lyu, L., Yu, H., & Yang, Q. (2023). Privacy-preserving collaboration in federated healthcare systems. *IEEE Transactions on Knowledge and Data Engineering, 35*(2), 189–202. DOI: 10.1109/TKDE.2021.3057850

Matsumura, Y., Yamashita, T., & Kitagaki, H. (2017). Mining association rules of combination medication patterns in medical prescriptions. *Journal of Biomedical Informatics, 68*, 138–148. DOI: 10.1016/j.jbi.2017.03.004

Muralidhar, A. (2015). The Sharpe ratio revisited: What it really tells us. *Journal of Performance Measurement, 19*(3).

Ordonez, C., Omiecinski, E., de Braal, L., Santana, C. A., Ezquerra, N., Taboada, J. A., & Cooke, D. (2001). Mining constrained association rules to predict heart disease. *Proceedings of the IEEE International Conference on Data Mining*, 433–440. DOI: 10.1109/ICDM.2001.989549

Patel, V. L., Shortliffe, E. H., Stefanelli, M., Szolovits, P., Berthold, M. R., Bellazzi, R., & Abu-Hanna, A. (2009). The coming of age of artificial intelligence in medicine. *Artificial Intelligence in Medicine*, *46*(1), 5–17. DOI: 10.1016/j.artmed.2008.07.017 PMID: 18790621

Pouriyeh, S., Vahid, S., Sannino, G., De Pietro, G., Arabnia, H. R., & Gutierrez, J. (2017). A comprehensive investigation and comparison of machine learning techniques in the domain of heart disease. *Computer Methods and Programs in Biomedicine*, *165*, 25–39.

Prados-Torres, A., Calderón-Larrañaga, A., Hancco-Saavedra, J., Poblador-Plou, B., & van den Akker, M. (2014). Multimorbidity patterns: A systematic review. *Journal of Clinical Epidemiology*, *67*(3), 254–266. DOI: 10.1016/j.jclinepi.2013.09.021 PMID: 24472295

Rai, N. S., Jain, S., & Jain, A. (2014). Mining interesting positive and negative association rule based on improved genetic algorithm. *International Journal of Advanced Computer Science and Applications*, *5*(1).

Rashid, M., Kwok, C. S., Gale, C. P., Doherty, P., Olier, I., Sperrin, M., Kontopantelis, E., Peat, G., & Mamas, M. A. (2017). Impact of co-morbid burden on mortality in patients with coronary heart disease, heart failure, and cerebrovascular accident: A systematic review and meta-analysis. *European Heart Journal. Quality of Care & Clinical Outcomes*, *3*(1), 20–36. DOI: 10.1093/ehjqcco/qcw025 PMID: 28927187

Sangma, J. W. (2020). Clustering-based hybrid approach for identifying associations in data. *PubMed*. https://pubmed.ncbi.nlm.nih.gov/32931587

Soria-Comas, J., & Domingo-Ferrer, J. (2021). Differential privacy in data mining for health information systems. *Computers in Biology and Medicine*, *134*, 104441. DOI: 10.1016/j.compbiomed.2021.104441

Thabtah, F. (2007). A review of associative classification mining. *The Knowledge Engineering Review*, *22*(1), 37–65. DOI: 10.1017/S0269888907001026

Wang, J., Li, Y., Zhang, Y., & Zhang, J. (2021). Scalable association rule mining for precision medicine. *Journal of Biomedical Informatics*, *118*, 103778. DOI: 10.1016/j.jbi.2021.103778

Wang, Y., Kung, L., & Byrd, T. A. (2018). Big data analytics: Understanding its capabilities and potential benefits for healthcare organizations. *Technological Forecasting and Social Change*, *126*, 3–13. DOI: 10.1016/j.techfore.2015.12.019

Zhang, Y., Wang, F., Hu, J., & Wu, X. (2022). Discovering multimorbidity patterns from electronic health records using association rule mining. *BMC Medical Informatics and Decision Making*, *22*(1), 95. DOI: 10.1186/s12911-022-01800-1 PMID: 35392890

Zhao, Y. (2024). A metaheuristic perspective on extracting numeric association rules. *Archives of Computational Methods in Engineering*. Advance online publication. DOI: 10.1007/s11831-024-10254-1

Chapter 3
Uncovering Hidden Patterns:
Association Rule Mining for Disease Detection and Treatment Planning in Healthcare

Arun Agrawal
http://orcid.org/0000-0001-7233-6660
Institute of Technology and Management, Gwalior, India

C. Umarani
http://orcid.org/0000-0002-9008-3350
Christ Academy Institute for Advanced Studies, Bangalore, India

Md Imtiyaz Ali
Vignana Bharathi Institute of Technology, Aushapur, India

Amol L. Mangrulkar
MCT's Rajiv Gandhi Institute of Technology, Mumbai, India

Mohsin Shaikh
http://orcid.org/0000-0002-9547-633X
Dr. Vishwanath Karad MIT World Peace University, Pune, India

Deepak Gupta
http://orcid.org/0000-0003-3929-1362
Institute of Technology and Management, Gwalior, India

Sujatha Somesula
CBIT, Pallavolu, India

ABSTRACT

Association Rule Mining (ARM) has become an important tool for uncovering hidden patterns and clinically meaningful relationships in large healthcare datasets. With the growth of electronic health records, administrative claims, and patient monitoring systems, ARM helps identify disease co-occurrences, multimorbidity patterns, medication risks, and factors influencing patient outcomes. This review examines

DOI: 10.4018/979-8-3373-6691-3.ch003

key ARM algorithms, recent methodological advances, and their applications in diagnosis support, drug safety, and precision medicine. It also highlights ongoing challenges related to data quality, integration, and clinical interpretability, while outlining future opportunities for improving patient management.

INTRODUCTION

The trend to data-driven decision-making in health-care systems is becoming global due to the growing availability of regularly collected information about patients in hospitals, clinics, diagnostic agencies, and in the general health services. The accumulation of the symptomatology, diagnostic tests, therapeutic histories, imaging studies, prescriptions, and longitudinal follow-ups per day have increased the size and accuracy of the corpus of data (Lyu, 2025). Therefore, the modern clinical activity is no longer dependent on the experience but it also encompasses the digital constructs which enable extraction of latent patterns of the dynamic datasets. Data -oriented health-care efforts will attempt to combine expertise in clinical and analytical disciplines, thus making diagnosis and treatment more accurate, timely and personal.

Medical data is enriched and made the detection of invisible, light relationships possible. Whereas the clinician can use signs and symptoms to arrive at a tentative diagnosis, the computational algorithms have the ability to execute some thousands of records simultaneously and identify co-occurrence rates, concomitant laboratory courses, and their prognostic qualities (Martínez-García & Hernández-Lemus, 2022). Most of these connections are so different that they are not easily observed conventionally being either weak or spread out into large bodies of data. Therefore, evidence-based approaches enable health-care professions to move towards evidence-based learning rather than every avenue being based on subjective interpretation, that way facilitating precision medicine when treatment modalities are customized to specific patient phenotypes instead of group-based stereotypes.

Introduction to Data-Driven Health-Care Systems

A data-driven healthcare system can be related to various diseases, and a laboratory value can be a different condition in different situations. Third, the decisions used in treatment are often based on interactions of factors, and not dependent variables: a pharmacologic agent can be effective only when combined with some other drug or a co-factor (Razzak et al., 2020).

Pattern discovery attempts to solve these complexities by determining co-occurrences, sequences of events and dependency structures (Lau et al., 2009). An example is a data may indicate that patients with a specific triad of blood pressure, glycaemic, and age parameters were found to have significantly high risk of a particular illness, and another data can show better efficacy of two medications when administered together with a particular patient group. The insights help clinicians to move past generalized assumptions to evidence-based accuracy.

In addition, pattern discovery can be used to counter misdiagnosis. In cases of unusual symptom mixes, clinicians should not be able to perceive their diagnostic respect at once. Pattern-mining systems have the capability of matching such combinations with past cases retrospectively and give early warnings and timely suggestions that minimize the diagnostic latency.

Significance of Association Rule Mining (ARM) In Disease Analysis

The most important pattern discovery tool relates to the Association Rules Mining (ARM), which is especially relevant since it is concerned with the identification of robust relationships between items in large datasets. In a health-care scenario, the items could be symptoms, diagnosis, lab results or pharmacologic agents. ARM generates rules such as: symptom A with symptom B tend to co-occur with symptom B, and therefore, disease X is probable, and as such are used to explain important combinations outside of two factors and their effects on clinical outcomes (Haug et al., 1994).

ARM is particularly useful in many-factorial diseases like diabetes, cardiovascular disease, malignancy and chronic respiratory diseases, which do not possess a single etiological determinant (Liu et al., 2025). Exposing the intersection of various risk factors, ARM provides comprehensive probabilistic information, such as depicting that a combination of smoking and specific genetic polymorphism and high-age group will result in a rapid increase in disease vulnerability. This type of granularity supports early identification and non-cognitive remedies.

In addition, ARM also helps in optimisation of therapy. Polypharmacy is often prescribed by clinicians and especially during the treatment of chronic illnesses. ARM is able to identify mutually beneficial drug regimen and identify a possible adverse drug interactions. These findings are over time incorporated into clinical decision-support system and help in steering off practitioners against unexpected complications.

Another advantage of ARM is that it is easily interpretable. Many advanced algorithms produce complex models that are difficult for doctors to understand. ARM produces simple "if-then" rules that match the natural reasoning style of clinicians. Because the rules are transparent, medical experts can evaluate and validate them. This makes ARM a practical tool for real-world healthcare applications.

FOUNDATIONS OF ASSOCIATION RULE MINING

Association Rule Mining (ARM) is one of the most widely used techniques for discovering hidden relationships in large datasets. It helps identify patterns that appear together and reveals how strongly they are connected. In healthcare, such patterns often relate to co-occurring symptoms, diagnostic indicators, and drug responses. ARM allows analysts and clinicians to examine these patterns in a systematic way and use them to support disease detection and treatment decisions. This section explains the basic concepts, types of rules, major algorithms, and the strengths and limitations of ARM within medical applications.

Fundamental Notions: Item-sets, Support, Confidence, Lift

The association-rule mining (ARM) is used to study the co-occurrence rates of items in a dataset. These products can be clinical manifestations, lab values, diagnosing codes, or medication treatment. The base construct is the item set, which refers to a group of items that co-exist (Kang'ethe, 2014). An example is a healthcare record that includes the item set fevers cough, or a more detailed assemblage of something like high blood pressure, chest pain, abnormal ECG. ARM aims at highlighting item sets that are repeated throughout the patient records, which reveals important trends.

Support measures the frequency of an item set in the whole database. When 200/2000 patient encounters show-up with fevers and cough, then the support is 10% of the whole group (2). As a result, support can be used to emphasize patterns ubiquitous and ostracize those combinations which occur infrequently and are unlikely to offer clinical implications. The greater the support value, the greater the dissemination of the pattern among the population.

Confidence tests the reliability of an association rule. A rule will usually have the form of: When A and B happen, the C happens (Scheffer, 2001). In medical lingo, it can be translated as follows: When a patient of symptom A and test results B presents, the likelihood of getting disease C is high. Confidence is the fraction number of time C has taken place when both A and B exist. The credibility is strong, which translates to a stable correlation that is worth the subsequent study.

Lift is a discriminative measure, which is used to test the rule which is out of the expectations in the independent rule. Analysing the empirical confidence against the prior probability of the consequent, lift measures the strength of the association (Sowan et al., 2025). A lift that is greater than one indicates a potentiated relationship, which exceeds chance, and a lift that is similar to one is marginally additional value. Lift helps investigators determine in the field of clinical analytics whether a symptom-drug pairing would provide real pathological meaning, or is simply the result of common co-occurrence.

These four concepts together which are frequency (support), reliability (confidence) and strength (lift) make it possible to detect meaningful, dependable patterns. The support distinguishes the frequency of occurrence, consistency by confidence, and lift to uncover the actual impact, so the derived rules can be assessed as statistically sound and clinically effective.

Association Rules Boolean, Quantitative, Temporal

Association rules can be categorized with the respect to the data modality and relational properties. The simplest category is the presence of binary attributes, presence or absence of an item. Boolean rules are used to deal with these attributes (David, 2007). Some examples would be; fever = yes or drug A prescribed = yes. Since many clinical variables are binary, types of Boolean rules are common across healthcare data and can be helpful in demonstrating patterns of co-occurrence among a symptom or a diagnostic code.

Quantitative rules are generalizations of Boolean rules, in which the numbers fields are real. These regulations work within intervals of measurements such as blood pressure, serum glucose, age or cholesterol (Shichkina et al., 2022). As an example, there can be defined a rule with the following form: If systolic blood pressure > 150mmHg and age = >50 years, then the threat of complication Y is high. Quantitative rules provide a more detailed granularity of knowledge, in that medical variations remain unrepresented in binary representations, and continuous variables can stratify the level of risk.

Chronology is added with the help of temporal rules. The health condition changes with time, and diseases are characterized by certain characteristics of manifestation in a sequence of symptoms (Bélair et al., 1995). Temporal rule mining perceives the sequence as well as time of occurrence. One such rule could be given as: in case of fatigue within the two weeks after weight loss, the chance of disease Y will be high. Temporal rules have a crucial role in explaining disease progression, dynamics of treatment, follow-up, and they are widely used in chronic disease management and patient pathway studies.

The type of rules is each used to achieve a different analysis effect: Boolean rules are used to express the co-occurrence at a single point in time; quantitative rules quantify relationships based on the measured values; temporal rules reveal the sequential and temporal correlations. Collectively, they make available a broad structure of investigating complex medical data.

ARM Algorithms: Apriori, FP-Growth, ECLAT

Association-rule mining is based on a number of algorithms. Apriori, FP-Growth, and ECLAT are the most popular of them: All three of them have a different approach to the discovery of frequent item-sets and the generation of rule (Srinadh, 2022).

The first and the most understandable algorithm is Apriori algorithm. It is an iterative process in which individual items meeting the minimum support threshold are identified, and larger item-sets are further built on top of the already identified ones (Nalavade & Meshram, 2014). Items causing the loss of the support criterion are further pruned at each iteration i.e. reducing the search space. Although Apriori is easy to understand and use, its high dependency on repetition of the database makes it computationally inefficient with huge data sets.

FP-Growth (Frequent Pattern Growth) is a method which justifies scans less extensively, which is more efficient than Apriori. FP-Growth represents item appearances in a sparse form using a highly compressed tree-like structure (the FP-tree) (Rana et al., 2025). Directly out of this tree, frequent item-sets are then extracted and candidate generation is not required anymore. The FP-Growth is therefore faster particularly in cases where there are many frequent patterns in the data set that can occur in particular cases in topic of health analytic where historical and quantity data matter greatly.

ECLAT (Equivalence Class Transformation) uses a vertical data structure, that is, each transaction is represented as a collection of record identifiers but not as a list of items. The intersections of these sets of identifiers yield frequent item-sets, which is effective when the data is dense (i.e. there are many frequent item-sets, but the dataset is not sparse) (Bakar et al., 2020).

Together, these algorithms provide a methodological flexibility to the analysts. Apriori is available on small to medium size datasets; FP-Growth is available on large datasets with a lot of patterns; ECLAT is the best in cases where a dense data set is present. Healthcare analysts should be able to maximize the speed and depth of their association-rule-mining efforts by ensuring ease of algorithm selection is matched to the properties of their data.

Recent Literature Evidence Supporting ARM in Healthcare

Recent literature reinforces the theoretical and practical relevance of Association Rule Mining (ARM) in healthcare by demonstrating its scalability, adaptability, and effectiveness across diverse clinical domains. Contemporary studies widely apply ARM to large-scale electronic health records (EHRs) to uncover complex multi-morbidity patterns, treatment associations, and combinations of risk factors that are often overlooked by conventional statistical techniques. These applications have proven particularly valuable in the analysis of chronic and lifestyle-related conditions, including diabetes, cardiovascular diseases, and metabolic disorders, where frequent disease co-occurrences and medication usage patterns play a critical role in clinical decision-making.

Beyond static co-occurrence analysis, recent research extends ARM through integration with temporal analytics and machine learning frameworks. Temporal ARM enables the identification of disease progression sequences and treatment response trajectories, offering insights into patient pathways and long-term outcomes. In addition, hybrid models combining ARM with clustering, deep learning, and clinical decision support systems have enhanced interpretability and predictive capability in healthcare analytics.

Methodological advancements in recent studies also address traditional ARM limitations such as rule explosion and computational inefficiency. Approaches including constraint-based mining, weighted association rules, and clinically guided pruning have been proposed to improve clinical relevance and reduce redundancy. Collectively, these developments confirm ARM as a robust and evolving analytical paradigm in modern healthcare research.

Strengths and Limitations of ARM in Medical Use-Cases

The association rule mining (ARM) has several advantages in the healthcare settings. ARM enables the discovery of latent associations which might be missed during a hand examination process, uncovering risk factors, clusters of symptoms and therapeutic outcomes. The algorithm produces easy to understand rules, which increase clinicians confidence and facilitates empirical validation. Notably, ARM does not rely on very strict assumptions about underlying data distributions, which is an interesting aspect of such comparison in the face of the irregular and heterogeneous nature of clinical data. Moreover, ARM helps in personalized medicine, by identifying patient subpopulations with similar features.

In spite of these advantages, ARM has a number of limitations. The tendency to produce too many rules is on the list of concerns; the large clinical repositories may produce thousands of candidate associations, a sizable portion of which are not clinically relevant. Therefore, effective distillation of clinically useful rules requires the Supreme Court judgement (Chernoff et al., 1995). The other issue is that ARM only deals in co-occurrence and not causal inference; the association between two symptoms does not presuppose a causal relationship. Lacking clinical judgment, these associations can give rise to false interpretations.

ARM also experiences problems with high-dimensional medical data. Combinatory explosion due to large attribute set makes the search space prohibitive in nature, which incurs heavy computational costs. Though algorithms like FP-Growth can reduce this burden, the interpretability problem is still not perfectly solved because the resulting rule sets may be cumbersome. Furthermore, the sensitivity of ARM to data quality (missing-ness, non-uniform data recording activity, and noise) amplifies the challenge as its presence can alter the support and confidence estimates. Such lack of data fidelity is widespread in the reality clinical databases.

Even though these shortcomings exist, ARM still has significant worth in the analytical fields of health care. Its simplicity in nature and interpretability make it a nice supplement to more complex causal or predictive models. As part of a knowledgeable domain and additional analytical analysis, ARM may provide actionable information which contributes to enhanced diagnostic and therapeutic decision-making.

To improve completeness, studies on Association Rule Mining in healthcare should clearly describe the benchmark datasets used, the evaluation metrics applied, and examples of real world clinical use. Benchmark datasets such as electronic health records, hospital databases, or publicly available clinical datasets help ensure transparency and allow comparison with other studies. Quantitative evaluation metrics including support, confidence, lift, and rule coverage are important for assessing the strength and reliability of the discovered rules. In addition, reporting practical deployment scenarios such as the use of Association Rule Mining in clinical decision support systems, patient risk identification, or hospital analytics platforms would demonstrate real clinical value. Including these details helps connect theoretical rule discovery with practical healthcare applications and strengthens the overall quality of Association Rule Mining research.

Scalability and interoperability are very important for using ARM (Advanced Analytics and Risk Management) in healthcare effectively. Scalability means that the system can grow and handle more data as hospitals, clinics, and patients generate large amounts of information from electronic health records, lab tests, medical devices, and wearable technology. A scalable ARM system can process this increasing data without slowing down, ensuring quick and accurate insights. Interoperability means that different healthcare systems, software, and devices can work together and share information easily. This allows doctors, nurses, and other healthcare providers to access complete patient information, improve coordination, and make better decisions. When ARM systems are both scalable and interoperable, they support real-time monitoring, predictive analysis, and personalized treatment plans. Challenges like differences in data formats, security concerns, and integration costs need to be managed for ARM to work successfully in healthcare.

While ARM offers significant benefits, such as identifying hidden patterns, improving decision-making, and enhancing efficiency, its practical limitations are often overlooked. High data volumes can strain the system, and noisy or inconsistent datasets may reduce the reliability of generated rules. Moreover, in complex healthcare or organizational settings, interpreting and applying these rules can be challenging, limiting their real-world effectiveness. Emphasizing only the advantages without acknowledging these constraints can give an incomplete picture. A balanced approach that considers both benefits and practical limitations is essential for leveraging ARM effectively.

HEALTHCARE DATA LANDSCAPE

The data in healthcare has been growing at an immense rate due to the digital systems recording patient data in hospitals, clinics, laboratories and imaging centres. These data are priceless in terms of detecting the disease, tracking the progress and structuring treatment plan because they reflect real clinical situations. Association rule takes advantage of such rich sets of data to detect such subtle trends that do not come out intuitionally. The viable and responsible use of ARM is thus only possible with a full comprehension of the healthcare data ecosystem. This section identifies the major type of data found in healthcare, the most common issue with the data, restrictions on the ethics and law, and the pre-processing and feature engineering of data prior to the actual deployment of the analytics.

Healthcare Data types: EHR, Laboratory Results, Metadata of Imaging, Prescriptions

A wide range of repositories provides the healthcare information. The Electronic Health Record (EHR) is the most common and it is a compilation of structured data (demographics, vital signs, diagnostic codes, procedures, allergies, and treatment regimens), combined with unstructured narratives created by clinicians (Wang et al., 2023). The data in EHR can be used to determine the trajectories of symptoms, disease process, and patient-specific risk profile. Another data source that is important is laboratory results. Such data sets represent the quantitative values, such as blood glucose, lipid levels, electrolytes, hepatic values, renal ones, and elements of infection in the form of numeric values that can be detected and allow the occurrence of abnormal figures on a single reading (Ehrenstein et al., 2019). Combination of ARM on laboratory data can indicate an early onset of diseases. Although imagine metadata is not a technology that requires raw image silicon, it provides context about the scan modality, technical settings, observations of the radiologist, and annotated results. Such metadata can also be analysed to make the identification of pathological changes and their progression in real-time faster. The prescription and medication records include drug names, dosage, frequency, duration and combinatorial therapy. ARM is able to both reveal the relationship between pharmacologic regimens and adverse events and identify best combinations of drug to a specific group of patients. All these data groups together create a unified base that when harmonised, will provide a comprehensive picture of the health of a patient and will cast light on the interaction between clinical manifestations, laboratory values, imaging results and treatment plans.

Data Problems: Values Missing, Noise, Imbalance, Heterogeneity

Although healthcare data is rich, it has many challenges. One of the problems is pervasive, i.e. it is the lack of those laboratory tests, vital measurements, or follow-ups in patient records because this work is skipped or not recorded, or systems are malfunctioning. These loopholes weaken the quality of the statistical metrics of ARM, which require correct frequency measures. Another complication is noise, patterns may be distorted by typographical errors, instrument errors or outdated information and produce spurious associations that are non-clinically valid. Rule discovery is also blocked by class imbalance; rare conditions or complications might not be found, and ARM selected to learn high-frequency patterns might miss clinically significant but low-frequency associations (Baryakova et al., 2023). Yet more complexity is introduced by heterogeneity: the data are obtained in different hospitals, regions, devices, and formats with different nomenclature, units, coding structures, and documentation traditions. It is difficult to ensure consistent referencing of diseases, tests, and treatments through such diverse sources and to make any reconciliation, cleaning, and standardisation is required. There is a dire need to address these challenges; otherwise, the outcome sets of the rules can present an inaccurate picture of the actual clinical conditions or continue spreading erroneous knowledge.

Ethical and Legal Concerns

Health information contains confidential and personal data. Ethical and legal protocols cannot be ignored to protect the rights of patients in the analytical activities. One of the main regulations is the Health Insurance Portability and Accountability Act (HIPAA). In spite of the fact that HIPAA is a United States-specific law, its structure has an impact on international procedures in the sphere of processing the data about healthcare. The Act emphasizes the security of the identity of patients, secure confidentiality in processing information, and a limitation to access confidential information (Shackelford et al., 2015).

Another mandatory condition is that of informed consent. The patients should understand how their information will be gathered, stored and used. They have the right to revoke the consent or limit the application of their data. Ethical research does not allow the use of patient data without the consent except in cases where the information has been anonymized in its entirety to benefit the study or the general health of the population.

Overwhelming importance is placed on the issue of privacy protection since health records often include recognizable information like names, address, contacts, medical histories, and information about the drugs. Illegal access may trigger abuse. Therefore, there is an extensive use of anonymization and de-identification methods. Such techniques cut or cover personal identifiers but retain the integrity of clinical data to be used in analysis.

The general ethics goal is to balance the issues of innovation and responsibility. Analytical services such as ARM have to be within the legal limits. Protecting the data, making it transparent and considerate of patients are crucial to maintaining the trust in healthcare analytics.

Pre-Processing/ Feature Engineering in Medical Dataset

The healthcare data will have to be pre-processed with care before the association rule mining is applied. Pre-processing improves the quality and reliability of final patterns that are discovered. Missing values are one of the critical steps that should be managed (Hossain et al., 2023). Depending on the type of data, techniques like models based imputation, forward or backward fill and mean substitution can be applied. Missing entries would not be ignored especially when patterns rely on accurate counts.

The minimization of noise is another critical activity. The wrong values, redundancy, and non-congruent formats should be fixed. Unification of units, sharing of similar codes and sifting out of unrealistic values make the data coherent and analysis ready.

It is also necessary that normalisation and discretization. A large variety of ARM algorithms work best with categorical data. When this is concerned, continuous variables, like blood pressure or cholesterol level, are frequently categorized into groups such as low, normal and high. The conversion produces interpretable patterns, which can be easily deciphered by the clinicians.

The critical role in assuring data quality is played by feature engineering. Inferable features could be derived indicators (e.g. risk scores, composite symptom indices, time between events, severity category) in the medical field. Such engineered features are capable of revealing the relationships, which the raw data may hide.

Lastly, the data integration is the process that consolidates the electronic health records, laboratory data, and imaging data, and prescription data in a single format. This global clinical image allows ARM to identify cross-domain patterns.

In general, the pre-processing and the feature engineering are the keystones to the plausible results of the analysis. In their absence, even the most sophisticated ARM algorithms can give erroneous or irrelevant clinically patterns.

ARM FOR DISEASE DETECTION

Association Rule Mining (ARM) has become an important tool in the determination of patterns of diseases in clinical data. ARM is used to discover co-occurring symptom sets, risk variables, lab values, and medication history that define patients in groups. Such interrelated patterns tend to sum up underlying disease processes or early warning signs that could be missed on regular clinical examination. The subsequent paragraphs discuss the role of ARM in assisting disease detection, describe early-warning associations, give exemplary cases of how ARM is applied to a total of major diseases, and compare it to the other forms of machine-learning that often find application in the context of predictive analytics.

Determining Co- Occurring Symptoms and Risk Factors

The detection of the disease is usually based on the significant combinations of symptoms and clinical indicators, but not on the petty observation. ARM should be efficient in this regard since it aims at establishing common item sets and drawing association rules attributing one group of items to another. These issues in the health care do include symptoms of fatigue, fever, or headache, laboratory results of hyperglycaemia or dyslipidaemia, risks of smoking, obesity, or old age (Rotaru-Zavaleanu et al., 2024).

ARM leads to the revelation of patterns in the form of statements like, patients who demonstrate A and B often also demonstrate C. Indicatively, in the context of metabolic disorders, the coincidence between the feeling of excessive thirst and frequent urination, could significantly be related to high fasting glucose levels. Such patterns can be examined with the help of analyses performed on large amounts of data, pointing to possible indicators of the presence or development of the disease.

The power of ARM lies in its ability to process enormous and multidimensional data involving many variables recorded in several encounters with patients. It is able to detect clinically intuitive combinations and surprise relationships. As an illustration, recurrent co-morbidity of mild forms of dizziness and palpitations during particular age groups can be indicative of early signs of cardiovascular impairment. What ARM does with its summaries of relationship measures as support, confidence, and lifts, is to guide the analysts to the most significant patterns.

Another important application applies to risk factor identification. ARM has the capability of revealing the links of lifestyle decisions, genetic identifiers, and outcomes of the diseases. Policies can prove that patients that have long sedentary lifestyle and high body mass index are susceptible to high blood pressure. Similarly, in lung-related disorders, ARM can identify independent symptom sets, which occur together in smokers. Such facts justify specific screening guidelines and help clinicians to identify individuals-at-risk before they develop serious symptoms.

Learning about Early-Warnings Relations

A key benefit of the Association Rule Mining (ARM) in the detection of disease is its ability to detect early-warning signals. These are minor patterns, which on their own might not seem of great clinical importance but once they co-occur they become meaningful. ARM is particularly effective when being used with large datasets, where early warning signs of a disease occur in far-flung and rare configurations (Yamamoto et al., 2023).

In chronic diseases, the early-warning relationships might include the small deviations in laboratory values, mild symptoms, or even small changes in vital signs. To use an example, gradual but continuous increases in blood pressure, which accompany increased stress values and sleep disturbance, may become a predisposing factor to hypertension. ARM allows uncovering such aggregations creating common outcomes that become the focus when analysed at the scale of thousands of patients records (Bays et al., 2022).

Infectious diseases Infectious diseases, the early-warning patterns may indicate the emergence of an infection. ARM can demonstrate that whole mild sore throat and light fatigue seem to be repeated two or three days before the manifestation of the more serious symptoms. These trends are priceless in the context of facility-wide health surveillance especially at the community level (Al-Halhouli et al., 2021).

ARM also helps in the explanation of disease progression. As an illustration, in cancer data, an early accumulation of biomarkers or a minor observation of imaging could indicate the onset of cancerous cell. When such associations have been identified, researchers are able to conduct further research, as well as combine the findings in the screening processes.

The other strength in ARM is that it supports temporal extensions. Temporal rules define the temporal development of symptoms, which allows identifying the patterns like symptom A then symptom B in one week predisposes the disease C. These policies balance the ability of clinicians to act sooner and allow families to spot the signs of danger earlier.

Case Study: Diabetes, Hypertension, Cancer and Infectious Diseases

ARM has been applied to a variety of disease situations of significant pathophysiological importance, with each case finding different benefits in pattern discovery.

Diabetes: ARM can be useful in diabetic datasets to identify combinations between the symptoms, lifestyle factors and laboratory values which lead to the diagnosis. Common trends consist of correlations between obesity, lack of physical activity, high levels of fasting glucose and family history. ARM can also detect some early symptoms like insensible thirst and slow-wound healing and marginally increased random glucose. The combinations help clinicians to diagnose pre diabetes and take preventive measures (Wang et al., 2020).

Hypertension: The development of hypertension is normally insidious. ARM is critical because it follows the identification of indirect and early-stage associations. Rules can show that patients with chronic stress, borderline blood pressure and poor sleep often develop overt hypertension in a period of many years. The trends in sodium intake, age and rising body-mass index also prominence. Varied sets of rules can make clinicians customize lifestyle-based counselling and emphasize screening programs (Iqbal & Jamal, 2023).

Cancer: ARM finds application in oncology to understand risk factors, collections of biomarkers, and imaging metadata. To illustrate, in breast-cancer data a occurrence like dense breast tissue with a definite age group and family predisposition to it may be indicative of an increased risk (Kumar & Joghee, 2025). In lung cancer, the association between long-term smoking, chronic cough and bizarre radiographs of the chest may be a rule. ARM is also used in finding hidden combinations of molecular markers which appear during early tumorigenesis.

Infectious Diseases: ARM is particularly beneficial in infectious-disease surveillance. It is able to identify trends of early spreading of pathogens in a population. The rules collected, especially during the outbreak of influenza, may show that the patients who come in with fever, sore throat, and sudden fatigue are temporally congregated over a small period of time (Murray & Cohen, 2016). ARM is also helpful to differentiate between mild and severe infections e.g. through the correlation of oxygen saturation, respiratory rate, and comorbidities. This feature serves the triage and early intervention protocols.

In all these diseases ARM provides clinicians with consistent and relevant combinations in patient data interpretation.

Comparison to other Machine-Learning Techniques in Prediction of Disease

Machine-learning strategies provide a continuum of disease prediction measures. ARM is differentiated by its transparency and ease of interpretation, unlike the models which can tend as opaque black boxes.

The methods include logistic regression, random forests, support vectors and deep learning, which are powerful predictors. They are able to handle high data of dimensions and achieve high performance levels. They, however, often produce complex models which cannot be easily used to justify the reasoning behind a prediction. Clinicians might thus be reluctant to embrace such outputs without explanations being clear.

On the contrary, ARM produces simple sets of rules, such as, If A and B, then C. These are rules which make sense, and between which clinical intuition is consistent. ARM does not make assumptions about data organization, which makes it flexible to different types of data. It also highlights patterns of co-occurrence, one of the patterns that cannot be easily revealed by many supervised models.

However, ARM has some drawbacks as compared to other machine-learning methods. Its ability to predict outcomes precisely may be hampered as it is oriented towards associations and not causality. ARM also can have a problem with very large variable sets where methods such as random forests can well work with high-dimensional data. Deep-learning-based models are useful in extracting patterns through unstructured inputs, including pictures and text, which ARM can aside find limited applications unless massive pre-processing is applied.

These differences notwithstanding, ARM and machine-learning techniques are complements to one another. Interpretable patterns that enhance clinical knowledge are discovered by ARM, and supervised models play valid predictive roles. When they are used together, both to create a strong system of analysis to detect and intervene early in case of the disease.

ARM FOR TREATMENT PLANNING

Association Rule Mining (ARM), has comes out as a central tool in explaining patient responses to various therapeutic interventions and also in defining drug-drug interactions in everyday clinical practice. The model of individualized treatment regimens frequently requires clinicians to balance a number of pharmacologic agents, comorbidities of the patient, adverse effects profile, and long-term outcome curves simultaneously. Modern clinical datasets have such a plethora of relationships most of which are obscure to standard tools of analysis. ARM helps in the uncovering of these covert connections and in effect, forms the basis of more clinical decisions being made. The main value of it is associated with its ability to identify regular patterns that are observed regularly throughout the history of patients, prescription history, and post-treatment follow-ups.

Patterns of Medication Responses

Ostensibly homogeneous diseases have heterogeneous pharmacologic responses in patients. An array of determinants (genetic predisposition, lifestyle factors, comorbid conditions and the pharmacokinetic variables) converges to influence therapeutic outcome. ARM is used to show the patterns of medication-response by analysing the patterns of improvement, relapse, or adverse events in cohorts of patients that receive drug combinations. As an example, ARM can also be used to prove how patients whose clinical presentation includes diabetes, comorbid obesity, and hypertriglyceridemia will always benefit using a specific oral antidiabetic combination, but the same treatment would not be optimal in patients with renal impairment. These insights are able to assist clinicians identify the subsets of patients in whom they are likely to accrue benefit of particular treatment methods. ARM also identifies delayed therapeutic reactions; others respond well during the acute stage and complications will arise after some months. ARM can identify longitudinal relationships between early drug reactions and later results by examining longitudinal data. Such relational rules guide the dosage modifications, timing, and the treatment period and thus enable hospitals to waste less effort in perfecting the standard procedures and reducing the extent of dependence on rule-of-thumb methods in the treatment of chronic diseases.

Side-Effects Pattern Discovery and Side-Effects Adverse Drug Reactions (ADRs)

The adverse drug reactions constitute one of the highest priorities of present-day medicine. Most of the ADRs are infrequent and appear in special circumstances which makes them difficult to detect during clinical trials. ARM helps in the study of patient large populations to reveal common relationships among pharmacologic agents and adverse side effects. As an example, ARM can demonstrate that a certain antibiotic has an increased tendency to increase hepatic enzymes in patients that are currently on some analgesics, or a certain oncologic agent regularly causes neuropathy in patients with vitamin deficiencies. Such trends allow the early detection and preventive measures. Hospitals might use the ARM-based ADR analyses to back such a decision as recalibration of the dosing guidelines, systematic observation, or simply prevent the use of dangerous combinations. ARM also follows cumulative drug effects including patients who are taking more than 1 medication at long durations. The identification of these interactions over the long term gives clinicians the powers to reformulate therapeutic regimens that reduce side-effects and maintain efficacy.

ARM in Clinical Pathway Optimisation

Clinical pathways formalize the series of administration of treatment, diagnoses, and protocols of specific diseases, thus guaranteeing prompt treatment and avoiding redundant services. ARM focuses on these pathways by determining the procedural steps, which have repeatedly been associated with better recovery, reduced admissions or fewer complications. To illustrate, ARM can also show that early Orthopaedic surgery physiotherapy shortens recovery in certain cohort of patients, and that post-admission diagnostic tests implemented the first 24 hours shortens treatment delays. These rules facilitate the work processes and minimize inter-department inconsistency. ARM may also be used to shed some light on the bottlenecks; processes that habitually result in delays during discharges can also be revealed and remedied by scheduling or resource allocation changes. Besides, ARM identifies alternative sequences of treatment which have worked out in specific groups of patients, thus informing the introduction of individualised treatment into mainstream protocols. Continuous implementation of ARM supports quality improvement efforts, helping institutions to identify best-practice protocols and revise the guidelines respectively, which eventually translates to improved patient satisfaction, patient outcomes, and resource use.

INTEGRATION WITH ADVANCED ANALYTICS

As a single method of identifying co-occurring patterns in healthcare data, the ARM has always been used almost independently. However, newer analytics are moving towards hybrid models where ARM is synergistically integrated with machine learning, deep learning, and sophisticated tools of visualisation. These integrations enable greater latent representations, promote greater accuracy of predictions and improve the accuracy of clinical judgment. With RBA insights coupled with the advanced computational forms, healthcare systems will be in a position to produce more detailed determinants and consequently improve better patient outcomes.

Hybrid ARM–Machine Learning Models in Healthcare

Hybrid models combine the predictive strength of machine learning and interior knowledge extraction facilities of Association Rule Mining (ARM). ARM identifies latent correlations between clinical indicators, such as symptoms, pharmacologic treatments and outcomes, and machine learning uses these correlations to improve its predictive models by using higher fidelity. The synergy resulting increases the accuracy of early diagnostics, level of risk stratification and maximization of therapeutic decisions. Practically, ARM generated antecedents are regularly reduced into feature vectors to be used by downstream classifiers. As an example, strong correlations between lifestyle determinants and pre-hypertensive manifestations can be represented using binary attributes as a statistical model, e.g., Random Forest, XGBoost, or Support Vector Machines, thus performing that task more effectively and faster than scanning an exhaustive raw variable set. In addition, this hybridisation also regulates overfitting by pitting machine-learning forecasts with empirical rule-based proofs, so the clinicians can outline subgroups of patients that should be examined more closely than others, personalize care guidelines, and determine which interventions have the most promising success prospects.

Deep Learning-based Feature Extraction

Deep learning plays a significant role in deriving complex forms of data among modalities like radiographic images, voice recordings, genomic sequences and huge volumes of observational data. Together with ARM, deep architectures originally encode high-dimensional sensory data into compact feature embedding's that may be utilized to seed rule-mining processes. This method is especially important in data where metadata, electronic health records, or sensor logs are structured in intricate non-linear forms, unseen by the more traditional statistical approaches. In practice, salient features, such as tumour morphology, texture gradient and boundary aberrations, can be distilled using convolutional networks by applying recent scans to magnetic resonance imaging; the resulting embedding are then consumed by ARM engines to find associations between oncologic phenotypes, genetic variants, therapy responses, and survival rates. The obtained regulations provide a more detailed representation of patient paths and increase the accuracy of clinical care. In its turn, ARM can serve as a dimensionality -reducing filter, which picks the most informative attributes among large sets of biomedical data. Motor training deep models on these carefully curated feature sets results in higher performance, fewer parameters, faster convergence and enhanced interpretability.

Rule Pattern Visualization Techniques

To make the voluminous rule sets generated by ARM useful to clinicians, it is important to visualize them. Normal visual encodings include heatmaps, node-link diagrams, parallel coordinate systems, matrix layouts, and interactive dashboards which can be used to bring out salient associations, cluster relationships, and often co-occurring antecedents. Heatmaps, such as, can quickly be used to evaluate support and confidence measure whereas node-link diagrams display hierarchical dependency schemes amongst clinical objects. Directly above platforms such as Tableau or Python libraries (e.g., Plotly, Bokeh), interactive dashboards can be created in which end-users can filter rules by cohort features, diagnostic features or pharmacologic agents and direct their decision-support efforts to the most contextually appealing patterns and speed-up clinical judgment.

ARM as a DSS part in CDSS

Clinical Decision Support Systems (CDSS) are evidence-based recommendations systems that are offered to practitioners and the integration of ARM into the systems enhances it by the addition of rules that reflect real-life practice patterns. Such regulations emphasize the areas of early warning indicators, typical risk synergies, interactions between drugs and the effective lines of treatment. A CDSS can also warn clinicians of an excessive pharmacologic interaction in their prescription, or propose confirmatory diagnoses based on common trends observed among similar groups of patients. Since the ARM-based guidelines are understandable, clinicians can have insight into the logic behind algorithmic recommendations, which leads to a greater level of trust and more personalized, safer care.

IMPLEMENTATION FRAMEWORK AT A U.S. LOCAL HOSPITAL

An empirical model is also necessary when implementing ARM in the active practices of healthcare. The medical information is multidimensional and requires strict control to guarantee its reliability, transparency, and integrity. It consists of a sequence of steps that leads to a systematic work that results into the following stages: (i) data gathering (ii) pre-processing (iii) rule mining (iv) validation. The components are presented in details below.

Workflow: Data Collection Data Pre-processing Rule Mining Validation

The arm of the pipeline starts with the acquisition of heterogeneous data which includes electronic health records, laboratory information systems, pharmacy management databases, imaging archives, and bedside monitoring devices. A unification of these dissimilar repositories is needed to obtain one cohesive analytical data set. There are other steps of pre-processing, including imputation of missing data, de-duplication, coding schema normalization and inconsistencies. The processes involved in feature engineering such as discrete variables of continuous variables, class imbalance management, attribute selection based on clinical usefulness are critical since ARM is vulnerable to noise and data heterogeneity. Having passed through data curation, frequent-item set algorithms (e.g. Apriori, FP-Growth, ECLAT, etc.) are then used to produce candidate association rules that represent co-occurring clinical entities. Statistical relevance, clinical plausibility, and interpretability are determined by the last validation process, which uses hypothesis testing to access the rules, expert review, and cross- dataset replication to access them.

Threshold choice of Medical Rules (Support, Confidence, Lift).

The decision of support, confidence and lift thresholds are paramount in retrieving quality medical rules, especially when the phenomena of clinical interest are likely to be rare. In medical data, support thresholds are typically set intentionally low to allow the detection of rare but possibly very crucial patterns (e.g., particular interactions of drugs). There are higher levels of confidence required, compared to commercial applications, to increase the accuracy of the recommendations and minimise the chances of making false inferences. The lift which measures the non-random association between the variables is interpreted to be a signal of a meaningful clinical correlation; a lift value beyond unity points to positive correlation beyond baseline prevalence. Through establishing appropriate threshold calibration, it is possible to have ARM deliver statistically sound and clinically meaningful rules, therefore making the placement of data-driven wisdom and evidence-based practice consistent.

There is no official clinical validation or review process involved, since the decision-making relies solely on the individual's personal judgment and experience, or even more on the subjective interpretation of the raw numbers collected.<|human|>No formal clinical validation and expert review There is no formal clinical validation and expert review involved in this, as the decision-making is based purely on personal judgment and experience of the individual, or even more on subjective interpretation of raw numbers obtained.

The rules are reviewed by clinical experts such as physicians, pharmacists and expert public health specialists after statistical validation. This, in turn, establishes the fact that the identified associations are medically understandable and aligned with what is known. Professionals also investigate inconsistencies, threats or outdated trends. The rules which suit the demands of clinical review can be implemented in decision-support systems, patient risk management, and treatment model. These joint assurances would strengthen the trust in ARM-based systems and increase their adoption in hospitals.

Tools and Platforms: Python, R, WEKA, Apache Spark.

There are many tools that support ARM in the medical sphere. The use of python is widespread because libraries, including mlxtend, pandas, and PySpark, are also available to manipulate large datasets. R has solid statistical back-up through packages such as arules and arulesViz. WEKA offers an easy to use interface on Apriori and FP-Growth, and is therefore appropriate to academic research and small scale hospital studies. In case of high volume of data, Apache Spark can offer distributed processing capabilities that can efficiently process millions of records using Spark MLlib. These tools enable the researchers and other healthcare analysts to implement ARM models, scale them and integrate them to the existing clinical workflow.

REAL LIFE SCENARIOS AND CASE STUDIES

Association Rule Mining (ARM) is no longer at the very frontier of investigative research, it is currently in use in hospitals, national health programmes and clinical research centres. Its main strength is that it exposes hidden relationships in large medical datasets, the relationship which is difficult to discover by a manual approach. Case studies provided below demonstrate the ways in which ARM enhances patient care, operational planning and long-term health management in real-life scenarios.

Development of the system would take into account the following insight: hospital readmission rates have not yet declined due to the quality of care provided.<|human|>Development of the system would consider the following finding: the hospital readmission rates have not yet decreased because of the quality of care offered.

Avoidable readmissions are among the most important goals of hospitals. Incomplete treatment, lack of a proper follow-up strategy, medication errors, or underlying problem have led to frequent readmissions. ARM helps in the identification of symptom, diagnosis and treatment combinations that keep recurring to cause repeat visits. As an example, ARM would show that patient discharges with congestive heart failure without follow-up electrolyte test have high readmission rates in the seven days after discharge. Moreover, it can indicate that some antibiotic and analgesic combinations increase the risk of readmission because of the side effects. These lessons will be used to create fine-tuned discharge procedures, better surveillance of high-risk groups, and more individualized follow-up measures. In the long term, this pattern identification reduces redundant admissions and maximises the use of resources.

ARM of Chronic Disease Management

Diseases like diabetes, high blood pressure, asthma, kidney disease, etc. are those that require chronic monitoring and regular therapeutic restructuring. ARM enhances chronic disease management through identification of habitual behaviours in the patient, medication reactions, and risk of complications. The applications of ARM in diabetes care (such as the identification of links between frequent high glucose spikes, irregular medication adherence, and poor dietary habits) can also be used. It can also show that oral antidiabetic agents that are better in certain age groups exhibit reduced effectiveness in patients of renal impairment. ARM would unravel in hypertension, salt consumption, discrepancy of exercise, and non-adherence to medication with intermittent high blood pressure. The results can assist clinicians to develop individualised management and education interventions in different patient groups. Besides, ARM may aid in avoiding the development of the complication in time by providing information on which combinations of lab values are followed by the disease, prior to its appearance.

Trends in ICU Treatment Plans

Intensive Care units produce voluminous data, such as ventilation, continuous vital signs, dose of medication, and laboratory. ARM helps to realize the patterns of treatment that contribute to the recovery or reduce complications. An example is that ARM can show that ventilator parameter adjustment in the early phase along with electrolyte correction within the appropriate time frames can prevent respiratory deterioration in particular groups of patients. It is also able to identify the links between specific sedative decisions and faster stabilisation during postoperative instances. These insights can be used by hospitals to optimise ICU procedures and streamline interventions that yield positive results uniformly. The analysis of the trends among several patients can help the clinicians to have a more profound knowledge of the most successful order of interventions, especially in time or situation-sensitive cases.

The governmental health services are concerned with large and heterogeneous groups of people, which makes ARM a useful tool to identify the emergent trends. ARM aids in surveillance to establish cluster of symptoms, patterns of infection, environmental triggers, and geographic dissemination. In the event of an outbreak of an infectious disease, ARM may emphasize common sources of exposure or combinations of symptoms that commonly occur at the beginning of the affected population. To illustrate, the ARM can detect early links between fever, musculo-skeletal pain, and certain neighbourhood clusters during the influenza seasons and therefore allow an immediate response by the health authorities. ARM has also been useful in tracking non-communicable diseases by clarifying the relationship existing between lifestyle and socioeconomic status and occurrence of a disease. Such understanding will empower the policymakers to establish specific awareness campaigns, distribute their resources effectively, and develop preventive actions.

HARDSHIP AND THE FUTURE PROSPECTS

Although the use of ARM has proved to be potential in the health care industry, there are obstacles limiting its widespread use. Medical knowledge is per se complicated with numerous regulations and with constant transformation that makes it more difficult to find the rules and integrate them into clinical practice. At the same time, the up-and-coming technologies, including IoT devices, wearables, and federated learning, provide new chances to use more precise and timely as well as non-invasion analytics. With a subtle understanding of these issues and opportunities, the future of ARM-based healthcare systems will be paved.

In this context, it is required that the data produced by the software is as interpretable as it can be, and is trusted clinically as well.

Ensuring Interpretability and Clinical Trust.

The data generated by the software must be as interpretable as possible and must also be clinically trusted. One of the main issues with the application of ARM in the healthcare sector is the ability to make clinicians understand and believe in the generated rules. Nurses and doctors are guided by logical thinking and scientific facts, and, therefore, any policy that affects diagnosis or provision of care must be easily comprehensible. Complex or very large sets of rules can also confuse the users and hinder uptake. Future studies should hence focus on streamlining redundant rules, development of better visual explanation as well as integrating rule summaries that emphasize clinical relevance. Clear and understandable models will create confidence and encourage acceptance in hospital settings.

High-dimensional medical data management.

Healthcare data often consist of hundreds of variables such as the laboratory results, drug histories, imaging characteristics, and demographic data. Such data is very dimensional, which makes effective rule mining difficult and those irrelevant patterns proliferate. As a result, feature selection, dimensionality reduction, and clinical filtering cannot be excluded in order to cope with this complexity. Future improvement can be holistic in terms of hybrid systems that combine Association Rule Mining (ARM) and deep learning methods to extract salient features before generating rules. In addition to this, it will also be necessary to have efficient algorithms and distributed processing models that would handle large datasets without losing the accuracy of analysis.

Streaming Health Data Mining Streaming Rule Mining in Health.

With the emergence of the remote monitoring systems and hospital sensors, there is increased pressure on real or time analytics. Traditional ARM algorithms work with fixed sets of data and fail to adaptively modify rules. However, continuous monitoring is required in the emergency care and intensive care unit. Real-time ARM techniques should be able to read streaming data, update patterns quite fast and find early warning signals as they appear. This requirement can be met by incremental rule-mining and online learning. The ARM with the real-time data pipelines installed in future healthcare will, perhaps, foresee instances of sudden deteriorations, and raise awareness of upcoming abnormal tendencies amid clinicians.

Opportunities on IoT, Wearable Health Devices, and Federated Learning.

The Internet-of-Things and wearable devices are constantly producing health information, including heartbeat rate, glucose levels, oxygen levels and activity patterns. This information provides possibilities that ARM could determine the onset of risky factors, lifestyle stimulations, and behavioural trends. At the same time, the privacy laws limit data exchange between hospitals. The federated learning offers a system through which ARM can be offered to multiple institutions without sensitive data leakage. Aggregation of patterns can be shared in hospitals instead of raw records and, therefore, provide protection to the patient privacy and reduces the quality of analysis. The addition of ARM to these new technologies will allow upcoming years to offer more customized care, more powerful disease prediction, and more increased national health knowledge.

CONCLUSION

This chapter has discussed the Association Rule Mining (ARM) as a capable tool used to reveal hidden associations in any complex healthcare data. The discussion has described how ARM goes beyond the conventional analyses to portray valuable co-occurrences between symptoms, treatments, and outcomes by articulating its concepts of conceptualization, algorithms, applications, and the relevant steps of implementation. These results can assist the clinicians in comprehending patient behaviour, predicting risks, and enhancing individual and system decision-making. ARM significantly contributes to enhancing precise health care by making it effectively possible to conduct personalised diagnosis and determine the effects of specific treatment combinations, and to timely detect possible complication occurrences. This ability to handle large amounts of clinical data empowers hospitals to identify patterns that otherwise could not be identified by manual review, improve evidence-based practices and operational effectiveness in chronic disease management, ICU planning, medication safety, and public health surveillance. In the future, the power of ARM can only get bigger with increasing data-driven healthcare. Combining it with machine learning, IoT gadgets, wearable sensors, and federated learning will bring the creation of the real-time privacy-sensitive systems that will be able to produce dynamic insights. This advancement will make detecting the disease earlier and pathing it to individual treatment process as well as continuous monitoring of the patient easier. With algorithms becoming increasingly accessible and expandable, ARM will remain among the core pillars of the development of intelligent, proactive, and patient-centred healthcare solutions.

REFERENCES

Al-Halhouli, A. A., Albagdady, A., Alawadi, J. F., & Abeeleh, M. A. (2021). Monitoring symptoms of infectious diseases: Perspectives for printed wearable sensors. *Micromachines*, *12*(6), 620. DOI: 10.3390/mi12060620 PMID: 34072174

Bakar, W. A. W. A., Man, M., Man, M., & Abdullah, Z. (2020). i-Eclat: Performance enhancement of Eclat via incremental approach in frequent itemset mining. *Telkomnika*, *18*(1), 562–570. DOI: 10.12928/telkomnika.v18i1.13497

Baryakova, T. H., Pogostin, B. H., Langer, R., & McHugh, K. J. (2023). Overcoming barriers to patient adherence: The case for developing innovative drug delivery systems. *Nature Reviews. Drug Discovery*, *22*(5), 387–409. DOI: 10.1038/s41573-023-00670-0 PMID: 36973491

Bays, H. E., Agarwala, A., German, C., Satish, P., Iluyomade, A., Dudum, R., Thakkar, A., Rifai, M. A., Mehta, A., Thobani, A., Al-Saiegh, Y., Nelson, A. J., Sheth, S., & Toth, P. P. (2022). Ten things to know about ten cardiovascular disease risk factors–2022. *American Journal of Preventive Cardiology*, *10*, 100342. DOI: 10.1016/j.ajpc.2022.100342 PMID: 35517870

Bélair, J., Glass, L., an der Heiden, U., & Milton, J. (1995). Dynamical disease: Identification, temporal aspects and treatment strategies of human illness. *Chaos (Woodbury, N.Y.)*, *5*(1), 1–7. DOI: 10.1063/1.166069 PMID: 12780147

Chernoff, M. C., Wang, M., Anderson, J. J., & Felson, D. T. (1995). Problems and suggested solutions in creating an archive of clinical trials data.... *Controlled Clinical Trials*, *16*(5), 342–355. DOI: 10.1016/0197-2456(95)00049-6 PMID: 8582152

David, J. (2007). Association rule ontology matching approach. *International Journal on Semantic Web and Information Systems*, *3*(2), 27–49. DOI: 10.4018/jswis.2007040102

Ehrenstein, V., Kharrazi, H., Lehmann, H., & Taylor, C. O. (2019). *Obtaining data from electronic health records....* AHRQ.

Haug, P. J., Gardner, R. M., Tate, K. E., Evans, R. S., East, T. D., Kuperman, G., Pryor, T. A., Huff, S. M., & Warner, H. R. (1994). Decision support in medicine: Examples from the HELP system. *Computers and Biomedical Research, an International Journal*, *27*(5), 396–418. DOI: 10.1006/cbmr.1994.1030 PMID: 7813202

Hossain, M., Devnath, A., & Karmokar, P. (2023). *Handling Missing Values and Outliers....* Diabetes Classification Accuracy.

Iqbal, A. M., & Jamal, S. F. (2023). *Essential hypertension. StatPearls*. StatPearls Publishing.

Kang'ethe, S. M. (2014). Discovering medical diagnosis patterns... (Doctoral dissertation).

Kumar, R. M. R., & Joghee, S. (2025). A Review on Integrating Breast Cancer Clinical Data. *Current Treatment Options in Oncology*, *26*(1), 1–13. DOI: 10.1007/s11864-024-01285-2 PMID: 39752094

Lau, J. M., Iochpe, C., Thom, L. H., & Reichert, M. (2009). *Discovery and analysis of activity pattern co-occurrences....* ICEIS.

Liu, L., Wang, X., Gui, M., Ju, F., Cao, L., & Bi, B. (2025). Investigation of multimorbidity patterns.... *Scientific Reports*, *15*(1), 25741. DOI: 10.1038/s41598-025-09926-8 PMID: 40670483

Lyu, G. (2025). Data-driven decision making in patient management: A systematic review. *BMC Medical Informatics and Decision Making*, *25*(1), 239. DOI: 10.1186/s12911-025-03072-x PMID: 40598137

Martínez-García, M., & Hernández-Lemus, E. (2022). Data integration challenges for machine learning in precision medicine. *Frontiers in Medicine*, *8*, 784455. DOI: 10.3389/fmed.2021.784455 PMID: 35145977

Murray, J., & Cohen, A. L. (2016). Infectious disease surveillance. *International encyclopedia of public health*, 222.

Nalavade, K., & Meshram, B. B. (2014). Finding frequent item-sets using Apriori algorithm.... *IJCAIT*, *6*(1), 84–92.

Rana, S., Mondal, M. N. I., & Islam, M. R. (2025). Unveiling Purchase Patterns... *ECCE 2025*.

Razzak, M. I., Imran, M., & Xu, G. (2020). Big data analytics for preventive medicine. *Neural Computing & Applications*, *32*(9), 4417–4451. DOI: 10.1007/s00521-019-04095-y PMID: 32205918

Rotaru-Zavaleanu, A. D., Lungulescu, C. V., Bunescu, M. G., Vasile, R. C., Gheorman, V., Gresita, A., & Dinescu, V. C. (2024). Occupational Carpal Tunnel Syndrome.... *Frontiers in Public Health*, *12*, 1407302. DOI: 10.3389/fpubh.2024.1407302 PMID: 38841666

Scheffer, T. (2001). Finding association rules that trade support optimally against confidence. *PKDD*, 424–435.

Shackelford, S. J., Proia, A. A., Martell, B., & Craig, A. N. (2015). Toward a global cybersecurity standard of care.... *Tex. Int'l LJ*, *50*, 305.

Shichkina, Y., Petrov, M., & Roza, F. (2022). Determination of significant parameters.... *Mathematics*, *10*(7), 1133. DOI: 10.3390/math10071133

Sowan, B., Zhang, L., Matar, N., Zraqou, J., Omar, F., & Alnatsheh, A. (2025). A novel lift adjustment methodology... *Decision Analytics Journal, 100582.*

Srinadh, V. (2022). Evaluation of Apriori, FP-growth and Eclat.... *International Journal of Health Sciences*, •••, 7475–7485. DOI: 10.53730/ijhs.v6nS2.6729

Wang, M., Tan, Y., Shi, Y., Wang, X., Liao, Z., & Wei, P. (2020). Diabetes and sarcopenic obesity.... *Frontiers in Endocrinology*, *11*, 568. DOI: 10.3389/fendo.2020.00568 PMID: 32982969

Wang, W., Ferrari, D., Haddon-Hill, G., & Curcin, V. (2023). Electronic health records as source of research data... *Machine Learning for Brain Disorders*, 331–354.

Yamamoto, H., Kayanuma, G., Nagashima, T., Toda, C., Nagayasu, K., & Kaneko, S. (2023). Early detection of adverse drug reaction signals.... *Drug Safety*, *46*(4), 371–389. DOI: 10.1007/s40264-023-01278-4 PMID: 36828947

Chapter 4
Healthcare Applications of Association Rule Mining in Disease Detection and Treatment Planning

Ashwini Manish Brahme
http://orcid.org/0009-0004-6283-5254
International Institute of Management Science, Savitribai Phule Pune University, India

Sagar Rajendra Kulkarni
Mumbai University, India

Shivaji D. Mundhe
International Institute of Management Science, Savitribai Phule Pune University, India

Manasi Sagar Kulkarni
Pillai College of Engineering, New Panvel, India

ABSTRACT

The evolution of health informatics through HER led to an overwhelming influx of data within healthcare organizations. These systems now house vast and varied datasets including patient profiles, medical histories, diagnostic results, admission details, and personal health metrics managed by a wide array of professionals. A critical area of focus is the prediction and monitoring of upcoming diseases

DOI: 10.4018/979-8-3373-6691-3.ch004

increasingly spreading across regions. There are various parameters like population, global travel, international trade, viral transmission, and limited awareness of timely medical intervention. These dynamics have intensified the impact on public health; several key elements must be considered: Geographic distribution, Victim count and impact, Treatment pathways. There is need to focus: the pre-processing of unstructured and heterogeneous data, to uncover frequent patterns and correlations by applying association rule mining, to generate the patterns from diseases, symptoms,individuals, locations, medications, to generate knowledge discovery through association rule mining.

INTRODUCTION

The adoption of electronic health records (EHRs) within health informatics has greatly increased the amount of information handled by healthcare organizations, often overwhelming them with data. These platforms gather a wide range of records—such as patient demographics, admission details, and administrative information—managed by specialists from different fields. Consequently, healthcare executives are seeking effective strategies to structure and leverage this expanding data environment to deliver precise and timely medical services. Clinicians frequently face challenges in linking patient histories to critical health conditions, identifying symptom patterns and underlying causes, and determining appropriate treatment options. An escalating issue is the emergence and spread of infectious diseases across regions, fuelled by factors like population growth, international travel, global commerce, and the swift transmission of viruses. These circumstances have intensified pressures on public health systems, highlighting the pressing need for predictive tools and proactive approaches to disease control.

Figure 1. Structured and unstructured data

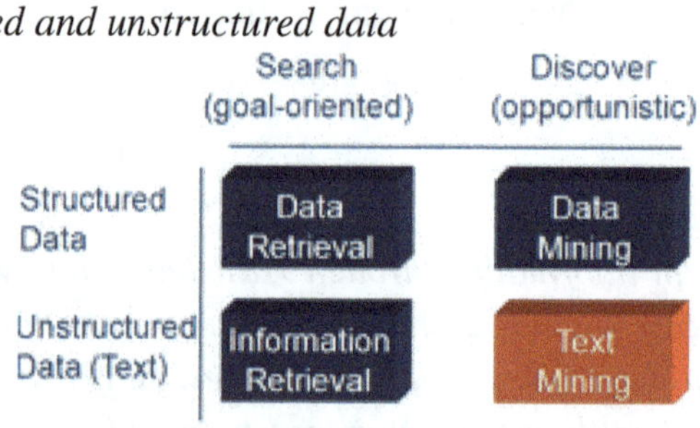

The primary objective of this chapter is:

1. To focus on the pre-processing of unstructured and heterogeneous data
2. To uncover frequent patterns and correlations by applying association rule mining (ARM),
3. To generate the patterns from parameters as diseases, symptoms, affected individuals, locations, medications, and treatment protocols—ultimately facilitating faster and more accurate clinical decisions.
4. To generate knowledge discovery using association mining

NEED OF PRE-PROCESSING HEALTHCARE DISEASES DATA

Healthcare faces several critical hurdles for unstructured, semi structured data processing and generative the effective patterns from the corpus amount of data, robust association rules, and effective knowledge discovery from the data and better decision making for healthcare organizations and stakeholders. (Prabavathy & Sumathi, 2013) This will lead towards the need of healthcare data processing for the following aspects:

- **Efficient Document Retrieval**: Identifying relevant and valuable information from massive datasets which is challenging with respect to heterogeneous data
- **Data Format Diversity**: Biomedical content available online spans structured, semi-structured, and unstructured formats, necessitating the use of advanced data mining techniques to process and analyze it effectively.
- **Discovering Relationships**: A primary aim of healthcare analytics is to identify significant links among illnesses, symptoms, treatments, preventive strategies, and patient groups.
- **Analytical Challenges**: Ongoing studies address problems such as classification, clustering, text modelling, information extraction, and detecting hidden trends within large datasets.
- **Data Transformation**: Converting unstructured text into formats suitable for analysis is a complex process that demands thorough pre-processing.
- **Multilingual Analysis**: Medical information must often be refined and interpreted across multiple languages.
- **Domain Knowledge Integration**: Embedding clinical expertise into data-mining algorithms is vital for producing accurate and context-sensitive outcomes.
- **Personalized and Autonomous Systems**: Developing applications that tailor insights to individual patient profiles and function independently is an emerging focus.

- **Managing High Dimensionality:** The vast scale and diversity of healthcare data create challenges in terms of scalability and system performance.
- **Complexity of Medical Language**: Clinical texts are often intricate, making them difficult to parse and interpret effectively.
- **Ambiguity and Context Dependence:** Correctly understanding medical terminology requires contextual awareness, which traditional mining techniques often struggle to achieve

1. Related Work

A KDD is step by step process and includes various steps specifically data selection, pre-processing, and transformation. Sumathy and Chidambaram (2013) focused on information retrieval feature of text mining. Text mining includes two major phases one is text refining and another is knowledge distillation. The paper also elaborates text mining applications, challenges and limitations in various domains (Babanejaddehaki et. al., 2025). A data mining tool WEKA is adopted for predictions of Dengue diseases (Shakil et al., 2015).

The researcher has compared different algorithms and suggested that Naïve Bayes classifications technique is useful for Dengue diseases prediction (Badawy et al., 2023). The paper described on the diversity and heterogeneous corpus data is the biggest challenges of test mining and information retrieval. A critical aspect in textual data mining is pre-processing, stemming and indexing is highlighted (Ibrahim et al., 2017). This proposed research seeks to apply text mining techniques with an efficient pre-processing approach in one of these areas, aiming to advance text mining methodologies and address its existing challenges (Kulkarni & Mundhe, 2017).

The research paper "Framework for Knowledge Discovery from Journal Articles Using Text Mining Techniques" highlights various applications of text mining and knowledge discovery derived from journal articles. It distinguishes between text mining and data mining, emphasizing the critical role of text mining across multiple fields. The paper outlines several key applications, including bioinformatics, customer profiling, trend analysis, anti-spam email filtering, event tracking, news agency text classification, web search, and patent analysis. The text mining comprised of text processing, transformation, feature selection, filtering, lemmatization, stemming, and index term selection. The researcher developed an algorithm and workflow to model an automated text mining system as part of this study (Mandal, 2013).

The system is designed and focused on various parameters of diseases where 12 disease were focused by the researchers to compare the doctor's diagnosis and system diagnosis to check the accuracy and efficiency of diseases, symptoms, causes and medications (Moral et al., 2014). The main challenge in biomedical text data and information mining lies in the evolving and complex nature of terminology and language within biological data. This field focuses on extracting meaningful information from texts related to biology, medicine, and chemistry. To explore relationships between proteins, genes, and diseases, the researcher employed techniques such as information extraction, retrieval, indexing, text classification, and categorization. These methods were applied to analyze articles, abstracts, and discussions found in databases like PubMed, Oxford, and others (Moral et al., 2014).

A research article by El-Sappagh, et al. (2013) titled "Data Mining and Knowledge Discovery: Applications, Techniques, Challenges and Process Models in Healthcare," describes about integrating KDD and HER could improve patient outcomes, lower medical errors, and increase patient safety by reducing undesired practice variation. KDD aids in identifying patterns and hidden linkages from various parameters in the data. In order to provide an analysis and demonstrate efficacy, such as by predicting the ideal dosage of medications, this study elaborate applications of knowledge discovery, text mining, data mining in the domain of healthcare industry by comparing causes, symptoms, and treatment plans.

Amin et al. (2014) focused on research entitled "Extract Association Rules to Minimize the Effects of Dengue Using a Text Mining Technique" which explores the application of XML for information retrieval and presents an architectural model for a text mining system. This system focuses on text processing, association rule mining, and visualization. The researcher developed the GRAW Algorithm used for association mining using XML files for dengue diseases (Ojo & Adeyemo, 2012).

The researcher Shakil et al. (2015) conducted study on prediction of Dengue diseases describes and explores the various techniques of data mining used to forecast dengue cases through the WEKA platform. It evaluates the effectiveness of five different algorithms namely REP Tree, J48, SMO, etc. by applying them to a dengue-related dataset. The researchers utilized these algorithms to assess their effectiveness in predicting the occurrence of dengue. The various text mining techniques, challenges, applications and tools are discussed by the researcher it has observed that there is need of effective Pre-processing in any one of the area and try to advancement in the text mining techniques (Kulkarni & Mundhe, 2017). Machine learning (ML) and deep learning (DL) are transforming traditional healthcare services by leveraging healthcare data as a key component. AI methods enhance disease diagnosis, predict healthcare trends, and analyze patient data by linking clinical records. The study serves as a valuable resource, advancing healthcare predictive analytics research and supporting future academic efforts. Text mining progress includes methods to classify articles on drug-drug interactions, detect catalytic protein sites in biomedical literature, and expand health-related taxonomies with consumer-friendly medical synonyms in biomedical research (Prabavathy & Sumathi, 2013).

The data from internet sources will be carefully evaluated and disseminated for both public awareness and commercial utilization, contributing to knowledge expansion and supporting valuable practical applications using web mining (Prabavathy & Sumathi, 2013). The effectiveness of text mining as a tool for analyzing free-text data, such as medical histories found in electronic medical records (EMRs). It aids in improving diagnostic accuracy and formulating hypotheses by leveraging past medical histories while considering age- and gender-specific conditions. The suggested approach and results have the potential to significantly improve healthcare information systems, both in research applications and clinical decision-making contexts (Ramon-Gonen et al., 2023).

The study carried out for predictive diseases outbreaks in terms of demographic, climate, density, vaccinations, classical classification for epidemic disease and infected demographics of these diseases. The researcher has used Backpropagation methods comprised of acquisition, extraction, classification, feature selection and outbreak prediction and identifies the correlation of epidemic diseases factors. Further the research carried out on diseases outbreak detection and forecasting comprised of prediction using conventional data sources and social media, internet sources used for collecting diseases information and using mathematical time series method and machine learning time series method is used for diseases categorization. The outbreak prediction is based on the various factors data sources, size, real-time data accessibility, type of data, demographics, and services provided by the healthcare at that location, etc. Therefore it is essential to process the text mining from corpus data.

Ramon-Gonen et al. (2023) particularized in his study on practical use of text mining for digital health records by applying text mining techniques and patients history which results in the detailed form of diagnosis.

2. Healthcare Data Mining

Data Mining Techniques

This is interdisciplinary filed comprised of pattern identification, statistical methods, computing, machine learning, neural networks data visualization, etc. It involves the application of analytical methods to uncover patterns, correlations, or relationships within large datasets. The overarching aim is to extract valuable insights or knowledge from data repositories also named as knowledge discovery. This process, commonly known as Knowledge Discovery in Databases focuses on identifying novel and actionable information within a specific context or application area.

According to Fayyad et al. (1996), data mining encompasses six core functions:

A. **Classification** – Developing models that categorize data in predetermined groups or classes.

B. **Regression** – Predicting constant numerical values depends on input data.
C. **Clustering** – Grouping data into distinct clusters or categories that share similar characteristics.
D. **Dependency Modelling / Association Rule Mining**– Identifying significant relationships or dependencies among variables.
E. **Anomaly Detection (Deviation Detection)** – Recognizing unusual or significant deviations within the data.
F. **Summarization** – Generating concise representations or summaries of data subsets.

Figure 2. Data mining and knowledge discovery from database (KDD)

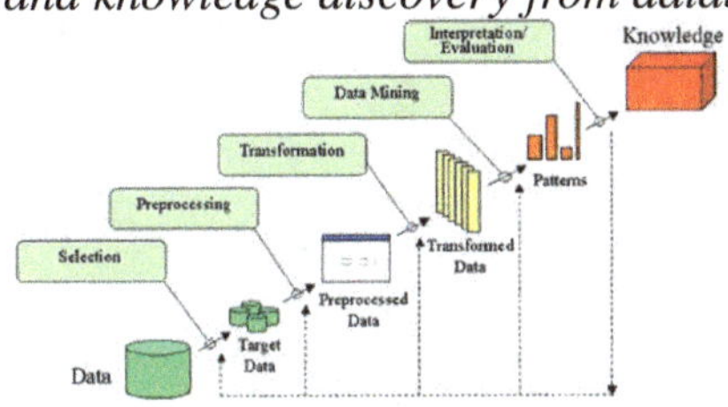

Data mining is classified as supervised and unsupervised learning. In unsupervised learning, analysis begins without any predefined model or hypothesis. Algorithms are applied directly to raw data, allowing patterns and structures to emerge organically. The methods of data mining namely clustering, association mining fall under this category; as they aim to uncover hidden relationships or groupings within datasets without prior labelling.

Conversely, supervised learning involves constructing a predictive and analytical model before the data analysis begins. Then it is refined by applying algorithms to estimate its parameters based on known input-output pairs. The primary goal here is to forecast specific outcomes or classify data into predefined categories. Common approaches in supervised learning include classification, regression analysis, and the development of artificial neural networks.

Figure 3. Data mining techniques

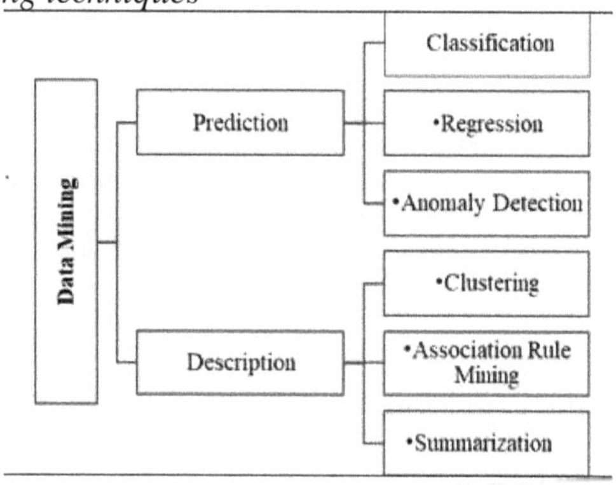

A. Classification

Classification stands as a fundamental approach within data mining, rooted in the principles of machine learning. As a form of supervised learning, it involves assigning data instances to predefined categories based on input features. The primary aim is to accurately group data objects according to shared characteristics or patterns.

To achieve this, classification leverages a range of computational and statistical techniques as DT-decision tree, support vector machines (SVM), Bayesian inference, neural network and association-based models. Each method provides a distinct approach to building predictive models capable of generalizing from training data to new, unseen instances.

For instance,

- Countries may be categorized based on climatic conditions such as tropical, temperate, or arid zones.
- In the healthcare domain, classification is frequently used to group patients by disease type, enabling more targeted diagnosis and treatment planning.

B. Clustering

Clustering refers to the analytical process of grouping data items based on shared attributes or similarities. Unlike classification, where categories are predefined, clustering allows the data itself to determine the structure of the groups. This technique is a form of unsupervised learning, as it does not rely on labelled datasets or prior assumptions about group membership.

The data is grouped into clusters; various clustering methodologies exist, including hierarchical approaches (both agglomerative and divisive), partitioning algorithms, density-based models, grid-based techniques, and model-driven strategies.

For example,

- In a library setting, books can be automatically grouped by genre or subject matter to streamline access for readers.
- In healthcare, clustering can be used to categorize diseases based on their nature—such as viral, bacterial, or genetic—supporting more efficient diagnosis and treatment planning.

C. Regression or Prediction

Regression technique is applied for identifying relationship among the terms. The various applications of predictions like crop, flood, weather, natural climates, stock market, price, market, diseases pandemics predictions and many more. It works on past and current dataset and predict what the possibility will be of or chances of a particular aspects.

Regressions is comprised of three techniques as linear, nonlinear and multivariate.

Example: In healthcare, the diseases, early prediction, parameters predictions, demographics prediction, pandemic prediction can be carried out.

D. Association Rule Mining

It is used to find relation between the variables or parameters. There are diverse applications of Association rule mining such as healthcare, sales, marketing, sentimental analysis, social media, market analysis as well as market basket analysis, etc.

For Example:

- If customer is purchasing product *A* then maybe he/she can purchase product *B* (If *bread* is purchased then *butter* will also be purchased).
- In medical / healthcare sector, the diseases are comprised of various parameters as diseases, symptoms, impact, demographics, remedial measures etc. in the line of these Parameters association rules are generated in the form of IF --- THEN like IF <Fever, Cough> THEN <Flue>

E. Summarization

It is also named as generalization. Categorization; it takes the data or information available and summarise it in the form of compressed data.

For example: in healthcare the patients information can be summarised so that easily his/her history can be taken for further diagnosis.

F. Anomaly Detection

Anomalies refer to significant difference among the patterns of data from expected or typical behaviour. Anomaly detection is widely applied in telecommunication abuse monitoring, cyber security for identifying network breaches, fault diagnosis in engineering systems, analysis of medical and public health records, financial frauds. It used in industrial monitoring, image analysis, other fields where recognizing results to timely interventions or deeper insights.

▪ Challenges of Data Mining Techniques

- Data mining techniques often struggle to process highly diverse and complex datasets due to limitations in adaptability and representation.
- One major obstacle is the fragmented nature of data sources.
- Analyzing structured data tends to be a simpler task, whereas uncovering meaningful information from unstructured or partially structured sources poses considerable difficulty.
- Handling large-scale, relational datasets with intricate interdependencies poses considerable computational and analytical difficulties.
- Incomplete or noisy data hampers the discovery of meaningful patterns, reducing the reliability of outcomes.
- Extracting useful knowledge from heterogeneous databases—those with varying formats and schemas—requires advanced integration strategies.
- Many data mining algorithms face limitations in scalability and performance, especially when applied to massive datasets requiring efficient and timely analysis.

▪ Advanced Data Mining and Challenges for Healthcare

Data mining identifies uncovering hidden, valuable insights from vast datasets also known as Knowledge Discovery from Databases, it represents a collaborative discipline that integrates principles from database systems, statistical analysis and machine learning. As the maple applications in data mining results into the various challenges and pitfalls. Due to the advancement in the technological era researchers have developed innovative approaches to mining complex data types. These include specialized techniques such as image mining, content mining, text mining, video mining, and web mining, each tailored to extract meaningful patterns from specific formats. The different techniques used for structured data, typically organized in relational databases. However, the increasing prevalence of unstructured and semi-structured data—such as textual documents, multimedia content, and web data—necessitates more advanced analytical tools. Text mining is a key solution for analyzing textual information, drawing upon a blend of machine learning, natural language processing, information retrieval, clustering, categorization, advanced data mining, and visualization techniques. This convergence makes text mining a distinctly multidisciplinary domain. Text data mining primarily aims to extract key elements by pinpointing commonly used words and ideas in documents, and to uncover associations like links between patient reported symptoms that enhance comprehension and guide informed decisions.

3. PRE-PROCESSING OF DISEASES HEALTHCARE DATA

3.1 Text Mining of Diseases and Treatment Planning

Text mining is nothing but mining meaningful insights from unstructured or semi-structured textual information or data by applying the related techniques. It is considered an advanced form of data mining tailored specifically for text-based information. This approach integrates elements from information retrieval, statistical analysis, computational linguistics, and artificial intelligence. Text data mining, intelligent text analysis, or knowledge discovery in text are also referred as text mining. The study mentioned by Kulkarni and Mundhe (2016) to analyze disease-related news and health information using text mining has four steps as Text *Transformation*, Text *Pre-processing*, *Data Mining Techniques Application*, *Visualization and Knowledge Extraction*.

1) Text Transformation

The data related to viral infectious diseases is collected from verified sources; this information is primarily in unstructured textual format, it must be converted into a structured layout to facilitate efficient processing. The transformation phase restructures the raw text into a format suitable for analysis, improving the effectiveness of information retrieval and subsequent data mining tasks.

2) Text Pre-Processing

Text pre-processing is the initial and crucial phase in the text mining; to streamline this process, data is converted into XML format. Pre-processing involves several steps such as filtering irrelevant content, tokenization, removing common stop words, and applying stemming techniques. Additionally, all text is standardized to lowercase, and special characters (e.g., @, #, $, %, etc.) are stripped out to data cleaning for further analyse

3) Data Mining Techniques

The different techniques of data mining applied in the healthcare domain to uncover patterns, predict outcomes, and support clinical decisions. These techniques include:

- Classification Models (such as Decision Trees and Naive Bayes): Used to categorize diseases based on patient data, helping in accurate diagnosis and risk assessment.
- Clustering Methods (like K-Means): Helps categorize patients based on shared health traits, supporting customized treatment plans and focused medical strategies.
- Association Rule Mining (including Apriori and FP-Growth): Applied to discover meaningful connections among symptoms, diagnoses, and treatments, revealing frequent co-occurrences in patient records.
- Regression Techniques: Employed to estimate disease progression or predict treatment effectiveness over time, based on historical data.
- Text Mining & Natural Language Processing: These approaches analyze unstructured textual data—such as clinical documentation, medical literature, and health-related news—to extract valuable insights and support evidence-based decision-making.

4) Visualization and Knowledge Extraction

Visual representation of mined data helps uncover hidden trends, relationships, and anomalies not represented in the textual information; word clouds, bar charts, heatmaps, and network graphs are commonly used to display:

- ✓ Frequently occurring symptoms or diseases
- ✓ Co-occurrence of medical terms
- ✓ Geographic distribution of disease outbreaks
- ✓ Temporal patterns in health-related events

These visuals enable healthcare professionals, researchers, and policymakers to quickly grasp complex insights and act accordingly.

Knowledge extraction involves identifying meaningful patterns, associations, and concepts from corpus textual data. In the context of healthcare, this includes:

- ✓ Detecting symptom-disease relationships
- ✓ Recognizing treatment protocols and outcomes
- ✓ Mapping disease progression across regions or populations
- ✓ Extracting key terms and medical things using natural language processing

The unstructured text converted into structured knowledge for healthcare systems which enhances predictive modelling, improve patient care, and support evidence-based practices.

3.2 Need of Data Diseases Data Pre-processing

Healthcare data is in heterogeneous and complex in the form of missing values, inconsistent formats, and duplicate entries and in unstructured format due to this there is need of data pre-processing. There are ample number of challenges of healthcare data pre-processing including intermediate data, Multilingual, NLP, corpus data, context sensitive data; Also there is difficulty in the identifying relationship and finding patterns from unstructured and semi-structured data . Due to these challenges there is need to the pre-processing of data and then apply the data mining techniques to further pattern discovery, rule generations and decision making etc.

Healthcare data is often noisy, incomplete, in multiple format which is stored at different format and locations for the same pre-processing removes unnecessary information, removes errors, fills missing values and convert the data into the understandable format for further processing. The pre-processing steps are follows:

- **Data Cleaning:** Process of removal of incorrect, incomplete, inaccurate data and replacing the missing data.
- **Data Integration:** Multiple heterogeneous sources of information integrated
- **Data Reduction:** Large volume data is compressed into smaller amount for easy analysis.
- **Data Transformation:** Data is transformed into appropriate form which is suitable for mining process.

The pre-processing of healthcare dataset regarding the viral highly frequent occurring viral diseases are considered from the digital / online news archival of English newspapers. Influenza (Flu), Dengue, Chikungunya, Swine Flu, Diarrhea selected for healthcare diseases information mining and association rule generation. The data mining in healthcare domain is possible for structured (row and column) format data while as heterogeneous data mining is complex task in health domain, different stakeholders to process the same and generate the effective results and decision making

Figure 4. Clustering of diseases

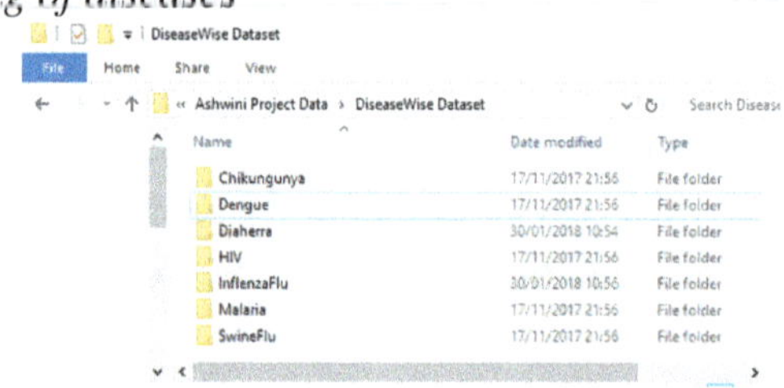

The healthcare data pre-processing of healthcare domain with respect to the selected diseases and their treatment planning is categorized as tokenization, Stop word removal, Filtration, Term Frequency, Inverse Document Frequency (TF-IDF) and stemming.

3.2.1. Tokenization

Tokenization plays significant role in NLP comprised of splitting the textual information or data into words, characters, phrases, special characters, notations and symbols. These are considered as token and used for input for further data processing.

To carry out the tokenization of healthcare data or information for the selected viral diseases the following algorithm is used.

Algorithm: Tokenization

Input: Online News articles of viral diseases from various English-language newspapers.

Output: A structured list of tokens derived from the textual content of disease-related news.

Steps:

1. Initialize the Process

- Create a database table named token to store extracted words.

2. Select Disease wise Directory

- Begin with the folder labelled "Dengue" containing relevant HTML files.

3. Process Each HTML File

- Loop through all files indexed from 0 to n:
  - a) Read and display the current file name.
  - b) Set a counter to zero to track the number of valid tokens.
  - c) Extract the main content from the body section of the webpage:
  - i) Read each word from the selected section.
  - ii) Apply a validation function (tokenizer) to check the word:
  - If the word contains punctuation, symbols, or special characters, skip it and continue scanning.
  - Otherwise:
  - Start inserting valid words into the token table.
  - Increment both the token counter and row index.
  - iii) Continue scanning words until end of section.
  - d) Move to next section - webpage and repeat the above steps until the entire file is processed.
  - e) Advance to the next HTML file and repeat steps a through d until all files in the directory are completed.

4. Close the Current Directory

5. Switch to Another Disease Folder

o Change the directory to "Chikungunya" and repeat the same process for all files.

6. Stop

Figure 5. Tokenization of online diseases news

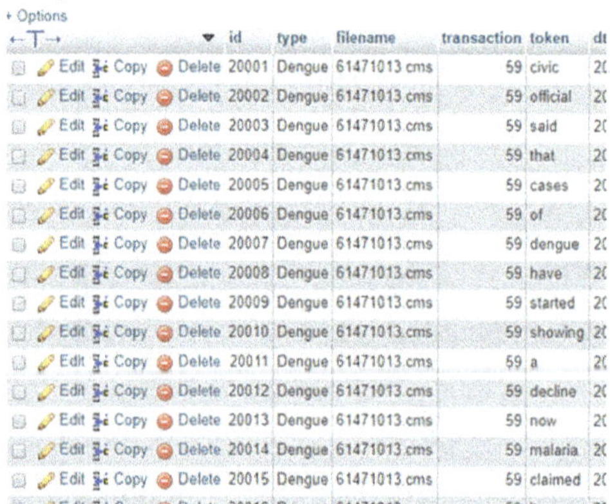

+ Options

	id	type	filename	transaction	token	dt
Edit Copy Delete	20001	Dengue	61471013.cms	59	civic	2(
Edit Copy Delete	20002	Dengue	61471013.cms	59	official	2(
Edit Copy Delete	20003	Dengue	61471013.cms	59	said	2(
Edit Copy Delete	20004	Dengue	61471013.cms	59	that	2(
Edit Copy Delete	20005	Dengue	61471013.cms	59	cases	2(
Edit Copy Delete	20006	Dengue	61471013.cms	59	of	2(
Edit Copy Delete	20007	Dengue	61471013.cms	59	dengue	2(
Edit Copy Delete	20008	Dengue	61471013.cms	59	have	2(
Edit Copy Delete	20009	Dengue	61471013.cms	59	started	2(
Edit Copy Delete	20010	Dengue	61471013.cms	59	showing	2(
Edit Copy Delete	20011	Dengue	61471013.cms	59	a	2(
Edit Copy Delete	20012	Dengue	61471013.cms	59	decline	2(
Edit Copy Delete	20013	Dengue	61471013.cms	59	now	2(
Edit Copy Delete	20014	Dengue	61471013.cms	59	malaria	2(
Edit Copy Delete	20015	Dengue	61471013.cms	59	claimed	2(

3.2.2. Stop Word Removal

The common words like a, an, the, who, when, where has least importance in the sentences such words named as stop words. These stop words were removed from the tokens to reduce the datasets and consider only important words for further processing. The 700 stop words were removed from online diseases news datasets.

Examples: who, when, where, a, an, the, some, at, in, is, he, she, where, too, to etc.

Table 1. List of stop words

A	as	certainly	especially	hadn't	indicates
a's	aside	changes	et	happens	inner
Able	ask	clearly	etc	hardly	insofar
About	asking	co	even	has	instead
Above	associated	com	ever	hasn't	into

continued on following page

Table 1. Continued

A	as	certainly	especially	hadn't	indicates
according	at	come	every	have	inward
accordingly,	available	comes	everybody	haven't	is
be	awfully	consequently	everything	he	it
After	therefore	consider	everywhere	how	latterly
Again	became	contain	exactly	help	it's
against	because	containing	example	hence	its
Ago	Become	contains	except	her	itself
don't	becomes	corresponding	hence	here	just
All	becoming	been	far	here	couldn't
being	definitely	followed	few	hereafter	so
Allows	before	course	fifth	hereby	keep
Almost	beforehand	currently	first	herein	keeps
Also	below	despite	follows	hi	known
although	beside	department	for	him	henceforth
Always	besides	did	former	himself	last
Am	best	didn't	formerly	his	lately
Among	better	different	forth	hither	later
amongst	between	do	four	hopefully	latter
An	beyond	does	from	how	latterly

3.2.3. Filtration

The stop words are removed from dataset by keeping the residual terms used for further processing for minimizing time, memory, and focusing only on relevant data.

Stop Word Removal Algorithm

Input: A collection of tokenized words [stop words].
Output: A refined set of keywords [eliminated stop words].

Steps

1. **Initialize Stop Word Repository**
    - o Load a comprehensive list containing commonly used stop words (e.g., “is,” “the,” “and,” “of”).
2. **Access Tokenized Data**

- o Retrieve the set of words generated during the tokenization phase.

3. **Filter Tokens**
   - o For each word in list of token:
     - ■ Compare it against list of stop word
     - ■ If a match is found, discard the word from token set.
4. **Repeat Filtering**
   - o Continue the comparison process until all stopwords removed from tokens list.
5. **Complete the Process**
   - o Finalize the cleaned keyword list for further analysis or processing.

Figure 6. Remaining tokens excluding stop words

←T→				id	type	filename	transaction	token
☐	Edit	Copy	Delete	1	SwineFlu	7-yr-old-dies-swine-flu-taking-toll-pune-81-3821	1	pune
☐	Edit	Copy	Delete	4	SwineFlu	7-yr-old-dies-swine-flu-taking-toll-pune-81-3821	1	year
☐	Edit	Copy	Delete	5	SwineFlu	7-yr-old-dies-swine-flu-taking-toll-pune-81-3821	1	old
☐	Edit	Copy	Delete	6	SwineFlu	7-yr-old-dies-swine-flu-taking-toll-pune-81-3821	1	boy
☐	Edit	Copy	Delete	7	SwineFlu	7-yr-old-dies-swine-flu-taking-toll-pune-81-3821	1	lost
☐	Edit	Copy	Delete	9	SwineFlu	7-yr-old-dies-swine-flu-taking-toll-pune-81-3821	1	battle
☐	Edit	Copy	Delete	11	SwineFlu	7-yr-old-dies-swine-flu-taking-toll-pune-81-3821	1	swine
☐	Edit	Copy	Delete	12	SwineFlu	7-yr-old-dies-swine-flu-taking-toll-pune-81-3821	1	flu
☐	Edit	Copy	Delete	13	SwineFlu	7-yr-old-dies-swine-flu-taking-toll-pune-81-3821	1	taking
☐	Edit	Copy	Delete	15	SwineFlu	7-yr-old-dies-swine-flu-taking-toll-pune-81-3821	1	city
☐	Edit	Copy	Delete	16	SwineFlu	7-yr-old-dies-swine-flu-taking-toll-pune-81-3821	1	toll
☐	Edit	Copy	Delete	21	SwineFlu	7-yr-old-dies-swine-flu-taking-toll-pune-81-3821	1	health
☐	Edit	Copy	Delete	25	SwineFlu	7-yr-old-dies-swine-flu-taking-toll-pune-81-3821	1	pune
☐	Edit	Copy	Delete	26	SwineFlu	7-yr-old-dies-swine-flu-taking-toll-pune-81-3821	1	municipal
☐	Edit	Copy	Delete	27	SwineFlu	7-yr-old-dies-swine-flu-taking-toll-pune-81-3821	1	corporation

Figure 7. Remaining tokens excluding stop words

←T→				id	type	filename	transaction	token	d
☐	Edit	Copy	Delete	41419	Malaria	59725632.cms	130	limits	2
☐	Edit	Copy	Delete	41421	Malaria	59725632.cms	130	vellayil	2
☐	Edit	Copy	Delete	41422	Malaria	59725632.cms	130	ward	2
☐	Edit	Copy	Delete	41425	Malaria	59725632.cms	130	city	2
☐	Edit	Copy	Delete	41426	Malaria	59725632.cms	130	corporation	2
☐	Edit	Copy	Delete	41427	Malaria	59725632.cms	130	additional	2
☐	Edit	Copy	Delete	41428	Malaria	59725632.cms	130	district	2
☐	Edit	Copy	Delete	41429	Malaria	59725632.cms	130	medical	2
☐	Edit	Copy	Delete	41430	Malaria	59725632.cms	130	officer	2
☐	Edit	Copy	Delete	41431	Malaria	59725632.cms	130	dr	2

3.2.4. Term Frequency, Inverse Document Frequency (TF-IDF)

In text mining, *TF-IDF (Term Frequency, Inverse Document Frequency)* is a statistical measure used to identify the significant word from corpus. It helps in identifying terms that are significant from particular document while reducing the weight of commonly used words across multiple documents. (Bhujade, V, *et. al.* (2011))

A) Term Frequency (TF)

Term Frequency refers to how often a specific token available in a single document. It is calculated number of times the term appears divided by the total number of words in that document.

Formula:

$TF(t_i,d_j)$= Number of times term t_i appears in document d_j/ Total number of terms in d_j

B) Inverse Document Frequency (IDF)

Inverse Document Frequency identifies unique a term is in collection of documents. If a term is available in multiple documents, then IDF value is lower, indicating it may be not much used in different documents.

Formula:

$IDF(t_j)=\log_2 (|C|/N_{tj})$

Where:

- $|C|$ is the total number of documents in the corpus
- N_{tj} is the number of documents in which term t_j appears at least once

C) TF-IDF Calculation

The TF-IDF score is obtained by multiplying the term frequency and inverse document frequency:

$TF\text{-}IDF(t_i,d_j)= TF(t_i,d_j) \times IDF(t_i)$

For example: a document contains 100 words, and the term *"Swine Flu"* appears 4 times.

$TF=4/100=0.04$

Now, consider corpus of 10,000 documents, where "Swine Flu" appears in 1,000 of them. The inverse document frequency is:

$DF=\log_{10}(10{,}000/ 1{,}000) = \log_{10}(10) =1$

So, the TF-IDF score for "Swine Flu" in that document is:

$TF\text{-}IDF=0.04\times1=0.04$

This score indicates the relative importance of the term "Swine Flu" within the specific document compared to its occurrence across the entire collection. A higher TF-IDF value suggests that the term is more distinctive to the document.

4.2 Challenges of Data Pre-Processing in Healthcare

- *Transitional Data Structures* Handling data in formats that bridge raw input and structured output during processing.
- *Refinement across Multiple Languages enhancing* and standardizing text content that originates from diverse linguistic sources.
- *Incorporating Subject Matter Expertise* Embedding domain-specific insights for better correctness in relevance of analysis.
- *High-Dimensional Data Challenges* Managing datasets with numerous variables and attributes that require advanced computational techniques.
- *Complexities in Language Understanding*: Understanding and working through the complexities of human language, such as its grammar, structure, and meaning
- *Handling Ambiguity and Contextual Variations*: Particular term having several meanings depending on their usage and surrounding context.
- *Uncovering Semantic Connections* Identifying meaningful links between keywords, phrases, and underlying concepts within the data.
- *Patient Data Sensitivity* Medical information is highly personal and must be handled with strict confidentiality. Ensuring secure access and ethical use of patient data is essential in healthcare analytics.
- *Varied Formats of HER* : Healthcare records and information is stored in multiple formats across different systems, making standardization a challenge. Effective data mining requires converting these diverse formats into a unified structure.
- *Bias in Datasets Leading to Unfair Predictions* Imbalanced or non-representative data can skew predictive models, resulting in misleading outcomes. Addressing bias is crucial to maintain fairness and accuracy in healthcare decisions.
- *Inaccurate and Discriminatory Outcomes* Predictive algorithms may produce incorrect or biased results if not properly trained. Such errors can lead to unequal treatment recommendations and compromise patient care.
- *Integration with Clinical Workflows* Analytical tools must align with existing medical procedures to be practically useful. Seamless integration ensures that insights are actionable and enhance clinical efficiency.

- *Customized Medications and Therapies* Data-driven approaches enable tailoring treatments to individual patient profiles. Personalized medicine improves effectiveness and reduces adverse reactions.
- *Analysis of Medical Images and Drug Response* Advanced techniques are used to interpret diagnostic images and assess medication impact. This supports early detection and informed treatment planning.
- *Handling Heterogeneous Data Sources* Managing a wide range of healthcare information devising from laboratories, medical equipment, and patient documentation which requires heterogeneous data integration to enable thorough and accurate analysis.
- *Extraction of Relevant Features from Data* Identifying key variables from complex datasets helps in building accurate predictive models.

4. STEMMING

- It involves transforming word into original form which is helpful to reduce grammatical forms, nouns, adjectives, verbs, adverbs etc.
- Example: supporting, supportive, supported, = support

Need of Stemming

- Suffixes alter the interpretation of words even when the root remains unchanged.
- Failure to eliminate suffixes can lead to unclear or misleading association rules.
- Extra suffixes increase data complexity and consume additional memory resources.
- Removing suffixes helps clarify the meaning and reduces linguistic ambiguity.
- This process supports the generation of accurate and relevant association rules.
- Extracting the correct stem ensures consistency in word representation.
- It allows for precise calculation of term frequency of stem or word.
- Minimizing redundant terms improves the efficiency of information retrieval.
- Reducing data volume helps conserve system memory and storage.
- Stemming techniques
- There are basically three techniques of stemming Truncating, Statistical, Mixed these are classified as:

Figure 8. Stemming techniques

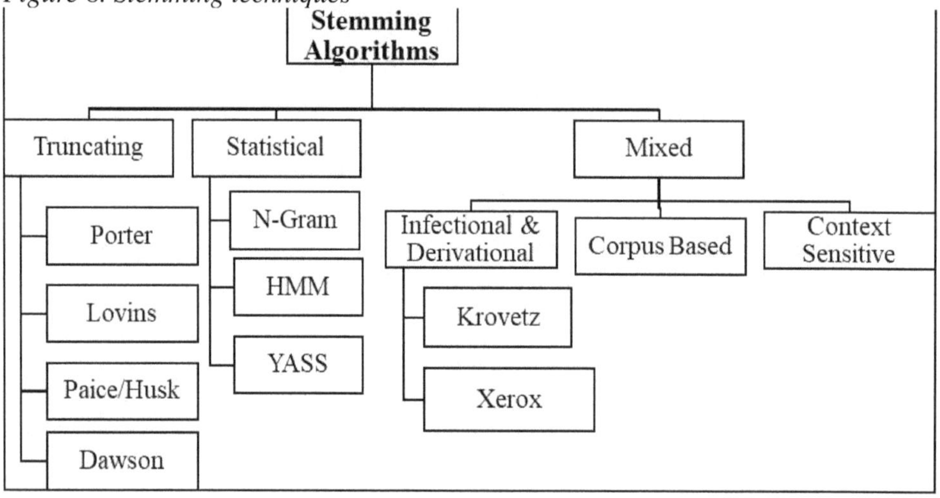

5. APPLICATION OF STEMMING TECHNIQUES FOR HEALTHCARE DATA PRE-PROCESSING

The study of Brahme et al (2022) designates that, there are truncating and mixed stemming techniques which are used for removing affix comprised of prefixes and suffixes. The Porter, Lovins, Paice/Husk, and Krovetz techniques are implemented on infectious diseases English news. Porter's Stemming is developed by Martin Porter in 1980, having is 5 steps and 60 rules for suffixes stripping Lovins Stemming is by Julie Beth Lovin's in 1968 contains 249 suffixes, 29 conditions and 35 rules for suffix removal .Paice/Husk Stemming formed by Charis Paice and Gareth Husk in 1980 comprised of 120 rules, it functions as a conflation stemmer. *Krovetz is developed* **by** Robert Krovetz in 1993 to handle inflectional suffixes consist of 3 steps and various number of rules. These stemming algorithms works only on English language.

6. ASSOCIATION RULE MINING

The study Brahme (2025) elaborated an association rule mining in healthcare is applied to study viral diseases and the factors that influence their spread. It explores how seasonal variations affect transmission patterns, the role of climate shifts in triggering outbreaks, and the ways medical professionals monitor and manage infection-related data. The research also examines whether healthcare systems receive timely alerts about emerging outbreaks, the forecasting tools and data sources they rely on, and how these help anticipate which regions may be impacted and what preventive measures should be taken. Furthermore, it highlights areas most vulnerable to viral spread and emphasizes the importance of predictive analytics in enabling healthcare institutions to prepare for and respond to epidemics more effectively. One of the major challenges in this field is uncovering meaningful links among critical components such as diseases, symptoms, patient groups, geographic locations, and available treatments or vaccines. Identifying these connections is essential for improving clinical decision-making and ensuring accurate treatment strategies. To support this, text mining techniques are employed to analyze both real-time and archived digital information, including online news portals, health bulletins, and medical publications. The central objective is to design a strong stemming algorithm that enhances information retrieval. Alongside this, the study aims to establish association rules that expose interdependencies among key terms, thereby strengthening the understanding of complex healthcare data relationships.

Ultimately, it aims to build a comprehensive knowledge discovery system capable of predicting frequent viral outbreaks, pinpointing their geographic origins, and suggesting preventive actions.

The best example of association rule induction is market basket analysis represented as IF-THEN as follows:

IF <Conditions> THEN <Conclusions>

Association rule mining (ARM) relies on two key metrics: *Support* and *Confidence*.

- *Support (P Q)* refers to the probability that both item sets P and Q appear together in a dataset.
- *Confidence (P Q)* measures the likelihood that item set Q appears in transactions that already contain item set P.

Mathematically, confidence can be expressed as:

Confidence (P ⇒ Q)=Support count (P ∪ Q)Support count (P)

Where:

- *Support count (P Q)* is the number of transactions that include both P and Q.
- *Support count (P)* is the number of transactions that include item set P.

Association rule mining generally consist of two primary steps

- *Frequent item sets Identification*: consistent of different attributes /items/ parameters co-occurs in dataset more frequently than a set minimum threshold.

- *Generating robust association rules*: Rules are generated from commonly occurring item combinations that satisfy the required thresholds for support and confidence

There are two techniques:

1) Apriori Algorithm and
2) FP Growth Algorithm

Apriori Algorithm is devised by Agrawal and Srikant (1995) which indicates that how a particular term is linked and associated with other. *Apriori Algorithm* used for the same, which is designed to discover frequent item sets through a candidate generation approach. The algorithm is named for its use of prior knowledge about item set properties and follows a step-by-step, level-wise strategy to refine and identify frequent patterns.

7. ASSOCIATION RULE MINING FOR DISEASES

Association rule mining plays a vital role across multiple stakeholders in the healthcare ecosystem. These include physicians, specialists, medical officers, clinical practitioners, diagnostic laboratories, patients, hospitals, public health organizations, government agencies, the World Health Organization (WHO), and media outlets such as newspapers, television, and health-focused websites. Within healthcare institutions, hospitals, and organizations like WHO, association rule mining is applied to forecast the spread of infectious viral diseases and to analyze demographic trends linked to transmission. A major challenge lies in extracting valuable insights from large, diverse, and complex healthcare datasets. To address this, the proposed knowledge discovery framework enhances strategic decision-making, supports preventive health initiatives, and enables local authorities to carry out timely interventions while shaping effective public health policies. By leveraging this system, medical professionals, healthcare experts, and government bodies gain actionable insights for controlling viral infections, refining treatment approaches, and implementing remedial measures. The framework also identifies crucial patterns—such as affected regions, symptoms, disease severity, treatment options, and preventive strategies—through the analysis of vast amounts of unstructured data. The association rules derived from infectious disease information are equally important for the general public and media platforms. They help raise awareness about emerging viral threats and contribute to public health education through newspapers, broadcast channels, and online health resources.

8.1. Overview of Association Rule Mining in Healthcare

Association rule mining is a technique applied to discover repeating trends, valuable correlations, and relationships among groups of items stored in different types of databases, such as transactional and relational systems. Within the broader domain of data mining, it is well regarded for its capacity to reveal important associations between variables across large datasets. The primary objective is to generate reliable rules that emphasize noteworthy and relevant connections, guided by defined evaluation measures. By uncovering hidden patterns, this approach supports improved decision-making and boosts operational effectiveness across diverse industries.

8.2. Applying Association Rule Mining on Healthcare Dataset

For example, in the healthcare domain, association rules can be applied to detect common symptom groupings that point to particular illnesses. A rule such as

{Fever, Cold, Bodyache} ⇒ {Influenza-Flu} OR {Fever, Cold, Bodyache} ⇒ {Dengue} if the mentioned symptoms are there then there will be Influenza-Flu or Dengue disease. It is useful for medical professionals, aiding in accurate diagnosis and informed treatment decisions.

8.3. Association Rule Generation Through FP Growth Technique

FP-Growth (Frequent Pattern Growth) is a data mining method that identifies frequent itemsets without the need to generate candidate sets, unlike the Apriori algorithm. It uses a compact data structure called an FP-tree to represent transactions and mine patterns directly.

The steps involved in FP growth are:

a) **Data Preparation:** Healthcare data is first restructured into a format suitable for transaction analysis. Each transaction typically includes elements such as patient symptoms, diagnoses, prescribed treatments, and other relevant medical details.
b) **FP-Tree Development:** An FP-tree is constructed by arranging items according to how frequently they appear. This compact structure efficiently represents the dataset and reveals recurring patterns.
c) **Frequent Pattern Discovery:** The FP-tree is explored the frequently occurred itemsets and meet the predefined support criteria. These itemsets reflect commonly associated medical attributes.

d) **Rule Formation:** association rules generated using the patterns and item sets which are derived that meet the required confidence level. These rules highlight strong correlations between different healthcare factors.

The dataset of viral infectious diseases in processed in Excel file, includes information of infectious diseases names, symptoms, frequency, demographics, impact. The information is transformed from nominal values into a binary format to facilitate analysis. Using the FP (Frequent Pattern) Growth, minimum support, confidence thresholds are applied to identify frequent patterns. Subsequently, association rules are derived, and these rules are visualized using the RapidMiner tool.

Figure 9. Association mining through rapid minder

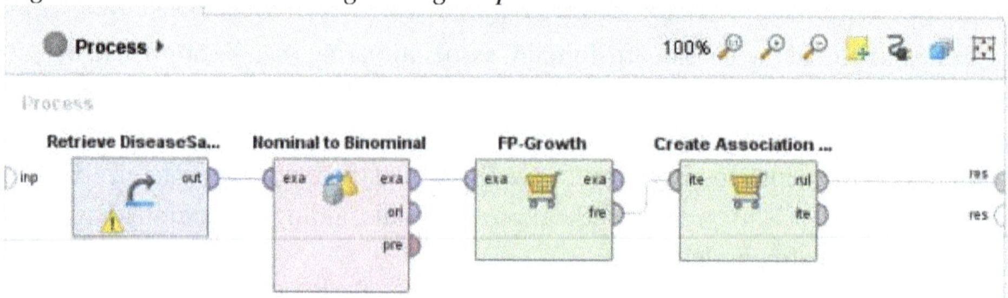

- [Symptoms = swelling, fever, headache, feeling-sick, dry-mouth, joint-ache] --> [Disease = Mumps] (confidence: 1.000)
- [Disease = Mumps] --> [Symptoms = swelling, fever, headache, feeling-sick, dry-mouth, joint-ache] (confidence: 1.000)
- [Symptoms = fever, chills, cough, soar-throat, runny-nose, bodyache, headache, fatigue, vomitting] --> [Disease = InfluenzaFlu] (confidence: 1.000)
- [Disease = InfluenzaFlu] --> [Symptoms = fever, chills, cough, soar-throat, runny-nose, bodyache, headache, fatigue, vomitting] (confidence: 1.000)
- [Symptoms = fever, jointpain, headache, musclepain, joint-swelling, rash] --> [Disease = Chikungunya] (confidence: 1.000)
- [Disease = Chikungunya] --> [Symptoms = fever, jointpain, headache, musclepain, joint-swelling, rash] (confidence: 1.000)

- [Symptoms = cough,coryza,runny-nose, fever, sneezing, rash, boadyache, watery-eyes, Soar-Throat] --> [Disease = Measles] (confidence: 1.000)
- [Disease = Measles] --> [Symptoms = cough,coryza,runny-nose, fever, sneezing, rash, boadyache, watery-eyes, SoarThroat] (confidence: 1.000)
- [Symptoms = chills, fever,coughing,sore-throat,runny-stuffy-nose,body-aches,fatigue, nausea,vomiting] --> [Disease = Swine Flu] (confidence: 1.000)
- [Disease = Swine Flu] --> [Symptoms = chills, fever,coughing,sore-throat,runny-stuffy-nose,bodyaches,fatigue, nausea,vomiting] (confidence: 1.000)
- [Symptoms = abdominal-pain, nausea, vomiting] --> [Disease = Diarrhoea] (confidence: 1.000) [Disease = Diarrhoea] --> [Symptoms = abdominal-pain, nausea, vomiting] (confidence: 1.000) [Symptoms = Rash, Red-spot, Soar-throat, high-fever, vomitting, headache, tiredness, Painfull-Blisters] --> [Disease = Chickenpox] (confidence: 1.000)
- [Disease = Chickenpox] --> [Symptoms = Rash, Red-spot, Soar-throat, high-fever, vomitting, headache, tiredness, Painfull-Blisters] (confidence: 1.000)
- [Symptoms = Nausea, vomiting, Dehydration, Muscle-cramps, abdominal-pain] --> [Disease = Cholera] (confidence: 1.000)
- [Symptoms = High-Fever, Abdomen-Pain, vomiting, cold, headache, rash] --> [Disease = Dengue] (confidence: 1.000)
- [Disease = Dengue] --> [Symptoms = High-Fever, Abdomen-Pain, vomiting, cold, headache, rash] (confidence: 1.000)
- [Symptoms = Fever, Headache, Agitation, Vomiting, Confusion] --> [Disease = Rabies] (confidence: 1.000)
- [Disease = Rabies] --> [Symptoms = Fever, Headache, Agitation, Vomiting, Confusion] (confidence: 1.000)

  Etc.

8.4 Identifying Diseases Patterns Through Association Mining

Association mining serves as an important method for analyzing large-scale healthcare datasets to reveal repeating trends and significant relationships. It helps in identifying clusters of symptoms, commonly diagnosed conditions within particular demographic groups, and frequently prescribed treatment combinations.

The *Association Induction Tool* simplifies the process of generating rules by:

- **Handling healthcare transactions:** Each patient record is treated as a transaction that includes clinical details such as symptoms, diagnoses, and medications.

- **Applying support and confidence measures:** User-defined thresholds are used to eliminate less relevant patterns, ensuring that only the most meaningful associations are preserved.
- **Delivering clear rules:** The tool produces straightforward and actionable insights, for example: *"Patients presenting both fever and fatigue are likely to have a viral infection."*

For this study, an open-source association rule generator developed by *Christian Berget* was utilized. The tool offers a user-friendly graphical interface and employs the *Apriori algorithm* to detect valuable associations. In the analysis, the researcher concentrated on the top 1,000 distinct tokens ranked according to their *TF-IDF scores* to ensure the most relevant terms were examined. Using this dataset, the tool rapidly produced a substantial volume of association rules—specifically, 41,708 rules were generated in just 6.673 seconds.

Figure 10. Association rule using induction tool

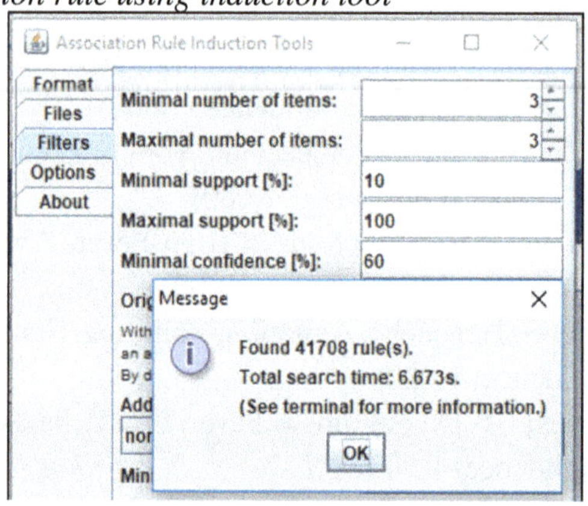

The association rules are expressed numerically, including support and confidence values, and they illustrate how different token IDs are interconnected

Figure 11. Association rule generation in numerical format

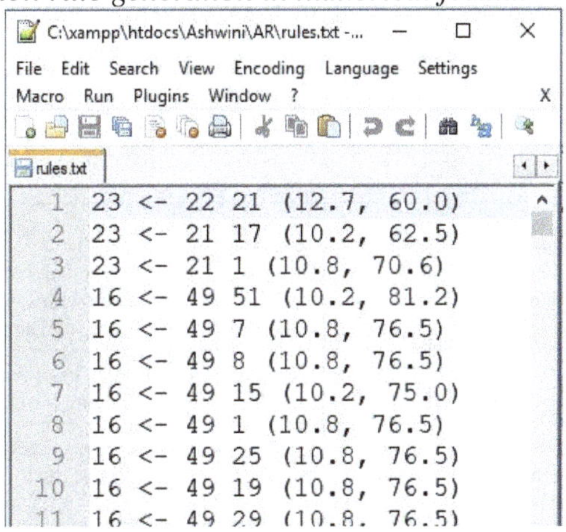

The association rules are presented using numerical identifiers for tokens. For instance, the rule 23 <- 21 17 (10.2, 62.5) suggests that token ID 23 is linked to token IDs 21 and 17, with a support value of 10.2 and a confidence level of 62.5%. This relationship can also be expressed as: IF <23> THEN <21, 17>, or the reverse. However, interpreting these rules using only token IDs can be confusing, as it requires constantly mapping each ID to its corresponding token name; token IDs are replaced with their actual names for robust rule generation as shown below:

Figure 12. Association rules with token

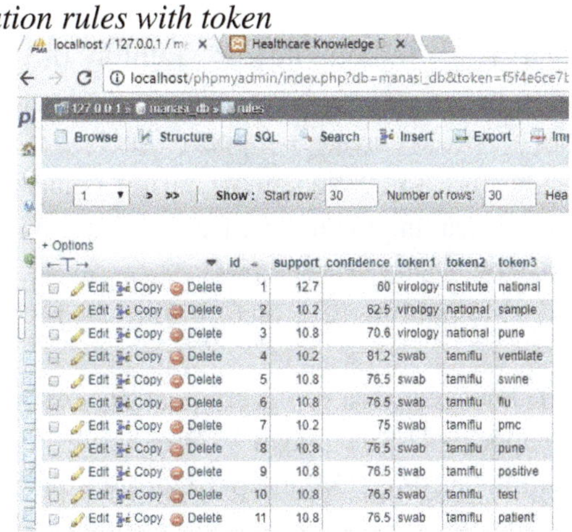

id	support	confidence	token1	token2	token3
1	12.7	60	virology	institute	national
2	10.2	62.5	virology	national	sample
3	10.8	70.6	virology	national	pune
4	10.2	81.2	swab	tamiflu	ventilate
5	10.8	76.5	swab	tamiflu	swine
6	10.8	76.5	swab	tamiflu	flu
7	10.2	75	swab	tamiflu	pmc
8	10.8	76.5	swab	tamiflu	pune
9	10.8	76.5	swab	tamiflu	positive
10	10.8	76.5	swab	tamiflu	test
11	10.8	76.5	swab	tamiflu	patient

As shown above Rule no. 4 represents, swab ← *{tamiflu, ventilate}* with a support value of 10.2 and a confidence level of 81.2%. This suggests a mutual association among these tokens. A selection of such rules, support and confidence with detailed interpretations, is in the table below.

Table 2. Association rules of viral diseases

Sr.no.	Association Rule	Support	confidence	Interpretation
Rule 5	{swab}<- { tamiflu, swine } or { tamiflu, swine } <- { swab}	10.8	76.5%	there is relation of swab is taken/ tested for related with swine flu diseases and need Tamiflu medicine
Rule 178	{pmc } <- { tamiflu, flu } or { tamiflu, flu } <- { pmc }	10.8	94.1%	PMC area has a higher number of flu patients, highlighting the need for Tamiflu medication.
Rule 395	{platelet} <- {count, dengue} or {count, dengue} <- {platelet}	11.5	72.2%	The rule suggests that if patient is having dengue, their platelet count should be monitored.
Rule 1845	dengue} <- {mosquitoes, breede} or {mosquitoe, breede} <- {dengue}	12.1	68.4%	It outcomes dengue diseases take places due to mosquitoes breede.

These above rules of selected tokens display both the antecedent and consequent as well as support and confidence metrics. The rule generation tool evaluates the user-defined support and confidence thresholds against the precompiled values of the selected keywords. Only those keywords that meet or exceed the specified thresholds are included in the final set of association rules. Some more rule can be interpreted as:

- **Rule 175:** {January} ← {Tamiflu, flu} or {Tamiflu, flu} ← {January} highlights a connection between the tokens "January," "Tamiflu," and "flu," represented as either this rule carries a support value of 10.8 and a confidence level of 70.6% indicating a notable pattern during January there was a higher incidence of flu cases leading to an increased demand for Tamiflu with a confidence of 70.6%.
- **Rule 178:** {p.m.} <- { tamiflu, flu } or { tamiflu, flu } <- { pmc }

The rule mentioned above reveals a strong connection among the tokens "PMC," "Tamiflu," and "flu," supported by a value of 10.8 and a confidence level of 94.1%. This indicates that within the Pune Municipal Corporation region, there was a significant number of flu cases, leading to a high demand for Tamiflu medication.

- **Rule 395:** {platelet} <- {count, dengue} or {count, dengue} <-{platelet}

The rule indicates a link between platelet count and dengue, supported by a value of 11.5 and a confidence level of 72.2%. This suggests that when dengue is suspected in a patient, monitoring their platelet levels becomes essential for proper assessment.

- **Rule 1845:** {dengue} <- {mosquitoes, breede} or

{mosquitoe, breede} <- {dengue}

The rule suggests a connection among the tokens "dengue," "mosquitoes," and "breeding," supported by a value of 12.1 and a confidence level of 68.4%. This implies that dengue cases are linked to mosquito breeding activity, highlighting the importance of controlling breeding grounds to prevent the spread of the disease.

- **Rule 3173**: { fever } <- { viral, health } or { viral, health }<-{ fever }

The rule highlights a relationship among the tokens "fever," "viral," and "health," supported by a value of 12.1 and a confidence level of 68.4%. This suggests that viral fever significantly affects health, indicating a meaningful association between these factors.

8.4. Challenges in Association Rule Mining

- Efficiently identifying relevant and valuable documents from massive datasets remains a key challenge.
- Biomedical data available online exists in diverse formats—structured, semi-structured, and unstructured—necessitating the use of data mining for better analysis and decision making.
- A central goal in healthcare analytics is to uncover connections among diseases, symptoms, medications, preventive measures, affected individuals, and other related factors.
- Contemporary text mining research addresses issues such as document classification, clustering, semantic representation, information extraction, and uncovering hidden patterns.
- Challenges include handling intermediate data formats, refining multilingual text, integrating domain-specific expertise, and enabling personalized, automated mining processes.
- Additional complexities arise from the high dimensionality of data, the intricate nature of human language, and the presence of ambiguity and context-dependent meanings.

- Not every generated rule holds clinical relevance. A key difficulty lies in eliminating insignificant or non-useful associations while ensuring that the retained rules are clear and practical for healthcare professionals to interpret.
- Medical and disease-related information continually evolves with the emergence of new conditions, updated treatments, and revised guidelines. As a result, association rules built on outdated datasets may lose their validity over time.

9. KNOWLEDGE DISCOVERY THROUGH ASSOCIATION RULE MINING

The association rules produced are applied to generate valuable insights in the healthcare sector. The system is designed to operate on multiple parameters such as type of disease, mode of transmission, affected population groups, severity levels, and geographic distribution. When a specific disease is selected, the system evaluates and displays patterns showing how it spreads, which communities are most impacted, the regions where it is concentrated, and the overall scale of its effects.

Beyond pattern recognition, the system delivers practical guidance—highlighting the need for vaccination, suggesting preventive measures, and offering expert recommendations. It also predicts frequently occurring epidemic diseases, allowing healthcare professionals and public authorities to take proactive steps, implement timely interventions, and manage potential outbreaks effectively. This capability is illustrated through its graphical interface, demonstrated with diseases such as Dengue and Chikungunya.

9.1. Framework for Pre-Processing of Healthcare Data and Knowledge Discovery

Figure 13. Healthcare data pre-processing and association rule mining

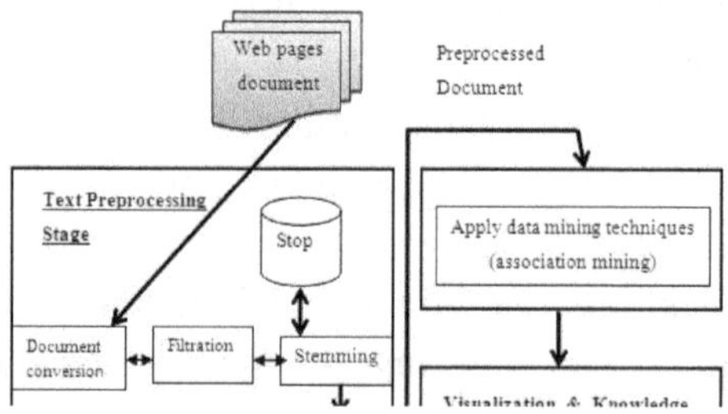

The huge data of viral diseases is available internet in various formats and sources. Manually examining the vast amount of healthcare data to produce actionable insights and accurate disease predictions—particularly regarding specific regions, affected populations, impacts, treatments, and remedies—is not feasible. A major research challenge lies in harnessing text-based information for effective knowledge discovery. Extracting key terms and identifying semantic relationships among them requires the use of *Natural Language Processing (NLP)*. To address these needs, a knowledge discovery system has been developed that applies text mining techniques for healthcare analysis, as illustrated in the figure above.

The primary goals of the proposed application and framework include:

- **Efficient Document Retrieval:** Locating relevant and valuable documents from large datasets on viral infectious diseases.
- **Enhanced Information Extraction:** Capturing critical data with greater accuracy and efficiency.
- **Revealing Hidden Patterns:** Identifying associations and uncovering latent rules within extensive textual records.
- **System Training:** Preparing the system to recognize diseases, symptoms, transmission methods, demographic factors, and preventive measures.
- **Disease Spread Prediction:** Identifying locations of highly frequent diseases

The following parameters of selected viral infectious diseases are taken for training the prolapsed knowledge discovery system.

Table 3. Selected diseases parameters

Diseases	Dengue, SwineFlu, Chikungunya, Malaria, Influenza Flu, Diarrhea
Spread By	Water, Mosquito, virus, food, bug, viral, H1N1, bacteria
Victims	People, children, girl, boy, worker, man, men, women, patients, person
Impact	Death, fever, ill, vomit, forehead ache, nose, cough, cold, throat, brain, face, arm, stomach, cancer, organ, swell, eye, depress, headache
Location	Pune, PCMC, Kothrud, Chinchwad, Pimpri, PMC, Maharashtra, Corporation

The diseases information with respect to diseases, spread by, victim, Impact and Location is mapped and the system is trained for healthcare knowledge discovery for the predictive analysis. After training the system the knowledge discovery results the highly frequent diseases, spread by, precautionary measures and it also predicts the geographical location of that highly frequent diseases.

9.2. Predictive ANALYSIs of Diseases, Outbreaks, and Precautionary Measures

A Knowledge-Based System holds great importance in the medical field due to the complexities and information extraction from heterogonous data used for decision making. Its primary goal is to identify patterns within large-scale medical data and utilize these patterns across different parameters which is beneficial for healthcare institutions, medical practitioners, professionals, and government bodies in implementing effective interventions and solutions.

This study gathered unstructured data related to specific diseases from English-language newspapers and applied text mining to generate patterns from the vast and complex dataset. The developed knowledge discovery system was evaluated by healthcare professionals, including doctors, practitioners, and medical staff. The system has ability to predict widely prevalent diseases, identify affected geographic regions, suggest preventive actions, and measure the accuracy and relevance of its outputs represented in the figures that follow.

Figure 14. Knowledge discovery system for selected diseases

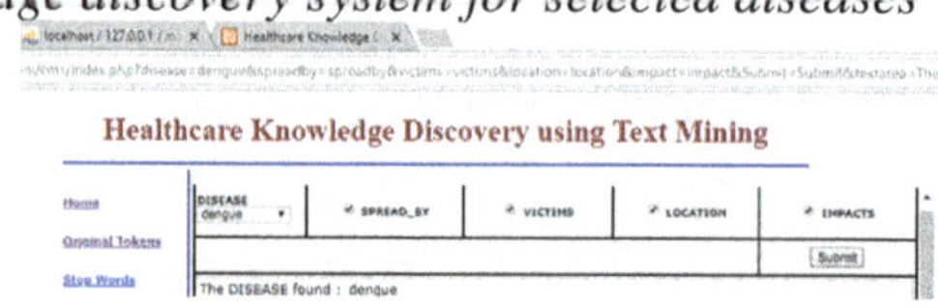

Figure 15. Knowledge discovery system for selected diseases

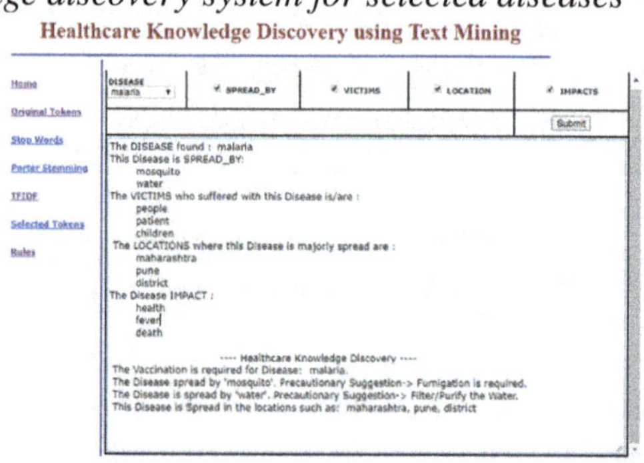

Suggestions for Healthcare: Diseases detection and treatment planning

- ✓ Health authorities should prioritize monitoring viral disease outbreaks and identifying regions with high transmission rates.
- ✓ Media outlets, including newspapers, social platforms, healthcare portals, online government related can use the system to raise public awareness and issue timely alerts about potential disease outbreaks.
- ✓ Medical institutions, healthcare professionals, and practitioners should actively promote preventive measures for infection diseases to educate the public.
- ✓ The healthcare designed and developed system should be adopted by key stakeholders—such as hospitals, physicians, medical experts, government bodies, and health organizations—to forecast disease spread and pinpoint affected areas.
- ✓ Daily operations and decision-making processes in clinics, hospitals, medical domain, and health experts get the significant perceptions provided by these intelligent systems.
- ✓ Physicians are encouraged to use online resources, including news platforms and medical websites, get the pandemic and epidemic information and share that knowledge with the community.
- ✓ Healthcare institutions can improve their ability to analyze textual and unstructured data, uncovering patterns that support more informed and effective strategic decisions.

10. CONCLUSION

Online data exists in vast volumes and often appears in structured or semi-structured formats that are complex, diverse, and sometimes ambiguous or sensitive in nature. Given this variability and scale, there is a clear need for robust text mining methods and efficient data processing techniques to enhance information extraction and facilitate meaningful knowledge discovery. This necessity forms the foundation and driving force behind the current research initiative. The outcome of the study is processing of unstructured corpus healthcare data, to discover the relationships and hidden patterns effectively from the massive healthcare data, to train the system for better knowledge discovery and predict the diseases outbreaks.

As healthcare continues to evolve toward data-centric models, association rule mining stands as a cornerstone for intelligent, evidence-based care. Its applications in disease detection and treatment planning underscore the transformative impact of data mining in medical practice.

The designed system is significant for predicting the highly contagious diseases outbreaks and their geographical locations comprised of association rule generation through the corpus data and knowledge discovery through the rules. The various stakeholders of healthcare domain like doctors, medical officers, healthcare experts, hospitals, and healthcare departments will be able to use the system to raise awareness about high-frequency diseases and their locations useful for the society and decision-making.

REFERENCES

Agrawal, R., & Srikant, R. (1995, March). Mining sequential patterns. In *Proceedings of the eleventh international conference on data engineering* (pp. 3-14). IEEE. DOI: 10.1109/ICDE.1995.380415

Amin, A., Talib, R., Raza, S., & Javed, S. (2014). Extract association rules to minimize the effects of dengue by using a text mining technique. *International Journal of Computer Science and Mobile Computing*, *3*(4), 394–400.

Babanejaddehaki, G., An, A., & Papagelis, M. (2025). Disease outbreak detection and forecasting: A review of methods and data sources. *ACM Transactions on Computing for Healthcare*, *6*(2), 1–40. DOI: 10.1145/3708549

Badawy, M., Ramadan, N., & Hefny, H. A. (2023). Healthcare predictive analytics using machine learning and deep learning techniques: A survey. *Journal of Electrical Systems and Information Technology*, *10*(1), 40. DOI: 10.1186/s43067-023-00108-y

Bhujade, V., Janwe, N. J., & Meshram, C. (2011). Discriminative Features Selection in Text Mining Using TF-IDF Scheme. *[IJCTT]. International Journal of Computer Trends and Technology*, *1*(3), 277–280.

Brahme, A. (2025). Association rule mining and information retrieval using stemming and text mining techniques. *Journal of Information Systems Engineering & Management*, *10*(18s).

Brahme, A., Kulkarni, S., & Kulkarni, M. (2022). To Devise and Implement Effective Stemming Algorithm for Text Mining and NLP for Healthcare Management. *JOURNAL OF MANAGEMENT & ENTREPRENEURSHIP*, 163

El-Sappagh, S. H., El-Masri, S., Riad, A. E.-D., & Elmogy, M. (2013). Data mining and knowledge discovery: Applications, techniques, challenges and process models in healthcare. [IJERA]. *International Journal of Engineering Research and Applications*, *3*(3), 900–906.

Fayyad, U., Piatetsky-Shapiro, G., & Smyth, P. (1996). From data mining to knowledge discovery in databases. *AI Magazine*, *17*(3), 37–37.

Ibrahim, N., Akhir, N. S. M., & Hassan, F. H. (2017, October). Predictive analysis effectiveness in determining the epidemic disease infected area. In AIP conference proceedings (Vol. 1891, No. 1, p. 020064). AIP Publishing LLC. DOI: 10.1063/1.5005397

Kulkarni, A., & Mundhe, S. (2016). A theoretical review on text mining: Tools, techniques, applications and future challenges. *International Journal of Innovative Research in Computer and Communication Engineering*, *4*(11), 19225–19230.

Kulkarni, A., & Mundhe, S. (2017). Data mining technique: An implementation of association rule mining in healthcare. *International Advanced Research Journal in Science. Engineering and Technology*, *4*(7), 62–65.

Moral, C., de Antonio, A., Imbert, R., & Ramírez, J. (2014). A survey of stemming algorithms in information retrieval. *Information Research*, *19*(1), n1.

Ojo, A., & Adeyemo, A. (2012). Framework for knowledge discovery from journal articles using text mining techniques. *African Journal of Computing and ICT*, *5*(2). www.ajocict.net

Prabavathy, K., & Sumathi, P. (2013). Text mining: Interpreting knowledge discovery from biomed articles. *The SIJ Transactions on Computer Science Engineering & its Applications (CSEA), 1*(2), 33–36.

Ramon-Gonen, R., Dori, A., & Shelly, S. (2023). Towards a practical use of text mining approaches in electrodiagnostic data. *Scientific Reports*, *13*(1), 45758. DOI: 10.1038/s41598-023-45758-0 PMID: 37945618

Shakil, K.A., Anis, S., & Alam, M. (2015). Dengue disease prediction using weka data mining tool. *ArXiv, abs/1502.05167.*

Sumathy, K. L., & Chidambaram, M. (2013). Text mining: Concepts, applications, tools and issues-an overview. *International Journal of Computer Applications*, *80*(4). Advance online publication. DOI: 10.5120/13851-1685

Chapter 5
Deep Learning-Based Association Rule Mining for Healthcare Applications

Prithi Samuel
http://orcid.org/0000-0001-5648-8891
Computational Intelligence, School of Computing, SRM Institute of Science and Technology, India

C. Dhiya
http://orcid.org/0009-0005-0115-3572
SRM Institute of Science and Technology, India

G. J. H. Umesh
SRM Institute of Science and Technology, India

ABSTRACT

This chapter presents the Deep Association Rule Mining (Deep ARM) as a hybrid intelligence paradigm of precision healthcare. It focuses on how deep learning techniques (autoencoders, RNNs, GNNs, Transformers) can be integrated with classical association rule mining to surmount the challenges on complex clinical data. By learning rich latent representations before mining, Deep ARM is able to find concise high-quality association rules from high-dimensional, temporal and multimodal medical datasets. The framework suggested focuses on explainability and domain integration which can translate the neural patterns into interpretable clinical rules with biomedical ontologies. We talk about clinical utility (and not just accuracy) evaluation metrics, and we show how these metrics are used to predict

DOI: 10.4018/979-8-3373-6691-3.ch005

disease trajectories, optimal treatments, real time monitoring, and phenotyping of patients. Finally, we outline ethical, fairness, and privacy considerations and chart future directions toward causal, trustworthy clinical AI.

1. INTRODUCTION: THE CONVERGENCE OF DEEP LEARNING AND ASSOCIATION RULE MINING

1.1 Rationale for Hybrid Intelligence in Clinical Analytics

Healthcare is becoming data intensive yet must have interpretable insight. The classical form of association rule mining (ARM) offers human-readable patterns of "if-then" based on clinical data, but it is not very scalable to high dimensions and unstructured inputs. Deep learning is opaque and efficient at extracting complex features in images, text and signals. Deep ARM is a hybrid intelligence model that fuses the two worlds, the representational strength of neural models with the interpretability of rules. Such synergy solves the fundamentals of the medical AI tradeoff: the necessity of strong pattern discovery without affecting transparency. Deep ARM aims to provide accurate as well as explainable knowledge discovery by embedding information into latent spaces with deep networks and subsequently mining the latent spaces (Miotto et al. 2018). E.g., an autoencoder can reduce the lab results and vital of a patient into a code, based on which the explicit rules (high glucose + hypertension = kidney disease risk) can be obtained to be used in clinical decisions.

1.2 Data-Driven Discovery in Modern Medicine

In modern medicine, a number of data sources are being produced: electronic health records (EHRs) and diagnostic imaging data, genomics, and continuous monitoring streams, etc. at a scale never before seen. It is not feasible to mine meaningful patterns using the human hand. The personalized diagnosis and treatment has become highly dependent on automated, data-driven discovery of knowledge. But the healthcare sphere has the following stringent demands: the algorithm should be resistant to the or noise and heterogeneous data and to provide justification to gain the trust of clinicians. Transparency is also required by regulatory requirements (e.g. FDA, GDPR). Deep ARM satisfies these requirements by offering a pipeline in which deep models are used to deal with complexity (e.g. learning on time-series signals of ICUs or multimodal patient data) and rule mining is used to generate actionable insights. This approach can help uncover new co-morbidity patterns or early warning signals with raw EHRs, and bring discovery in epidemiology and precision health faster.

1.3 Research Objectives and Chapter Scope

This chapter does not limit itself to a survey, but rather suggests an organized model of Deep ARM in clinical analytics. This is followed by a review of the classical ARM basics and constraints, and finally, the introduction of deep representation techniques, which complement ARM. It describes a new hybrid architecture that can be used to integrate neural embeddings and symbolic rules. Then we draw up examples in medicine and explain technical implementation and resources. Ethical and trust concerns are tackled and new frontiers are investigated leading to a conclusion which leads to the direction of associations to causal insights. In the process, the focus is put on clinical relevance and explainability. This will be the goal of a unified vision of Deep ARM of transformative capability in clinical decision support and precise health.

2. FROM CLASSICAL ARM TO DEEP ASSOCIATION DISCOVERY

2.1 Revisiting the Foundations of Association Rule Mining

Association rule mining (ARM) is a data mining algorithm that discovers common and notable co-occurring patterns in transactional or binary data. A rule has the form *X* *Y*, where *X* (antecedent) and *Y* (consequent) are sets of items (e.g., symptoms, diagnoses, drugs). Key metrics include support (frequency of transactions containing *X* *Y*), confidence (P(Y|X)), and lift (P(Y|X)/(P(Y)*P(X))). As an example, an ARM between EHR data may show that patients with items {'chest pain', 'elevated troponin'} are highly likely to have other items, such as myocardial infarction. High support is used to mean the pattern is widespread; high confidence is used to mean that the implications are strong Berteloot et al. (2023); lift is used to mean the degree to which the rule goes beyond chance co-occurrence. ARM has a rich history in healthcare analytics to perform such tasks as identifying comorbidity patterns or drug-adverse event associations. Regular algorithms (Apriori, FP-Growth) produce all frequent item sets and rules that have over user-configured thresholds. Although helpful, traditional ARM presupposes the existence of data that are fixed, categorical transactions.

2.2 Structural Limitations of Traditional ARM

Classical ARM is challenged by a number of issues in clinical practice. First, dimensionality: contemporary health records consist of thousands of variables (lab results, genomic markers, sensor readings), which results in the proliferation of potential patterns of items and often millions of rules. This rule outburst imposes interpretation and calculation. Second, ARM is generally only about static transactions (e.g., diagnosis codes) but not about temporal dynamics. Patient data is longitudinal, sequence and timing of events are important (e.g. infection and then antibiotic treatment). ARM Standard cannot directly record sequences or time holes. Third, the traditional ARM is not good with continuous or unstructured data. Numbers and textual notes will require the values to be discrete or processed, which may not have a lot of nuance. Fourth, ARM produces rules that lack contextual semantics; it lacks the use of domain knowledge. As an illustration, it may suggest a rule concerning two conditions that lacks the identification of their clinical association by pathophysiology. Fifth, the rules can be quite fixed: they do not evolve as new incoming data arrives. Patterns may drift (new variations, treatment, or groups of patients) in rapid-paced clinical settings.

These drawbacks drive a switch in paradigm: we require ARM capable of managing high-dim, changing, multimodal medical data, and which can produce a set of clinically significant rules manageable.

2.3 Paradigm Shift: Learning Representations Before Mining

The suggested paradigm shift approach is to learn deep representations, then mine rules on representations. Deep neural networks have the ability to learn high-dimensional medical data at informative and compact embeddings. An example is an autoencoder that mono-, multi-, or multi-dimensional codes the feature vectors of patients into a lower-dimensional representation that encodes important code-co-occurrence relationships. Likewise, recurrent networks or Transformers coded temporal sequence of events into fixed-size vectors. GNNs are able to map the entities of a knowledge graph (e.g., patient-disease-drug) into embeddings. ARM can also be applied to the latent space, not to raw features, after having learned a neural representation. It has a number of benefits: it decreases noise and redundancy, dimensionality reduction based on latent concepts is minimized, and it may expose compressed relationships that cannot be observed in the sparse original data. Theory Ideas of Jiaming Cui et al. (2022), Shrestha et al. (2021) and Naidenova et al. (2022)

specifies that the network generalizes or smooths similar items, hence rule mining produces a smaller and stronger rule set.

As an example, a denoising autoencoder can be trained to understand that the latent code tendencies to have features such as smoking and respiratory failure go together. After which rule extraction determines that rule smoking equals respiratory failure has high-confidence, although the frequency of individual transactions might have been low. The rule discovery based on this neural representation is an answer to the sub-symbolic learning and the symbolic pattern mining. It basically permits the deep models to perform data pre-processing and feature learning with the structured interpretation to ARM. The outcome is a more scalable, flexible ARM capable of taking advantage of the modern neural architectures.

3. DEEP REPRESENTATION LEARNING AS THE NEW FOUNDATION FOR ARM

3.1 Autoencoder-Based Latent Rule Learning

Autoencoders are neural networks, which are trained on reconstruction of their inputs, and the low-dimensional bottleneck causes salient structure to be captured. In the case of ARM, an incomplete autoencoder (a bottleneck smaller than the input) is trained to learn a small set of codes of every patient record or transaction. In current research, it is shown that the encoding of the autoencoder can reveal co-occurrence patterns. Practically, categorical clinical data (e.g. one-hot symptoms, medications) are coded, and noise (denoising autoenceroder) may be added to enhance robustness. After training, rule extraction proceeds by probing the decoder: specific category values are "clamped" on input, and the decoder's output is observed. If setting input item X to 1 leads the decoder to strongly activate item Y in the output (above a threshold), one infers the rule X Y. A set of rules of neural derivation is obtained by systematically testing combinations of size to a given size.

There are merits of this latent-rule approach. Since the autoencoder is trained on global feature relationships, the mined rules can be of higher level and less redundant. In one case, the autoencoder can be a diagnosis "diabetes" in different symptom patterns, thus the rules reflect the main idea. Such techniques have been demonstrated to also use concise rule sets with similar or superior confidence to exhaustive ARM, methods such as ARM-AE (a previous method based on autoencoders) and Aerial+ have shown that such methods can find similar concise rule sets. Conventionally, with less rules, it is enough to address the rule explosion traditionally. [6] Nevertheless, there are still problems addressed by Sadati et al. (2019), Chen & Guo (2023) and Mienye & Swart (2025) when the autoencoder is overfitting and/or too powerful, there is a risk of acquiring spurious dependencies; the choice of architecture (layers, noise level) and rule pruning are essential.

Table 1. Comparison of representation models for ARM

Model Type	Data Handled	Key Feature	Example Use-Case
Autoencoder	Categorical & binary (via one-hot)	Compresses co-occurrences into latent codes	Mining latent symptom/drug co-occurrences
Variational AE	Same + regularized latent space	Captures distribution of patterns	Discovery of probabilistic patient subgroups
Binary AE	Bit-vector transactions	Optimized for sparse binary input	Retail or medical billing data association

Table 1 compares different deep learning models (autoencoders, VAEs, etc.) used for representation learning in ARM, highlighting their data handling and use cases.

3.2 Temporal Association Mining via RNNs and LSTMs

Clinical events are dynamic (doctor visits, lab tests, medication courses), and therefore, it is very important to capture temporal relationships. RNNs, in particular, Long Short-Term Memory (LSTM) ones are capable of processing event sequences and learning time-dependent relationships. Deep ARM: An RNN is utilized to encode the history of events in a patient into an ultimate hidden state (vector) that summarizes the sequence. This is implicitly coded in terms of time: e.g. the sequence in which the diagnosis and treatment took place. Temporal rules can be mined by observing the behavior of the RNN after it has been trained (to be used in reconstruction or prediction). As an example, using the input of half sequences and observing the hidden state or prediction of the output one can learn the relations such as: on event A hence future event B.

It can be performed by an LSTM encoder-decoder on sequential clinical data: the encoder acts on the previous events and the decoder predicts the following event (or sequence). The way attention mechanisms can bring to fore what past events were used to predict it indicates that there might be rules in sequence. Alternatively, the hidden state may be discretized or clustered, and standard ARM may be applied on these high-level patterns of states, to recognize common patterns. Considering an LSTM trained on ICU vitals by Rai et al. (2023), one might always go into a specific state when a patient is in a bad condition; a rule may be formed between patterns of vital signs and the results.

Temporal deep ARM has the ability of making associations not made by the static ARM. Ji et al. (2024) also showed a functional temporal association technique as a method to identify drug drug interaction signals using longitudinal EMR. Deep

ARM can produce sequential rules by time-warping deep learning with sliding windows e.g. antibiotic start within 2 days of fever ⇒ sepsis onset. Long Short-Term Memory networks can also be used with irregularly-sampled records: they can absorb time gaps or intervals between events and learn that some irregularity patterns are indicative of risk. In brief, RNNs/LSTMs complement ARM incorporating the time dimension into latent representations to reveal sequential medical rules to model the trajectory.

3.3 Graph-Based ARM Using GNNs and Knowledge Graphs

The networks of relationships are complex between patients, diseases, treatments, genes and hospitals. Graph Neural Networks (GNNs) can be used to model heterogeneous medical knowledge in the form of graphs, which allows the discovering of multi-hop associations. As an example, it is possible to build a patient-centered knowledge graph between individuals and diagnoses (ICD codes), medications (RxNorm), lab tests (LOINC), and phenotypes. The nodes refer to entities and the edges refer to interactions or relations (e.g. prescription, has diagnosis).

GNNs (e.g. Graph Convolutional Networks, GraphSAGE, Graph Attention Networks) are trained to embed nodes with the purpose of spreading information over edges. When training a GNN on a biomedical graph, it is possible to mine graph association rules in Deep ARM. As an example, when two disease nodes are brought near each other by GNN because there are many shared patients connections, it implies an association rule Disease A ⇒ Disease B in the context of the patient population. Additionally, there might be transverse of the knowledge graph (such as cross-domain rules e.g. gene-drug-disease paths). This can be compared to mining procedures in a knowledge graph: when the paths among nodes meet support/confidence requirements, they constitute association rules (e.g. patient genotype G and exposure E ⇒ adverse effect F) by Upadhyaya et al. (2024).

Interpretability is enriched with knowledge graphs (KG): these bases rules on an ontology. Indicatively, by connecting the rules that are discovered to concepts of SNOMED CT or UMLS, the reference of PatientAge > 65 and Hypertension ⇒ CardiovascularEvent implies that the reference is a standardized concept. Such ontologies can also be encoded into the GNNs as prior connectivity: e.g. graph nodes representing myocardial infarction and heart attack are connected thus the model will know that the two are the same. Recent studies of Healthcare KGs demonstrate that domain knowledge plays out to make inferences more robust.

Table 2. Graph-based approaches for ARM

GNN Type	Input Graph	Key Idea	Example Discovery
GCN/GAT	Patient–Doctor–Diagnosis graph	Aggregates neighbors to learn node features	Predict new patient–disease associations
R-GCN	Multi-relational KG (drugs, genes)	Models different relation types (e.g., treats, causes)	Detect drug–gene–disease triadic rules
GraphSAGE	Large population graph	Samples neighborhoods for scalability	Personal risk scores via local graph patterns

Table 2 details various graph neural network architectures, explaining how they process biomedical knowledge graphs for association pattern discovery.

By exploiting relational structure, graph-based ARM can find rich associations, such as comorbid conditions mediated by shared risk factors, or polygenic risk patterns. As an illustration, a GNN used on an ontology of diseases and patient data could reveal that Hypertension and Obesity often co-occur with Stroke and this is more than simple co-occurrence.

3.4 Transformer and Attention-Driven Association Discovery

The models and their self-attention mechanisms have transformed sequence modeling. In healthcare, Transformers may take as inputs all the history of a patient or multimodality (e.g. sequence of clinical codes). In contrast to RNNs, Transformers listen to each position in the input, and long-range dependencies are captured. In the case of Deep ARM, it implies that contextual associations between events or features that are distant to each other can be determined. It is possible to feed a sequence of visits (visit with diagnoses, lab, procedures) into a Transformer encoder and generate contextual embeddings of each visit; attention scores can be used to understand which previous visits affect a particular outcome.

The advantage is two fold. To begin with, Transformers inherently combine heterogeneous inputs through multi-head attentions: a single head may combine lab values with diagnoses, another one may combine imaging results with genomics. This produces attention-driven rules, like "Symptom X and Lab abnormality Y attended together by the model importantly Diagnosis Z." Attention weights are an inbuilt measure of importance of a rule candidate. Second, Transformer training on large clinical corpora (e.g. ClinicalBERT, BEHRT) provides the model with medical language information, thereby allowing fine-tuning with EHR data to provide subtle associations. E.g. a clinical BERT model could be conditioned to the fact that icd_E11 (Type 2 diabetes) can tend to co-occur with icd_I10 (Hypertension) and med_INSULIN over long patient courses, suggesting a rule on a higher level.

Interestingly, patient representation learning also has new models which are based on transformers. Hierarchical Transformer (e.g. Hi-BEHR) can use highly long input (years of visits). Such models together with post hoc rule mining can produce accurate phenotypes. As an example specified by Kaur et al. (2015), once all patient notes are encoded with ClinicalTransformer, common concepts identified by large attention with respect to an outcome can be converted into rules (e.g., mention and symptom A in notes and lab B abnormal next event C).

The main takeaway that can be made is that Transformers add contextual, long-range associations to the deep ARM toolkit. They can adapt well to complex EHR patterns in which significant predictors can be separated by long distances in time or modality. The attention scores provide a preliminary explainable indication which could be converted into formal association rules to be used by clinicians.

4. THE DEEP ARM FRAMEWORK: A NOVEL HYBRID ARCHITECTURE

4.1 Conceptual Design and Workflow

Figure 1. Conceptual workflow for deep ARM in clinical analytics

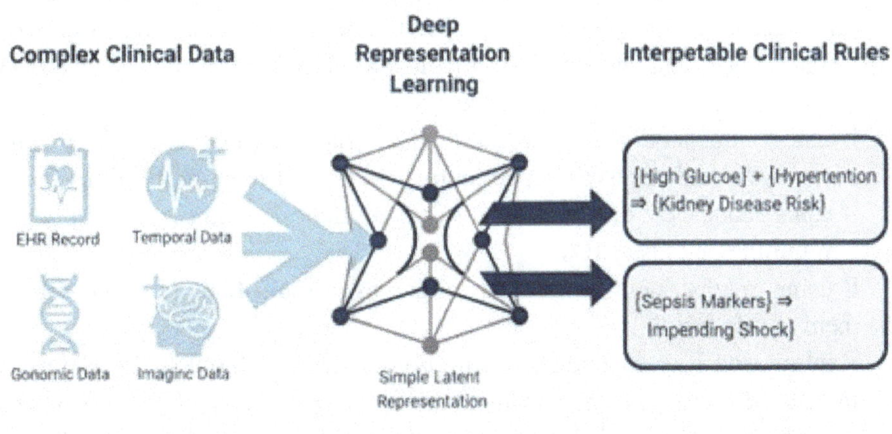

Figure 1 illustrates how complex multimodal clinical data, including EHR, temporal, genomic, and imaging information, are encoded through deep representation learning into latent features from which interpretable clinical association rules are derived.

A Deep ARM architecture integrates neural embedding modules with a symbolic rule mining component. A general workflow is:

- **Data Ingestion and Integration:** Collect multimodal clinical inputs (structured EHR tables, unstructured clinical notes, imaging features, genomic data). Perform standard preprocessing (e.g. one-hot encoding categorical codes, embedding text with word vectors, image feature extraction).
- **Representation Learning:** Feed data into deep models chosen by modality:
- *Autoencoders* for categorical demographics, ICD codes, lab categories.
- *RNNs/LSTMs* for patient timelines of events (visit sequences, time-series signals).
- *Graph Neural Networks* for knowledge graphs linking entities (patients-nodes, diagnoses, drugs).
- *Transformers* for long-range sequence data (full patient history, notes).

Each network outputs latent embeddings or reconstructions that capture underlying patterns.

- **Rule Extraction:** Apply an ARM algorithm on the latent space or decoder outputs. For example, use thresholding on decoder probabilities to derive rules (autoencoder approach), or mine frequent patterns among discretized neural activations. One can also treat neural predictions as new derived features and mine on them. In practice:
- If using autoencoders: freeze the model, generate "test vectors" by fixing some inputs and observe decoder outputs to form if-then implications.
- If using sequences: cluster hidden states or attention patterns and apply pattern mining on cluster IDs.
- If using graphs: identify frequent subgraphs or multi-hop paths and convert them to rule form.
- **Explanation Layer:** Translate neural outcomes into human-readable rules. For each discovered rule, map latent features back to original terms. This may involve referencing a domain ontology or semantic layer, ensuring rules use clinically recognized terms (e.g. mapping a neural node to "diabetes" rather than "autoencoder dimension 5").
- **Domain Integration:** Optionally, refine rules using biomedical knowledge bases. For instance, discard rules contradictory to known biology, or extend partial rules using ontology hierarchies (e.g. replace a specific drug name with a drug class concept).

- **Output and Feedback:** The final output is a set of association rules with metrics (support, confidence) and provenance (which embedding produced them). Optionally, the system includes a user interface for clinicians to review and annotate rules, feeding back into model refinement Badhon et al. (2019)

A high-level schematic of this Deep ARM pipeline is shown below:

- Data (EHRs, images, text) → Neural Embedding (AE/RNN/GNN/Transformer) → Latent Representations → Rule Mining Module → Human-Readable Association Rules → Clinical Knowledge Base (for domain alignment).

This workflow can be implemented as an end-to-end pipeline, e.g. using Spark for data integration and ARM libraries (MLxtend) in combination with PyTorch/TensorFlow neural components. It supports scaling to large datasets (GPU acceleration for neural training; distributed mining for rule generation). The architecture is modular: one can plug in different deep models depending on the application, and combine multiple rule sets (e.g. autoencoder-derived + sequence-derived) for richer knowledge.

4.2 Neural Rule Extraction and Explainability Layer

This "explainability layer" converts sub-symbolic activations into symbolic. Several strategies exist:

- **Output Probing:** Output Probing: Probes on the output probabilities of the decoder are sought to determine the outputs.This yield rules directly. The second strategy is the employment of model. inversion: create synthetic examples (through GANs or decoder) which maximize some. then obtain conditions, which such instances have in common.
- **Saliency and Attention:** In sequence models that are attention-based, the most attended is the highest one. events/features imply antecedents of rules. Our attention scores are added together on a large scale. patients in order to find regular patterns. As an illustration, when one pays attention to high blood. pressure" repeatingly causes "stroke" forecast, one thinks "Hypertension = Stroke" in rule form.
- **Concept Layer Interventions:** Add a bottleneck layer of human-concepts. (e.g. interim clinical tests) in the neural network. Analyze during training or after the training. what notions tend to be activated. This can be compared to

concept learning: hidden units can. are associated with established clinical determinants. Algorithms of Post-hoc Rule Extraction: DeepRED or LORE are tools that are capable of extracting. Splitting by systematically partitioning the input, the decision trees or rules of an educated network.

- **Post-hoc Rule Extraction Algorithms:** Tools like DeepRED or LORE can extract decision trees or rules from a trained network by systematically partitioning the input space. Adapted to ARM, such methods can generate if-then rules approximating the network's decision boundaries. For association rules specifically, one could train the network as a multi-label predictor and then use rule extraction on its learned decision logic.
- **Tracing Neuron Influence:** Track which input features most strongly influence a particular output through backpropagation gradients or layer-wise relevance propagation. Features with consistently high influence become part of a rule antecedent for that output class.

The overarching goal is that each discovered rule has a clear mapping to original clinical variables. For trust, it is crucial that this mapping be validated: e.g. when the network implies "fever ⇒ sepsis", we should ensure the word "fever" corresponds to a symptom concept. The explainability layer may cross-reference a clinical ontology to label latent variables. In practice, an expert review step is often included: clinicians examine the candidate rules for plausibility, further filtering or adjusting them.

4.3 Integration with Clinical Ontologies and Domain Knowledge

Embedding biomedical knowledge directly into Deep ARM enhances interpretability and reliability. Clinical ontologies are used, such as SNOMED CT (diseases, findings), RxNorm (drugs). LOINC (labs), and higher level knowledge bases (UMLS, Gene Ontology) are structured. domain context. Integration takes place in several points:

- **Encoding of features:** Encode raw data into ontology concepts prior to or during training. For instance, use SNOMED concept IDs instead of free-text diagnoses, ensuring that semantically similar terms share embeddings. One can also use ontological hierarchies as part of the model (e.g. graph edges in a GNN).
- **Regularization:** Impose constraints that latent representations respect ontological relations. For example, if two lab tests have a parent concept, their latent embeddings may be encouraged to be close. This helps the network focus on medically relevant groupings.

- **Rule Post-Processing:** After mining raw rules, use ontologies to filter or generalize them. A mined rule "aspirin ∧ acetaminophen ⇒ liver injury" can be compared against known pharmacology paths or drug class hierarchies. One might generalize it to "NSAIDs ∧ Painkillers ⇒ liver injury" if supported by data and ontology structure.
- **Domain Knowledge Graphs:** Link the discovered rules into a larger healthcare knowledge graph (KG). This permits the relational reasoning. For example, if an ontology connects hypertension to stroke through vascular pathology and it solidifies a rule HTN => human associates hypertension and stroke by the vascular pathology and it solidifies a rule HTN => Stroke" found in data. Likewise, knowledge-based reasoning tools (e.g. ontology-based. reasoning engines) have the capability to check rules with extant literature or unveil conflicting ones. knowledge (notifying the analyst about false positives).

We develop a layer of trust by matching Deep ARM output to existing biomedical schemas. Clinicians are likely to embrace rules presented using standardized terminologies. Besides, this integration may point to really new rules: ones involving the association of distant branches of ontology (e.g. between a genetic marker and a rare phenotype) can be pointing to discoveries. As a concrete example, embedding SNOMED concepts in an autoencoder means that a latent association among concepts has a direct interpretation in the ontology. Recent reviews on healthcare knowledge graphs show that using ontologies yields interpretable embeddings and supports discovery of phenotypic correlations.

4.4 Evaluation Metrics for Clinical Utility

Evaluating Deep ARM requires going beyond raw predictive accuracy to measures of clinical relevance and interpretability. Key metrics include:

- **Traditional ARM metrics:** *Support*, *confidence*, and *lift* remain fundamental. In Deep ARM, one assesses these on the underlying data distribution to ensure mined rules are statistically significant and not data artifacts.
- **Coverage:** The proportion of patients or records to which a rule applies. High coverage means a rule is broadly relevant; very narrow coverage rules may be less useful clinically, even if high confidence.
- **Rule Quality and Interestingness:** Conviction, Leverage or Chi. squared is used to measure the extent to which a rule is shocking or new in comparison with independence. In high lift (e.g. >2) or odds ratio analogs can be signs of potential clinical. importance.

- **Complexity:** The number of conditions (length of the antecedent) and the number of the rules must be few in order to be interpretable. We monitor mean antecedent size and mean number of rules - the less the better. Multi-objective performance (maximizing confidence and reduction of length) is frequently required.
- **Clinical Significance:** At the end of the day, the value of a rule is associated with practical value. Domain experts are able to tag rule relevancy or a clinical interestingness score. Surrogate metrics can be the presence of known risk factors or new associations in a rule.
- **Predictive Utility:** In a predictive model (e.g. rule-based classifier), such metrics as are useful. accurate, sensitive and specific rule set on held-out data is important. For sequential forecasting time-to-event prediction metrics (e.g. C-index, AUC over time) are relevant.
- **Stability and Robustness:** Rules are expected to be generalized across cohorts. We may compute what is the count of rules that are present when the model is retrained using alternate data splits (Jaccard) similarity of rule sets). Inter-site/cohort stable rules are more credible.
- **Efficiency:** We quantify the time of computation and memory consumption, in particular. because Deep ARM is intended to be better than exhaustive ARM. Metrics like time to mine k rules are informative concerning scalability.

Table 3. Example evaluation metrics

Metric	Purpose	Clinical Relevance Example
Support	Frequency of rule in data	Common comorbid patterns vs. rare events
Confidence	Strength of implication	Likelihood of an outcome given antecedents
Lift	Independence baseline comparison	Identifies non-trivial (synergistic) patterns
Coverage	Population coverage of rule	Ensures rule applies to significant patient subset
Antecedent Length	Simplicity of rule	Shorter (fewer conditions) is more interpretable
Stability Score	Robustness across datasets	Consistent rule in multiple hospital cohorts
Clinical Validity*	Expert judgment of relevance	Expert-validated vs. spurious associations

*Some metrics (like clinical validity) involve expert evaluation and may be qualitative.

Table 3 lists evaluation measures including support, confidence and lift which are critical in evaluating the clinical relevance and reliability of the discovered rules.

In short, Deep ARM analysis should be both statistically correct and cognitively practical. Our objectives include the rules that address key segments of patients, are very probable in event of triggering, and their rules are simple enough to be used by clinicians. This may usually involve trade-offs between model accuracy and interpretability which depend on domain knowledge

5. CLINICAL INTELLIGENCE APPLICATIONS

5.1 Disease Trajectory Prediction and Risk Stratification

Deep ARM has the potential to shed light on the disease development in individuals which is used to detect the disease in its initial stages. In case of chronic diseases (diabetes, renal disease, neurodegeneration), longitudinal EHR data include hints regarding future complications. We can discover such rules as (Obesity ∧ Family history of diabetes) ⇒ High risk of Type 2 Diabetes within 5 years with the application of Temporal deep ARM to patient history. RNN/LSTM encoders are trained to learn patient course and are capable of grouping similar progression patterns, ARM then extracts prototypical pattern of progression. As an example, ICU data may show that Day-1 Sepsis markers = Acute kidney injury Day 3. Transformer-based embedding (that takes into account both distant and recent events) can be used to stratify patients into risk groups. The found rules may serve as foundation of risk scores: e.g. a rule-based risk stratifier, which adds up the confidences of invoked rules to estimate heart failure onset.

Deep ARM helps in the development of phenotypes in population health. Knowledge of subpopulations (e.g. as in age hypertensives with pneumonia vs young diabetics with early nephropathy) can be gained by clustering patient embeddings. The characteristics of each group are defined by association rules. This enables focused screening: in case one rule states that a subset (such as patients between 55-70 years old and having obesity and high LDL) are likely to develop coronary artery disease, it will be possible to identify such patients and provide them with preventive care. Notably, deep models have the ability to learn numerous risk factors (labs, genetics, social determinants) into its latent space Karabulut et al. (2024), and it produces more evidence-based trajectories compared to hand-crafted risk models. Deep phenotyping studies have already generated novel high-risk cohorts and inclusion of ARM would give explicit rules that clinicians can rely on and trust to make early interventions.

5.2 Therapeutic Optimization and Drug Interaction Discovery

Deep ARM can be used to derive patterns in therapeutic reactions and drug interactions in the treatment planning. Indicatively, longitudinal treatment data may be mined to give personalized therapy rules such as: (Patient on Drug A ∧ Genetic marker X) ⇒ Better response to Drug B. Continuous measurements of drug activity (e.g. reduction of tumor, blood pressure management) can be modeled by deep learning and ARM can correlate these measurements with treatment practices or patient characteristics. Hybrid models predicting drug response based on molecular profiles have been applied in oncology; implementation in Deep ARM may reveal rules like BRCA1 mutation 0 high PD-L1 0 immunotherapy success.

The Deep ARM is also effective in pharmacovigilance. A traditional method to determine adverse drug reactions (co-occurrence of drug-event in post-marketing data) is association rule mining. With more profound embedding of the history of medications that patients have been taking and trends in lab results, higher-order interactions not covered by simple co-occurrence can be discovered. As an example, a GNN on a drug enzyme network would be able to suggest a hypothesis such as Drug C metabolized by enzyme Y 6 polymorphism Z 7 toxicity increased. Deep models are used to make sure that the complex patient contexts (comorbidities, dose adjustments) are taken into account. In addition, ARM on the latent space can be used to identify uncommon yet clinically relevant interactions. As an example, should a Transformer discover that the occurrence of late ICU events co-occurs with a series of two antibiotics, a rule such as (Antibiotic1 at T1 ∧ Antibiotic2 at T2) ⇒ Seizure risk may be generated, which may inform pharmacists to create a reminder or change treatment plans. To conclude, Deep ARM is used to streamline therapy using the experience of large-scale real-world treatment results and generalize the knowledge to explicit clinical guidelines and safety policies.

5.3 Real-Time Monitoring and Clinical Event Forecasting

The ability to forecast clinical events at the right moment becomes essential for saving lives in both acute care settings and chronic disease management. Deep ARM functions as a system which provides predictive surveillance systems to operate. The method requires ongoing application of temporal rule mining to process streaming patient data. The system would analyze vital sign streams using LSTM to detect rising trends and then ARM would analyze LSTM output or hidden state to generate the rule: "(RR↑ ∧ BP↓ ∧ WBC↑) ⇒ impending septic shock". The system identifies abnormal signal combinations through its network-based detection system and the extracted rules represent the discovered abnormal patterns.

The rules enable real-time alert generation because an ICU system would trigger an alert when it detects simultaneous absence of urine output and rising lactate levels and increased ventilation support because these conditions strongly predict cardiac arrest within the next few hours. The telemonitoring system for chronic disease management uses deep model rules to detect worsening heart failure through the pattern of weight gain exceeding 2 kilograms within three days combined with new atrial fibrillation which indicates heart failure exacerbation. The sequential association rules function as a knowledge base which enables clinical decision support by forecasting the consequent event whenever input data satisfies the antecedent conditions.

The forecasting process benefits from the assistance of graph models and transformer models. A patient-centric knowledge graph that receives real-time updates through current vital signs and historical data nodes enables GNNs to forecast upcoming events and association rules extracted from graph patterns such as deterioration subgraph motifs serve as understandable triggers. The combination of wearable sensors with IoT devices generates fast data streams which enables edge computing to operate lightweight Deep ARM pipelines that execute ongoing rule activation updates. The monitoring system predicts adverse events like ICU transfer and sepsis while providing explanations about the discovered associations which creates trust for clinicians to respond to the alerts.

5.4 Population-Level Phenotyping and Personalized Medicine

Deep ARM enables the discovery of phenotypes on a large scale which supports the development of personalized medical treatment plans. Unsupervised deep learning methods such as autoencoders and VAEs and clustering on embeddings can detect concealed patient subgroups through big data analysis (e.g. "silent MI subgroup" or "pediatric asthma subtype"). The association rules describe the unique characteristics of each phenotype. The rule extraction layer would generate the rule "(Type 2 Diabetes $\wedge$ Proteinuria) $\Rightarrow$ Rapid progression to ESRD" based on an embedding cluster which shows diabetic patients who develop kidney failure. The rules provide understandable definitions of phenotypes which enable doctors to detect and treat patients using specific methods.

Transformers and multimodal networks allow integration of diverse data for deeper phenotyping. The model needs to handle three different types of input data which include clinical notes in text form and X-ray images and laboratory test results. The model creates patient groups by identifying overall similarities between individual patients through its embedding process. It is the mining of the extracted data that will provide means of extracting intricate subtypes of these rules resulting in statements such as X-ray signs of fatty liver and gene variant V predicts Metabolic Syndrome subtype. The regulations allow precision medicine to carry out its work more efficiently since they perform two critical roles. The regulations set new standards of medical research and they identify certain population of patients who demand certain medical care.

Deep ARM at the population level also supports population health analytics. The integration of the rules across regions and groups of people identifies gaps in health.

An example of a rule will be Race: X combined with low Income level results in Decreased cancer screening rates which can be used to devise policy solutions. Deep embeddings embrace socioeconomic and demographic factors that allow ARM to present the way in which socioeconomic factors result in various outcomes thereby facilitating the formulation of equitable healthcare schemes. The Deep ARM system can work on various levels between individual patient care and the whole population health management through the developing of risk assessments and health profiles that can be used in the context of personal medical treatment as well as community health initiatives.

6. IMPLEMENTATION ECOSYSTEM FOR DEEP ARM

6.1 Technical Stack and Framework Integration

The construction of Deep ARM system presupposes the usage of new machine learning systems and data tools. Core components include:

- **Deep Learning Libraries:** TensorFlow/Keras and PyTorch provide flexible platforms for constructing autoencoders, RNNs, GNNs, and Transformers. Their graphics processing unit acceleration is essential in training of high-dimensional medical data. GNNs such as PyTorch Geometric or DGL facilitate the development of libraries.
- **Association Rule Mining Tools:** Python Libraries MLxtend or Spark MLlib. supply optimum Apriori/FP-Growth implementations of rule generation. These can be trained on normalized neural-data (e.g., binarized embeddings). Spark MLlib can handle large-scale mining in distributed fashion.
- **Data Processing and Pipelines:** Apache Spark or Hadoop are often used to preprocess large EHR datasets, enabling distributed feature engineering (e.g. creating transactional itemsets). Orchestration tools (Airflow, Kubeflow) manage end-to-end workflows.
- **Integration Frameworks:** Combining deep models with ARM rules can be done in a pipeline: for example, after training a PyTorch model on Spark cluster, outputs are passed to MLxtend. Alternatively, TensorFlow Extended (TFX) could orchestrate the pipeline including a custom ARM step.
- **Deployment:** For real-time applications, trained models can be exported (e.g. TensorFlow SavedModel, ONNX format) and served via REST APIs. ARM rules, once mined, can be stored in a rule database (e.g. Redis or SQL) and queried by a decision support application.

- **Scalability:** GPUs and TPUs (for TensorFlow) accelerate deep training. For ARM, distributed computing (Spark/Flink) allows mining on multi-terabyte EHR repositories. On the user side, rule-based inference is fast and light-weight, suitable for edge deployment in hospital systems.

An implementation process consists of these steps: (1) Data engineers employ Spark to perform cleaning and merging operations on various clinical tables; (2) Data scientists train a PyTorch autoencoder on Spark-managed data, save the latent representations; (3) Use MLxtend to run FP-Growth on the latent codes;(4) The rules need to be filtered and formatted before use; (5) Deploy a Flask app serving these rules for clinicians. The modular technology stack makes sure that there is the best-fit tool used in each step.

6.2 Datasets, Ontologies, and Benchmark Resources

The creation and assessment of Deep ARM needs abundant clinical datasets and ontologies. Key resources include:

Table 4. Key resources

Resource	Type	Description
MIMIC-III	ICU EHR Dataset	Free access to critical care database. Has approximately 53,000 ICU admissions ([?]40,000 patients) that contain highly-detailed data: demographics, hourly vital signs, laboratory tests, procedures, medications, notes, and outcomes. It is diverse and granular, allowing the study of the trends of critical illnesses.
eICU-CRD	Multi-ICU EHR Dataset	Multi-center ICU database (Philips eICU program) of more than 200,000 ICU admissions in the US (2014-2015). Vitals, care plans, severity scores (APACHE), diagnoses, and treatments. Applicable in the validation of rules in other hospital environments.
SNOMED CT	Clinical Ontology	Comprehensive medical terminology (>300,000 concepts, including diseases, findings, procedures). Organizes terms in hierarchies. Used to standardize EHR fields and interpret rule items.
RxNorm	Drug Vocabulary	Standard names and IDs for clinical drugs (includes mappings to many drug vocabularies). Enables normalization of medication data and alignment of drug-related rules.
OMOP CDM	Data Standard	Common Data Model for harmonizing observational health data. Defines standard table schemas (e.g. person, visit, drug_exposure) and vocabularies. Facilitates applying models/rules across different institutions.

Table 4 summarizes some of the major datasets and ontologies (e.g., MIMIC-III, SNOMED) utilized in deep. ARM, which is based on real-world biomedical information sources.

SNOMED UMLS (Unified Medical Language System) of code mappings, the LOINC lab code set, and open genomics datasets, such as the UK Biobank, are other useful resources. When developing Deep ARM, one typically uses MIMIC-III or eICU for proof-of-concept due to their public availability. Ontologies ensure that features fed into the models and rules are semantically consistent. For example, mapping ICD-9/10 codes in MIMIC to SNOMED allows rules to generalize across datasets.

6.3 Computational Acceleration and Deployment Strategies

Deep ARM systems must handle large-scale, sensitive health data, and often support real-time use. Key strategies include:

- **Cloud–Edge Hybrid:** Training deep models on cloud GPUs/TPUs (AWS, Google Cloud, Azure) for scalability; deploying rule-based inference at the edge (hospital servers) for low-latency decisions. For example, training an autoencoder on a large EHR in the cloud, then shipping a distilled rule set to bedside monitors.
- **Federated Learning:** In multi-institutional settings, data cannot be pooled. Federated learning enables distributed model training: each site trains on local data, shares model updates (not raw data). ARM could likewise operate in a federated way: individual hospitals mine local rules, then a central server aggregates and filters rule sets, as in federated association rule mining. Differential privacy techniques (adding noise to shared model updates) protect patient confidentiality.
- **Privacy-Preserving Computation:** Homomorphic encryption or. secure enclaves permit calculation of encryptedd data. This could allow joint rule mining between institutions without disclosing crude patient records.
- **Hardware Acceleration:** ardware Acceleration: Training deep networks is done using specialized AI chips (NVIDIA GPUs, Google TPUs). Computations with ARM (such as bit-vector operations in FPGrowth) can be optimized with CPU instructions (SIMD instructions) or parallel. An example is the RAPIDS and cuDF created by NVIDIA and used to execute data processing using a GPU.
- **Containerization and MLOps:** Docker and Kubernetes are two technologies used to deploy Deep ARM services (model serving, rule engines, databases) in clinical IT. Continuous integration pipelines are models/rules that are automatically updated as new data comes.
- **Benchmarking and Optimization:** In performance-critical environments (e.g. ICU alarms), the models and rules should be efficient. Neural models could be quantised and pruned to reduce their size; rule sets could be re-

duced to a top-k rule set. It is necessary to profile in order to have sub-second inferences.

With healthcare IT combined with modern ML infrastructure, Deep ARM can expand research prototypes to clinical system grade, with the requirements of computational acceleration and security requirements being satisfied.

7. ETHICAL, INTERPRETABILITY, AND TRUST DIMENSIONS

7.1 The Explainability Gap in Deep ARM

Deep ARM is an interpretable model but suffers a lot of challenges that make it not realize its potential. The complex form of neural networks enables them to extract arbitrary links between medical data that are mixed estimates. The rule extraction process requires a validation stage to decide whether the extracted rule is a true causal knowledge rather than a biased data. The neural architecture introduces a gap between the highly complex design and the simple laws that can be comprehended by human beings. Deep ARM needs to add particular explanation methods to solve this problem. The evidence for rules derived from neural models needs to include patient profiles and explanations which show how model features affect decision-making. The visualization tools operate automatically to display the specific inputs which determine each rule. The evaluation process requires experts to review and endorse rules before they can be implemented. Unexplained rules risk eroding trust (e.g. a rule predicting "acetaminophen ⇒ kidney injury" might be correct in data but clinicians will question its mechanism). The medical field requires doctors to understand data origins and model validation methods and rule development processes before they accept clinical applications.

7.2 Fairness, Bias, and Data Quality Considerations

Clinical data often reflect systemic biases (e.g. unequal care access, underrepresentation of minorities). The Deep ARM system learns rules through its operations which can lead to the unintentional creation of biased rules. The model identifies a valid pattern which states "Race = X leads to lower screening rates" yet this pattern creates fairness problems. The implementation of fairness metrics enables organizations to detect when rule support or confidence levels produce unequal advantages or damages to particular demographic segments. The process of bias mitigation requires two main approaches which consist of demographic parity enforcement in rule coverage and sensitive attribute removal during rule mining. Data quality emerges as the basic requirement. The presence of inaccurate or missing data in EHR systems leads to incorrect associations between information mentioned by Dehghani et al. (2023). The model will develop an incorrect association between test absence and medical conditions because it will learn from the non-random missing patterns in the data. The combination of imputation and outlier removal along with the validation process on separate data sets helps to prevent these problems. Additionally, rules must be audited for clinical plausibility: a high-confidence rule that defies medical logic should be flagged for scrutiny. The ethical deployment of Deep ARM systems needs both precise operation and equal treatment of all patients. The Deep ARM system needs to show its decision-making process for bias correction through example re-weighting which prevents discrimination against any patient group.

7.3 Federated and Privacy-Preserving Learning Paradigms

Clinical data requires absolute protection of privacy because it needs to be safeguarded. The solution for multi-site Deep ARM through federated learning eliminates the need for centralized patient record storage. Each hospital conducts its own local training of deep models which produces specific rules that get combined into a global rule set through the sharing of model parameters or aggregated rules. Technologies like Secure Multi-Party Computation (SMPC) or homomorphic encryption can further protect individual data during rule aggregation. The addition of noise through differential privacy mechanisms protects patient identities in the mining process. The privacy-preserving ARM enables organizations to work together on rare disease research through multi-center studies while keeping patient data protected under HIPAA and GDPR regulations. The system generates trust between organizations which participate in the model sharing process. A consortium could establish national sepsis risk patterns through encoded model weight sharing instead of EHR data exchange which safeguards patient privacy. The trustworthiness and ethical compliance of Deep ARM for multi-institutional healthcare analytics depends on transparent protocol practices which include privacy budget disclosure.

8. EMERGING FRONTIERS AND FUTURE RESEARCH DIRECTIONS

8.1 Multimodal and Cross-Domain Deep ARM

Future Deep ARM systems will need to fuse multimodal data. The dataset needs to contain structured EHR information together with X-ray and MRI imaging data and genomic data and wearable sensor data streams and patient-generated text including symptom diaries and social media posts. A transformer would be capable of learning cross-modal associations by processing medical notes and lab results together with genomic variants through joint encoding. A potential rule might be: "(MRI lesion pattern $\wedge$ gene mutation $\wedge$ symptom combination) $\Rightarrow$ Disease subtype". The integration of vision transformers for imaging features and natural language models for text and graph models for genomics will produce a combined latent representation which requires mining. The system will analyze medical data through cross-domain Deep ARM to integrate external information about environmental factors and socioeconomic status and purchasing habits to identify comprehensive health determinants. The combination of different fields leads to total understanding but it creates difficulties when trying to combine various representations and handle different levels of complexity.

8.2 Continual and Self-Adaptive Rule Learning

Healthcare operates as a constantly evolving system because medical advancements lead to new treatment options and healthcare guidelines transform and population demographics transform. The system needs to process data continuously because it needs to update its rules whenever new information becomes available. Research into continual learning (e.g. Elastic Weight Consolidation)can keep neural representations current without catastrophic forgetting. The system needs to perform two main functions when it comes to rule mining: it should apply incremental ARM algorithms to update existing rules with new cases and eliminate rules which have become obsolete. A self-adaptive Deep ARM system might detect when incoming data deviates (e.g. a novel virus) and trigger re-mining of associations by Raza et al. (2021) and Arumuga Perumal (2013). During an epidemic Deep ARM would create fresh rules which would connect patient information to the emerging disease. The learning process of Continual Learning includes On-Device Learning because smart medical devices can develop personalized care through rule adaptation for individual patients. Medical staff need to verify all adjustments through clinical evaluation and benchmark assessment to stop the drift problem from developing. The technique of real-time rule scoring and curation within interactive machine learning systems shows great potential to advance self-adaptation in machine learning.

8.3 Knowledge-Augmented and Human-in-the-Loop ARM

Human expertise continues to play a vital role in the workplace even though automated systems have taken over many tasks. The Deep ARM loop system of future systems will operate through human feedback, which will be integrated into its design. The neural model benefits from expert actions that label or modify discovered rules through splitting rules and merging conditions to improve its representation during supervised fine-tuning on rule annotations. Active learning serves as a method to identify rules with uncertain validity. These then require human evaluation so experts can concentrate on these specific cases. The field of knowledge-augmented learning continues to develop through the use of scientific literature and clinical guidelines as soft constraints. Biomedical text-mining models help prove the ARM rule through external evidence about the sequence of smoking before lung cancer development. The system operates as a collaborative platform because data mining produces hypotheses, which domain experts validate before the network learns from their confirmation. The goal of hybrid workflows is to unite artificial intelligence with human expertise to develop rules that healthcare professionals can use in their practice.

8.4 Towards Trustworthy and Regulatory-Compliant Clinical AI

Deep ARM needs to follow all clinical decision support software (CDSS) standards to meet regulatory requirements. The process requires exact record-keeping of algorithms and strict rule version management and system operation consistency. Researchers need to create methods which transform ARM-generated data into formats that people can understand while keeping all information traceable. The system would track data origins to show which specific data generated each rule and the exact patient conditions that make these rules applicable thus enabling FDA compliance. The system needs to handle incorrect usage by showing error messages when users input bad data and by displaying results with uncertainty measurements Shaoxiong et al. (2024). Deep ARM needs to move beyond correlation to establish causation by employing causal discovery methods such as constraint-based causal learning to detect which associations carry causal weight. The primary goal of medical AI requires the systems to be able to go beyond predicting risks and understanding the underlying causes that cause these risks. Before association-based models can be applied to clinical settings the validation and approval procedures will be established by regulatory organizations. Deep ARM will be shifting towards healthcare applications in a process that begins with pattern recognition to the mechanistic understanding.

9. CONCLUSION

9.1 Summary of Deep ARM's Transformative Potential

Deep Association Rule Mining is the recent algorithm of clinical data analytics that is an ultimate shift in the sphere. It combines rich representation learning and symbolic rule learning and thus overcomes major shortcomings of classical approaches. Deep ARM works on the basis of high-dimensional analysis of health data to generate simple rules that can identify significant medical patterns. The system provides real-time patient monitoring and phenotype definition, prediction and optimization of treatment of diseases using Deep ARM, and provides immediate clinical insights. The hybrid design of the system enables both power from neural models and explainability through rules which makes it suitable for critical healthcare environments. The system depends on every component which includes autoencoders and knowledge graphs to generate automated "if-then" medical knowledge from complicated data.

9.2 Strategic Pathway for Translational Implementation

Deep ARM requires collaboration between researchers and medical professionals to reach its goal of bedside application. The research teams need to team up with medical staff to create practical applications which they will then validate through their discovered rules. The trust in Deep ARM will develop through pilot studies which will test its integration with current clinical decision support systems by adding rule alerts to EHR interfaces. The adoption process will speed up through open-source platforms which provide accessible documentation of operational workflows. Healthcare data scientists together with clinicians require education about the process of creating and understanding neural-augmented rules during their training. The system needs multidisciplinary standards which link AI developers to informaticians and ethicists and regulators to maintain system robustness and safety. The rules about cancer risk assessment need to get approval from oncologists before they can influence medical practice because they need to match established oncology guidelines. Deep ARM will move from prototype stage to routine care through ongoing development based on actual clinical feedback which will enable its integration as an advanced analytics module within hospital data warehouse systems.

9.3 The Road Ahead: From Associations to Causal Insights

The future direction of clinical analytics will surpass association rules because it will operate through causal relationships instead of correlation based methods.

Deep ARM functions as an initial tool which produces ideas about medical results for patients. The upcoming advancement requires scientists to execute causal testing through structural equation models and counterfactual reasoning methods in order to determine if the identified relationship represents a direct cause. Chen et al. (2024) need to examine randomized trials and instrumental variables for causal confirmation when evaluating the association between Drug A and Outcome B. Research scientists actively investigate how causal inference methods combine with deep learning and ARM systems. The research will allow scientists to predict diseases through mechanisms which will generate explanations about disease processes which will enable them to develop treatments based on scientific explanations instead of statistical relationships. Deep ARM technology will develop to create clinical AI systems which provide both statistical outcome predictions and causal explanations for medical events. The core principle of AI in healthcare will emerge from the process of converting patterns into fundamental principles.

REFERENCES

Arumuga, P. (2013). Association rule mining and medical application: A detailed survey. *International Journal of Computer Applications*, *80*(4), 10–19. DOI: 10.5120/13967-1698

Badhon, B., Kabir, M., Xu, S., & Kabir, M. (2019). A survey on association rule mining based on evolutionary algorithms. *International Journal of Computers and Applications*, *43*(1), 1–11. DOI: 10.1080/1206212X.2019.1612993

Berteloot, T., Khoury, R., & Durand, A. (2023). *Association rules mining with auto-encoders*. arXiv. https://doi.org//arXiv.2304.13717DOI: 10.48550

Chen, S., & Guo, W. (2023). Auto-encoders in deep learning—A review with new perspectives. *Mathematics*, *11*(8), 1777. DOI: 10.3390/math11081777

Chen, Y., Ling, M., Liu, Y., Chen, X., Li, Y., & Tong, B. (2024). Enhancing MRI image retrieval using autoencoder-based deep learning: A solution for efficient clinical and teaching applications. *Journal of Radiation Research and Applied Sciences*, *17*(3), 100932. DOI: 10.1016/j.jrras.2024.100932

Cui, J., Zhao, S., & Sun, X. (2022). An association rule mining algorithm for clinical decision support. In *Proceedings of the 8th International Conference on Computing and Artificial Intelligence (ICCAI '22)* (pp. 137–143). Association for Computing Machinery. DOI: 10.1145/3532213.3532234

Dehghani, M., Yazdanparast, Z., & Mohammadi, M. (2023). *Discovering the symptom patterns of COVID-19 from recovered and deceased patients using Apriori association rule mining*. arXiv. https://doi.org//arXiv.2308.06763DOI: 10.48550

Ji, S., Li, X., Sun, W., Dong, H., Taalas, A., Zhang, Y., Wu, H., Pitkänen, E., & Marttinen, P. (2024). A unified review of deep learning for automated medical coding. *ACM Computing Surveys*, *56*(12), 306. Advance online publication. DOI: 10.1145/3664615

Karabulut, E., Degeler, V., & Groth, P. (2024). *AE SemRL: Learning semantic association rules with autoencoders*. arXiv. https://arxiv.org/abs/2403.18133

Kaur, J., & Madan, N. (2015). Association rule mining: A survey. *International Journal of Hybrid Information Technology*, *8*(7), 239–242. DOI: 10.14257/ijhit.2015.8.7.22

Mienye, I. D., & Swart, T. G. (2025). Deep autoencoder neural networks: A comprehensive review and new perspectives. *Archives of Computational Methods in Engineering*, *32*(7), 3981–4000. DOI: 10.1007/s11831-025-10260-5

Miotto, R., Wang, F., Wang, S., Jiang, X., & Dudley, J. T. (2018). Deep learning for healthcare: Review, opportunities, and challenges. *Briefings in Bioinformatics*, *19*(6), 1236–1246. DOI: 10.1093/bib/bbx044 PMID: 28481991

Naidenova, X., Ganapolsky, V., Yakovlev, A., & Martirova, T. (2022). Application association rule mining in medical-biological investigations [Journal information not specified]. *Survey (London, England)*.

Rai, V. K., Chakraborty, S., & Chakraborty, S. (2023). Association rule mining for prediction of COVID-19. *Decision Making: Applications in Management and Engineering*, *6*(1), 365–378. DOI: 10.31181/dmame0317102022r

Raza, A., Tran, K. P., Koehl, L., & Li, S. (2021). Designing ECG monitoring healthcare system with federated transfer learning and explainable AI. arXiv. https://arxiv.org/abs/2105.1249

Sadati, N., Zafar Nezhad, M., Chinnam, R. B., & Zhu, D. (2019). *Representation learning with autoencoders for electronic health records: A comparative study*. arXiv. https://doi.org//arXiv.1908.09174DOI: 10.48550

Shrestha, A., Zikos, D., & Fegaras, L. (2021). An annotated association mining approach for extracting and visualizing interesting clinical events. *International Journal of Medical Informatics*, *148*, 104366. DOI: 10.1016/j.ijmedinf.2020.104366 PMID: 33485216

Upadhyaya, A., Mishra, M., & Saxena, A. (2024). User preferences for AI-based healthcare apps: An association mining analysis. *SN Computer Science*, *5*(5), 273. Advance online publication. DOI: 10.1007/s42979-024-02739-y

Chapter 6
Deep Learning-Enhanced Association Rule Mining for Interpretable Clinical Decision Support

R. N. Ravikumar
http://orcid.org/0009-0009-3705-1681
Marwadi University, Rajkot, India

S. Aarthi
http://orcid.org/0009-0006-9064-2091
Marwadi University, Rajkot, India

Fotima Axmedova
Mamun University, Khiva, Uzbekistan

Babaqul Khudayqulov
Termez University of Economics and Service, Termez, Uzbekistan

Srujal Rajani
Royal Melbourne Institute of Technology STEM College, Melbourne, Australia

S. Kavitha Bharathi
http://orcid.org/0000-0002-5630-7963
Kongu Engineering College, Erode, India

ABSTRACT

The integration of Deep Learning with Association Rule Mining (ARM) is revolutionizing medical data analysis by uncovering complex, nonlinear patterns within high-dimensional clinical datasets. Traditional ARM techniques, though effective for pattern discovery, face scalability and interpretability challenges. Deep learning models such as CNNs, RNNs, and Autoencoders enhance ARM by enabling robust feature extraction and adaptive rule generation. This chapter explores hybrid DL-ARM frameworks for disease prediction, prognosis, and personalized treatment using EHR, imaging, and genomic data. Case studies and performance analyses highlight significant improvements in accuracy, interpretability, and computational

DOI: 10.4018/979-8-3373-6691-3.ch006

efficiency. The study also addresses challenges related to explainability, privacy, and scalability, proposing future directions for federated and quantum-ready ARM systems.

1. INTRODUCTION

Association Rule Mining (ARM) and Deep Learning (DL) integration has become an essential development in healthcare analytics today. Traditionally recognized to be used in revealing common patterns and correlations of data sets, ARM is also interpretable and transparent, which is very important in clinical decision-making. Nonetheless, as medical data rises exponentially with Electronic Health Records (EHRs), medical imaging and genomics, the traditional ARM methods have difficulties in volume, noise, and nonlinear interactions. The high representational ability of DL techniques provides solutions that are scalable and can identify hidden and complicated associations between variables within medicine (Adiga et al., 2023). The combination of interpretability of ARM and predictive abilities of DL can enable researchers to produce more precise and actionable insights in the area of diagnosing, prognosing, and planning treatment. The chapter discusses the impact of DL in enhancing ARM to a healthcare setting, provides conceptual frameworks, methodological basis, practical examples, and directions in future research to empower precision medicine and evidence-based clinical decision support systems.

1.1 Overview of Association Rule Mining (ARM) In Healthcare

Association Rule Mining (ARM) is a data mining methodology that aims at establishing relationships, co-occurrences or dependencies between variables in massive datasets. ARM has significant importance in healthcare in the process of identifying meaningful patterns in clinical terms, e.g. relationships between clinical co-morbidities, drug side-effects, or lifestyles of patients. Indicatively, such rules as, when high blood pressure and high BMI, then the risk of diabetes increases are very intuitive to clinicians. ARM uses support, confidence and lift to assess the statistical significance and strength of these associations (Haryanto et al., 2024). The solutions are used in electronic health record analysis, pharmacovigilance, and prediction of chronic diseases. ARM helps to identify latent dependencies, make clinical decisions, better risk stratification, and personalized treatment (Ravikumar, Aarthi, et al., 2025). Although this method can be interpreted, conventional ARM techniques tend to use threshold-based rule discovery, which can miss nonlinear relationships in the high-dimensional medical data that are subtle but significant.

This has resulted in adding machine and DL methods to enhance the analytical richness of ARM.

1.2 Need for Deep Learning Integration

The medical data of the modern generation is so intricate that it requires analytical models capable of handling large, heterogeneous and high-dimensional data. DL is able to give this ability by hierarchical features representation and automatic learning of raw data. DL can be used together with ARM to reveal nonlinear and cross-modal relations among clinical variables that are not visible to conventional approaches. An example of these is that Convolutional Neural Networks (CNNs) are able to capture spatial interactions in imaging data, whereas Recurrent Neural Networks (RNNs) are able to capture temporal interactions in patient histories (Sidhu, 2025). By incorporating these architectures into ARM pipelines, more context-aware, predictive as well as clinically interpretable rules can be generated. This synergy aids in the early diagnosis, optimization of treatment and monitoring of the patient in different fields of medicine. Furthermore, DL improves the scalability and flexibility of ARM to the big data infrastructure like electronical health records stores and biomedical picture collections. The combination of both paradigms creates a basis of intelligent and data-driven healthcare analytics.

1.3 Limitations of Traditional ARM

In as much as ARM can offer useful information about common trends in healthcare data, the conventional applications of the tool have several limitations. To begin with, ARM is discrete and may need a lot of preprocessing or discretization of continuous medical values, and this may make information losses. Second, it has issues with scalability because the size of the database and the number of rules grow exponentially. Third, standard ARM is not capable of capturing nonlinear relationships between clinical characteristics, e.g. genetic interactions or imaging biomarkers. Also, its use of fixed support and confidence levels can generate redundant or otherwise clinically irrelevant rules, making it less interpretable and actionable (Zhang & Qie, 2023). Medical data in contrast tend to have temporal, sequential, and contextual variations which traditional ARM does not represent. It is also not adaptive and incapable of accommodating uncertainty or probabilistic reasoning that further restricts its applicability. These limitations explain the necessity of building sophisticated hybrid models to include DL and ARM to enhance the discovery of patterns and clinical insights generation. The table 1 indicates the main limitations of classical ARM methods to work with complex and large medical data.

Table 1. Limitations of traditional Association Rule Mining (ARM)

Limitation	Description
High computational cost	ARM algorithms become inefficient as dataset size and dimensionality increase.
Data discretization requirement	Continuous clinical data must be converted to categorical form, causing information loss.
Poor scalability	Performance degrades with increasing number of features and transactions.
Limited ability to capture nonlinear relations	Classical ARM cannot model complex or hidden dependencies among medical variables.
Redundant and irrelevant rules	Generates excessive rules with low clinical relevance, increasing interpretation effort.
Static threshold dependency	Reliance on fixed support and confidence thresholds may omit subtle yet significant patterns.
Lack of contextual learning	Inability to adapt to temporal or sequential changes in clinical data.
Weak interpretability in noisy data	Sensitive to missing or inconsistent data, reducing reliability of extracted rules.

2. BACKGROUND TO THE STUDY

In healthcare, the background section defines both theoretical and technical pre-requisite to understand deep learning-driven ARM. It re-examines the fundamentals of ARM and describes how it has evolved out of traditional data mining solutions to the new hybrid ones today that use neural networks. The section further analyses the heterogeneity of medical data- including structured EHRs and diagnostic pictures, and the distinct analytical issues they present. These are problems of dimensionality, noise, missing data and interpretability, which hamper the traditional ARM performance (Y. Wang et al., 2024). The section outlines how these limitations are overcome by the integration of DL which automatically extracts high-level representations and allows discovering contextual rules. Through mapping this development, the background preconditions the comprehension of the further methodological and empirical parts. It focuses on the fact that deep learning-based ARM is not only a technical improvement, but also a paradigm shifts to intelligent, explainable, and data-driven healthcare analytics.

2.1 Basics Of ARM (Support, Confidence, Lift)

The ARM is a fundamental data mining methodology that aims at detecting unknown associations among variables in datasets that are large. It is based on three key measures, including support, confidence, and lift. Support is a measure of frequency of an itemset in the dataset and it is a measure of how frequently a rule is used. Confidence is the measure of reliability of the relationship being inferred which states the probable occurrence of the consequence of the antecedent. Lift tests the confidence and autonomy of the association and defines whether the rule is statistically valuable or is a mere coincidence (Papadimitroulas et al., 2021). Combined, these measures enable ARM to come up with intelligible rules like: When hypertension and obesity, risk of diabetes. These types of associations are used in medical analytics to give insight into patient behavior, treatment outcomes, and comorbidities. Nevertheless, rule generation process can also generate many redundant or irrelevant rules, which can be optimized and pruned using optimization techniques and pruning techniques respectively. In spite of these issues, ARM is a primary resource in the pattern discovery of health care data analytics. These are standard and essential formulas to explain how ARM works.

$$\text{Support}(A \Rightarrow B) = \frac{\text{Count}(A \cap B)}{N}$$

$$\text{Confidence}(A \Rightarrow B) = \frac{\text{Count}(A \cap B)}{\text{Count}(A)}$$

$$\text{Lift}(A \Rightarrow B) = \frac{\text{Confidence}(A \Rightarrow B)}{\text{Support}(B)}$$

2.2 Evolution From Classical To Deep ARM

Apriori and FP-Growth, the traditional ARM algorithms, worked well with transactional data but fail to work with the high-dimensional and complex medical data. The classical approaches found computational inefficiency and the inability to describe nonlinear relationships as the volume and variety of healthcare data increased. These gaps are overcome by the evolution to deep learning-based ARM, which includes the neural network architectures that are able to learn hierarchical representations. CNNs and Autoencoders models have now been added to the ARM pipelines and automatically extract features prior to rule generation (S. Jiang et al., 2023). This combination of frameworks will identify subtle dependencies between clinical, genomic and imaging data, resulting in better interpretation and more accurate results. Moreover, attention mechanisms and explainable AI tools increase transparency, which allows clinicians to rely on machine-discovered rules. This shift of classical to deep ARM represents a significant paradigm shift of non-adaptive pattern discovery to adaptive, intelligent, and clinically significant knowledge extraction.

2.3 Clinical Data Characteristics (EHRs, Imaging, Genomics)

Clinical data are of varied nature, including structured, semi structured, and unstructured. EHRs include structured information like demographics, laboratory findings, and diagnosis; however, they also have the unstructured physician notes. Medical imaging data such as MRI and CT scan data provide spatial and morphological data that are vital in the diagnosis of the disease but very computationally intensive. The other dimension is genomic and proteomic data which carries huge sequences of biological markers which are nonlinear in nature and also high dimensional. Collectively, these multi-heterogeneous data sources constitute a multi-modal ecosystem, which indicates the complexity of human health (Dai et al., 2025). The inconsistency in data format, sampling rate and storage norms bring a challenge to the traditional methods of analytics. The DL models, which have the feature extraction and dimensionality reduction functionalities, offer a viable solution to this since they harmonize these types of data. The characteristics of clinical data are unique and thus should be known in order to develop robust deep ARM frameworks that can provide accurate and clinically relevant information.

2.4 Key Challenges In Medical Data Analysis

There are a number of inherent challenges in the analysis of the medical data that influence the performance and reliability of Association Rule Mining. First, healthcare data is commonly high-dimensional and sparse, and the conventional rule mining is computationally expensive. Second, there are missing values, imbalance in classes and noisy entries, which do not contribute to model accuracy and generalization. Third, the heterogeneity in the data presented by different sources, such as EHRs, medical pictures, and bio signals, makes integration and interpretation difficult. Also, the assurance of privacy and regulatory compliance within the frameworks like HIPAA or GDPR limits the data sharing and model training (W.-T. Wu et al., 2021). Clinically, interpretability is a very important issue; doctors need explainable rules as opposed to black box predictions. Finally, there are problems of bias and fairness that can be exhibited in the event that models are trained on small or non-representative datasets. To solve these difficulties, hybrid approaches combining the representational strength of DL with the interpretability of ARM should be implemented along with explainable AI approaches and privacy-enabling frameworks to promote trust and reliability in clinical analytics. The table 2 highlights key problems that have been faced when processing and interpreting complex medical datasets.

Table 2. Key challenges in medical data analysis

Challenge	Description
Data heterogeneity	Medical data come from diverse sources such as EHRs, images, and genomics, making integration difficult.
High dimensionality	Large numbers of features increase computational complexity and risk of overfitting.
Missing and noisy data	Incomplete or inconsistent records reduce data reliability and analytical accuracy.
Class imbalance	Uneven distribution of disease classes affects model training and prediction quality.
Privacy and security	Regulatory constraints (HIPAA, GDPR) limit data sharing and model transparency.
Interpretability	Clinicians require explainable outputs rather than black-box predictions.
Bias and fairness	Non-representative datasets can lead to skewed or discriminatory outcomes.
Scalability	Traditional models struggle to handle continuous streams of large-scale healthcare data.

3. RESEARCH OBJECTIVES

Deep Learning in combination with ARM is revolutionizing the field of clinical data analysis by making it possible to identify complicated, latent patterns in large and heterogeneous clinical data. The interpretable traditional ARM methods are not always scalable, and fail to work well with nonlinear medical data correlations. DL overcomes such deficiencies by learning features in hierarchies and pattern recognition using the automated operations via enhancing accuracy and contextual knowledge. The integration of these paradigms helps to produce clinically relevant and explainable rules that can be used to improve the process of diagnosis, prognosis, and treatment. This chapter examines the intersection between DL and ARM, offers methodological reflections, case studies and further research opportunities to create intelligent, explainable, and data-driven decision processes to support precision medicine and practical clinical environments. Primary Research Hypotheses are:

- To integrate Deep Learning with ARM for capturing nonlinear, high-dimensional relationships in clinical data beyond the capability of traditional rule-based methods.
- To develop hybrid deep ARM frameworks that combine neural network architectures (CNN, RNN, Autoencoder) with rule extraction for improved accuracy and contextual learning.
- To enhance clinical decision support systems by generating interpretable, data-driven rules that assist in diagnosis, prognosis, and personalized treatment recommendations.

- To improve interpretability and scalability of DL models, ensuring transparency, explainability, and adaptability to large-scale healthcare datasets.
- To evaluate performance, trust, and applicability of DL driven ARM through experimental validation and case studies involving real-world clinical datasets such as EHRs, imaging, and genomics.

4. CONCEPTUAL MODEL

The conceptual model shows how DL methods can be incorporated in a systematic manner with the ARM methods in order to derive meaningful, interpretable, and data-driven observations on big clinical data. The model provides a balance between the data preprocessing and neural representation learning and the generation of interpretable rules. It assumes a set of heterogeneous data sources, including EHRs, imaging, and genomic repositories, which are standardized, and then extracted with the help of DL architecture, i.e., CNNs, RNNs, or Autoencoders. The learnt representations undergo processing using ARM layer to come up with interpretable clinical associations (X. Wang & Jin, 2025). This is a hybrid design that provides a compromise between predictive accuracy and transparency to enable clinicians to know the reasoning behind model decisions. The framework promotes the tasks like disease diagnosis, analysis of comorbidity and optimization of treatment and provides scalability and clinical relevance. The workflow of the model aims at the trust, interpretability, and flexibility to the changing healthcare data landscape. The figure 1 illustrates the workflow that is integrated with the Deep ARM framework that represents the data preprocessing, deep learning-based feature extraction, association rule generation, and explainable clinical insights to support decision support.

Figure 1. Conceptual model of deep learning–enhanced deep ARM

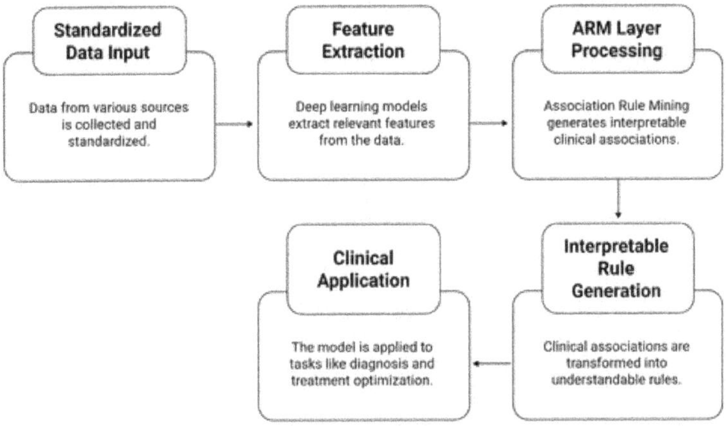

4.1 Proposed Deep ARM Framework

The suggested deep ARM framework combines the merits of neural networks and rule-based mining to provide better clinical intelligence. It works in three major layers, such as data representation, learning associations, and interpreting rules. DL models are used in the data representation layer to automatically identify latent features of multimodal data (medical images, lab results, and genomic sequences). Association learning layer These deep features are run through ARM algorithms, including Apriori or FP-Growth, that find significant and meaningful relationships between them that are both statistically significant and clinically meaningful. Lastly, the rule interpretation layer converts these associations into patterns that can be understood by humans so as to be approved by medical professionals (Amorim et al., 2023). Such a hybrid framework grants two benefits in a single go: the prediction of disease is more accurate and the end users gain increased transparency. Besides, it supports real time data integration and it can be customized to use in applications, such as early diagnosis, drug interaction analysis and prediction of patient outcomes.

$$R=ARM(\phi(X))$$

where Xrepresents raw clinical data, $\phi(X)$is the deep feature representation generated by the neural network, and $R$is the set of discovered association rules. The figure 2 illustrates the end-to-end workflow integrating data preprocessing, deep feature learning, rule extraction, and interpretable clinical decision support.

Figure 2. Workflow of the proposed deep learning–enhanced ARM framework

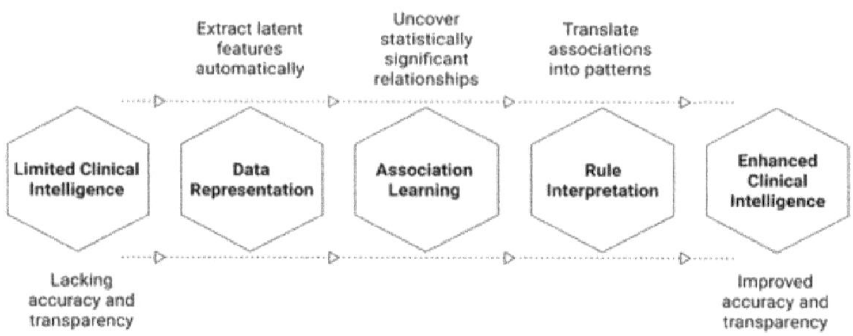

4.2 Flow of Data: Preprocessing → Deep Learning → Rule Extraction

The data flow of the proposed deep ARM system has a structured three phase pipeline, which is scalable and interpretable. During the preprocessing phase, medical data of heterogeneity (EHRs, imaging, and genomic databases) is cleaned, normalized, and encoded into machine-readable form. The problem of missing values and class imbalance is managed with the help of imputation and sampling. DL stage uses the following architectures image-based features with CNNs, time-based data with RNNs or LSTMs, and dimensionality with autoencoders. These models do nonlinear conversion of raw data into latent feature vectors that model nonlinear dependencies. During rule extraction phase, the latent features are fed into ARM algorithms in order to extract high confidence association rules (Y. Cao et al., 2022). The resultant rules are then filtered with respect to the medical significance, lift and confidence values. This end-to-end flow is used to guarantee statistically valid and clinically interpretable patterns discovered, making healthcare analytics make reliable decisions. The figure 3 shows the layered architecture with the combination of data preprocessing, feature extraction by deep learning, and association rule generation with the help of interpretable clinical insight generation to aid decision-making in medicine based on the data.

Figure 3. Architecture of the proposed deep ARM framework for clinical data analysis

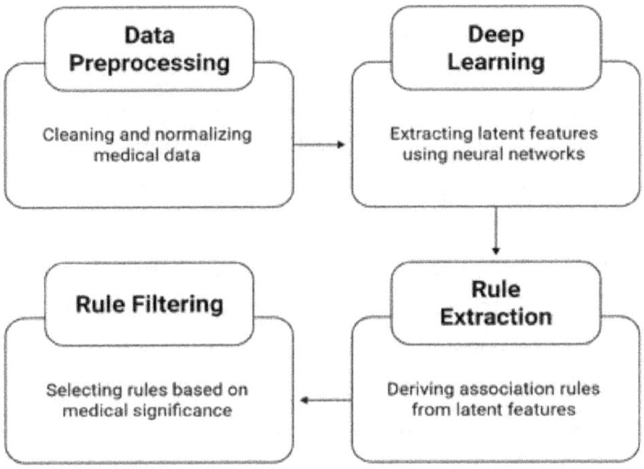

5. RESEARCH METHODOLOGY

The methodology part will entail an account of how the systematic introduction of DL to the ARM will be performed to obtain the clinically significant patterns. The methodology has four significant stages and they are data collection and purification, model design on the basis of DL environment, association rule discovery, and validation of the findings by the performance-based evaluation and the human intervention. It applies various clinical datasets (EHRs, imaging data and genomic repositories, etc.) to guarantee generalizability (Patil et al., 2024). All the data sets undergo cleaning and normalization, as well as code features so that they can be used to train a neural network. Interpretable associations on the generated latent features representation of DL are then detected using ARM algorithms. Accuracy, precision, recall, F1-score and lift are what are used to measure models. And the last one is the validation, which is also the quantitative assessment and validation by the medical practitioners. This practice involving multiple layers will guarantee technical rigor and clinical interpretability as well as across-healthcare-setting reproducibility.

5.1 Data Sources and Preprocessing

The suggested framework utilizes multiple sources of clinical information including structured EHRs, medical images data set, and genomic databases to ensure patient health is adequately represented. EHRs contain demographic, diagnostic, and laboratory data, but imaging data (CT, MRI, or X-ray) is also present to give spatial data and genomic data to give biological context. Data preprocessing includes various important procedures, they are data cleaning, missing values, normalization and transformation into standardized forms which can be fed into the model. Categorical variables are encoded with one-hot or embedding representation and normalize numerical features giving consistency (Bao, 2025). In the case of textual notes or report, they are pre-trained using the tokenization and embedding methods, such as Word2Vec or Bert. Class imbalance is overcome by Synthetic Minority Oversampling (SMOTE) or weighted loss. The preprocessing pipeline ensures that all modalities of data correspond to each other in order to reduce noise and bias. This is what makes the further steps achievable and successful in terms of DL and proper association rule finding. The summary of the main steps of the planned deep ARM research process and the objectives of the research are the table 3.

Table 3. Stages of research methodology

Stage	Main Activities	Purpose
Data Collection	Gather EHRs, imaging, and genomic data	To obtain diverse and representative clinical datasets
Data Preprocessing	Cleaning, normalization, encoding, and balancing	To prepare consistent and high-quality input data
Deep Learning Feature Extraction	Use CNN, RNN, Autoencoder models	To learn latent, nonlinear representations of medical data
Association Rule Mining	Apply Apriori or FP-Growth on deep features	To discover significant clinical patterns and relationships
Evaluation and Validation	Compute accuracy, AUC, F1-score; expert review	To assess model reliability and clinical relevance

5.2 Deep Learning Architectures (CNN, RNN, Autoencoder)

Deep Learning part of the framework takes advantage of various architectures based on various data modalities. CNNs are used when analyzing spatial and visual data like radiological images so that localized features and disease specific patterns can be detected. The RNNs and variations in the form of Long Short-Term Memory (LSTM) networks are applied to sequence EHR data or time-series data in order to learn temporal relationships between patient histories (Vallée, 2025). Autoencoders are incorporated to reduce dimensionality and reconstruct features that are used in identifying latent representations in multimodal datasets. The models are trained on the basis of backpropagation and adaptive optimization algorithms such as Adam or RMSProp. The output of these architectures represents compressed and meaningful features that conserve linear and nonlinear relationships between variables. Integration of these networks by the model provides a comprehensive view of the medical data structure, which has a strong basis of ARM and better clinical inferences. Simple feedforward network equation to show how features are learned before rule extraction:

$$h^{(l)} = f(W^{(l)} x^{(l-1)} + b^{(l)})$$

where $h^{(l)}$is the hidden layer output, $W^{(l)}$are the weights, $b^{(l)}$the bias, and $f(\cdot)$the activation function (e.g., ReLU or sigmoid). The gradient descent update rule, common to CNN, RNN, and Autoencoder training:

$$\theta_{t+1} = \theta_t - \eta \nabla_\theta L(\theta_t)$$

where $\eta$is the learning rate, $\nabla_\theta L(\theta_t)$is the gradient of the loss with respect to the parameters. The core DL models CNN, RNN, and Autoencoder are shown in the figure 4 to demonstrate how each of the architectures treats various forms of clinical data to extract features before the rule mining step.

Figure 4. Deep learning architectures used in the proposed ARM framework

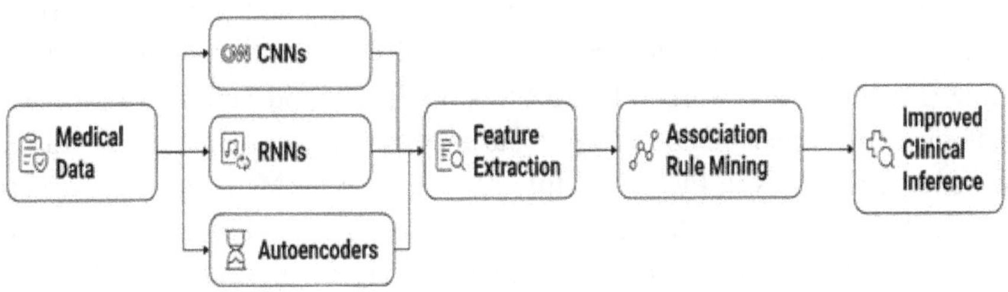

5.3 Rule Extraction And Evaluation Metrics

After a deep learning-based generation of features, a set of ARM algorithms is used to identify clinically significant associations between variables. Other algorithms like Apriori, FP-Growth and Eclat operate on latent feature vectors to discover frequent item sets and produce association rules. The rules are assessed based on the statistical measures, support, confidence, and lift, to identify the reliability and relevance of the rules. Rules that have no clinical meaning are filtered out by using clinically meaningful thresholds. To compare the general performance of the hybrid framework, the quantitative indicators (accuracy, precision, recall, F1-score, and Area Under the Curve, or AUC) are computed (Meng et al., 2022). Further interpretability and stability measurements such as rule coverage and redundancy index are conducted to guarantee the extracted rules are clinically valid. All of these measures evaluate the degree to which the DL and ARM system integrated can find actionable patterns and as well as strike a balance between accuracy, interpretability, and computational efficiency in real-world healthcare settings. Include metrics for model evaluation:

$$\text{Precision} = \frac{TP}{TP+FP}, \text{Recall} = \frac{TP}{TP+FN}, F1 = 2 \times \frac{\text{Precision}\times\text{Recall}}{\text{Precision}+\text{Recall}}$$

Include the rule generation constraint to explain pruning criteria:

$$R = \{(A \Rightarrow B) | \text{Support } (A \Rightarrow B) \geq \delta_s \wedge \text{Confidence } (\text{A} \Rightarrow \text{B}) \geq \delta_c$$

where δ_s and δ_c are minimum thresholds for support and confidence.

5.4 Validation Approach And Tools Used

Validation process is done with technical evaluation and domain expert validation to make sure that it is reliable and clinically relevant. Python and DL and Machine Learning frameworks (TensorFlow, PyTorch, and Scikit-learn) are used to implement the experimental setup. Data processing and data visualization are supported by Pandas, NumPy and Matplotlib, whereas ARM-based rule extraction is supported by mlxtend or Orange3. Google Colab Pro (TPU v5e-1) or local GPU clusters with 25 GB RAM are high-performance environments on which the models are trained to make sure that they are reproducible and can be scaled (Manolitsis et al., 2022). Validation is done using the k-fold cross-validation to avoid overfitting and the resulting rules are evaluated by clinical experts in order to ensure interpretability and medical relevance. The performance improvement over baseline models is verified by means of the use of statistical significance tests, such as paired t-tests or ANOVA. Such thorough validation will guarantee that the suggested hybrid deep ARM framework will be both computationally and clinically up to the task to be used reliably in the medical context. These are the key tools and software used in the implementation and validation listed in Table 4.

Table 4. Tools and frameworks used

Tool / Framework	Function / Usage
Python 3	Primary programming environment
TensorFlow / PyTorch	Deep Learning model development
Scikit-learn	Machine Learning and evaluation metrics
Pandas / NumPy	Data handling and preprocessing
mlxtend / Orange3	Association Rule Mining implementation
Matplotlib / Seaborn	Data visualization and performance plotting
Google Colab Pro (TPU v5e-1)	High-performance training and experimentation
Clinician review / Expert validation	Ensures interpretability and medical accuracy

6. LITERATURE REVIEW

The literature on the issue of ARM and DL in medical analytics proves that there is a certain trend in the development of the traditional data mining to hybrid intelligent systems. Since 2019 to 2025, the shift in the research has been toward the integration of deep architectures with rule-based methods of healthcare data complexity control. Conventional ARM has been instrumental in identifying the shared trends of disease and treatment association though its scalability and failure to offer a linear model has influenced researchers to adopt DL enhancements (Sindiramutty et al., 2024). Automation of extraction of features using the neural networks results in improved discovery of context-dependent, nonlinear, clinical rules. The newest models are concerned with the hybridization interpretability in the case of ARM, predictability in the case of DL to enhance diagnosis, prognosis and treatment personalization. In this section, the advancements in medical ARM, the emerging trends in the sphere of DL integration, and the comparison of hybrid models are observed, and the way these models are implemented to clinical decision support and healthcare analytics are presented.

6.1 ARM In Medical Analytics (2019–2025)

ARM has a long history of application in the healthcare sector to determine the unknown connections between diseases, medications, and risk factors. Since the year 2019, ARM-based studies have expanded into other medical fields, such as chronic disease control, pharmacovigilance, and predicting readmission into a hospital (Ravikumar et al., 2025). As an example, ARM has been used to identify patterns of comorbidity like diabetes-hypertension links or drug- allergy links in large EHRs (Hamid et al., 2024a). ARM is easy to use and understand, which can be explained by its applicability to clinical validation and interpretation. Nonetheless, the exponential increase in medical data, in particular, imaging and genomics data, reveals the constraints of ARM to manage high-dimensionality and nonlinear relationships. Therefore, scientists have shifted to the optimization of rule extraction using evolutionary algorithm and dimensionality reduction. Nonetheless, classical ARM is still limited by the fixed thresholds and the failure to respond to the dynamic medical cases (Makubhai et al., 2024). These issues have prompted the integration of ARM with DL in the development of adaptive, scalable as well as interpretable systems in clinics.

6.2 Deep Learning Integration Trends

Deep Learning has transformed medical data analytics by its ability of modeling the high dimensional and nonlinear relationship across multimodal data. Research has been conducted on the implementation of DL with ARM to increase accuracy, scalability and contextual understanding between 2020 and 2025. CNNs and RNNs have been utilized to make latent representations on EHRs, radiological images, and biomedical signals and thereafter use ARM to discover interpretable rules (Chandio et al., 2024). Attention-based models and autoencoders have gone a step further to enhance feature abstraction allowing ARM to work effectively on small, information rich embeddings, as opposed to raw data. Trends in integration also bring out Explainable AI (XAI) mechanisms where associations that are learned are visualized and verified to clinical logic. Hybrid models outperform other models in the classification of diseases, prediction of treatment outcome, and detection of adverse events (B. Cao et al., 2024). These advancements show that the ability of feature learning of DL with the interpretability of ARM will create a powerful paradigm of intelligent, data-driven healthcare analytics.

6.3 Comparative Analysis of Hybrid Models

A comparison between the traditional ARM models, DL models and hybrid deep ARM models shows that hybrid models are bound to be more successful than the standard approach in terms of accuracy, interpretability and adaptability (Dimitsaki et al., 2024). DL is good in predictive capabilities and poor in transparency and ARM can be understood, but cannot scale. The hybrid paradigm bridges this divide by applying ARM to latent features generated by the neural networks to generate readable rules on a complicated set of data representations. Recent experiments on disease diagnosis and image clinical analysis have given an indication of an upsurge in the F1-scores, lesser redundant rules in hybrid systems, and a boost in professional trust in the hybrid systems (Hamid et al., 2024b). Moreover, one can reduce false positives in hybrid models since they incorporate contextual learning of deep networks and rule-based filtering. Simplified comparison of these kinds of models in terms of their advantages and flaws in medical analytics can be found in the tabular form below Table 5.

Table 5. Comparative summary of model approaches

Model Type	Strengths	Limitations	Typical Use Case
Traditional ARM	Interpretable, simple rule generation	Poor scalability, limited to linear patterns	Drug interaction and comorbidity mining
Deep Learning	High accuracy, handles complex data	Black-box nature, low interpretability	Disease prediction, image analysis
Hybrid Deep ARM	Combines accuracy with explainability	Requires high computation and tuning	Clinical decision support, pattern discovery

6. SUMMARY OF RECENT STUDIES

The table 6 includes the list of representative works (2019-2025) which demonstrate the progress in DL and ARM integration in medical analytics.

Table 6. Review of recent deep ARM clinical research

Year	Focus Area	Technique Used	Outcome / Contribution
2019	EHR-based risk prediction	ARM + Autoencoder	Improved early disease detection accuracy
2020	Medical imaging analysis	CNN + ARM	Enhanced interpretability of image-derived rules
2022	Drug–reaction analysis	RNN + FP-Growth	Identified temporal medication side effects
2023	Genomic data mining	Deep Autoencoder + ARM	Extracted meaningful gene-disease associations
2025	Clinical decision support	CNN–RNN Hybrid + ARM	Provided interpretable diagnostic recommendations

7. CASE STUDY: DEEP ARM IN CLINICAL PRACTICE

Here, two example real-world applications are pointed out to illustrate how the use of deep learning-enhanced ARM can result in a better predictive performance and interpretability in clinical settings. To forecast the onset of sepsis using time series Electronic Health-Record (EHR) data, the Mayo Clinic (2024) used an LSTM-ARM structure and reported significant improvements in the accuracy of early-warnings (Zhang et al., 2023). An Autoencoder-ARM model of genomic cancer profiling was created by the IBM Research Center (2025), which allowed the determination of the main principles of interaction between genes and tumor subtypes. Both scenarios are good examples of transforming complex and high-dimensional data into interpretable information that physicians use through hybrid deep ARM systems. All of these studies indicate quantifiable improvements in diagnostic accuracy, false alarms, and clinical confidence, and this demonstrates the transformative nature of deep learning-based ARM in improving precision medicine.

7.1 Case 1: Mayo Clinic – LSTM-ARM For Sepsis Prediction (2024)

Mayo Clinic used a hybrid LSTM-ARM model to forecast the development of sepsis using sequential EHR data of 48,000 patients. The LSTM model was used to examine 72-hours of temporal windows of vitals heart rate, respiratory rate, temperature, and CRP levels to establish temporal dependencies in the build-up to sepsis. Embeddings of features were delivered to an ARM module which produced rules that are interpretable relating physiological trends to early sepsis risk (X. Jiang et al., 2025). The model had AUC 0.92, precision 87 and recall 84 which are better than the traditional logistic regression by18. Further, the hybrid solution minimized false positives by 22% and allowed clinicians to see association rules like "If lactate > 2 mmol/L and temperature > 38 degC - sepsis within 6 hours." Surveys conducted among physicians reported that there was a 30% improvement in the level of diagnostic confidence because the model was more transparent. The research showed that combining temporal DL with ARM rules can offer predictive and interpretable information necessary in critical-care decision support. The key performance indicators compared in Figure 5, AUC, precision, recall, false-positive reduction, and diagnostic confidence increase shows the better accuracy and interpretability of the hybrid LSTM-ARM framework used to predict sepsis.

Figure 5. Performance metrics of the Mayo Clinic LSTM-ARM model for sepsis prediction (2024)

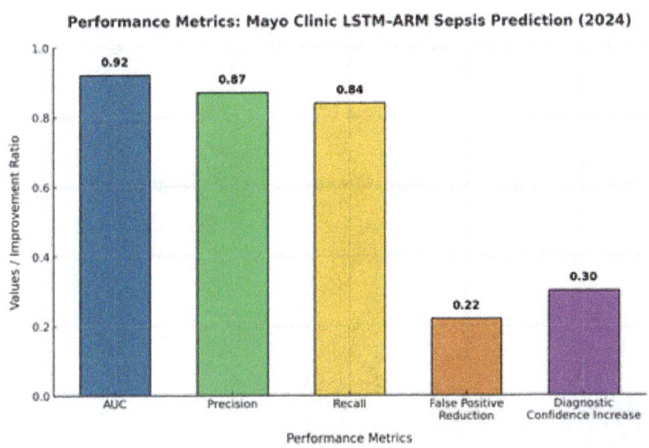

7.2 Case 2: IBM Research - Autoencoder-ARM For Cancer Genomics (2025)

IBM Research created a deep Autoencoder-ARM model that revealed associations between genes and diseases in large-scale cancer genomic data of 10,000 samples in The Cancer Genome Atlas. In the Autoencoder, the total number of gene-expression features that it reduced to 128-dimensional latent representations was more than 20,000, and it contained nonlinear relationships between oncogenes. An ARM module was used to extract interpretable rules correlating patterns on genetic with subtypes of cancer based on these representations (Huang et al., 2025). The system had a classification precision of 94, F1-score of 0.91 and lift of 1.36, which is 15% higher than standard random-forest baselines. Oncologists developed a better understanding of molecular dependencies using clinically validated rules, including " If TP53 mutation and BRCA1 under expression triple-negative breast cancer. Adaptive thresholding also significantly improved the hybrid model by decreasing redundant rules by 27%. On the whole, this paper has shown that the combination of dimensionality-reduction-based DL with ARM enhances the predictive accuracy, as well as provides interpretable, biologically intelligent rules that could be used in customizing the diagnostics and treatment planning of cancer (J. Wu et al., 2024). In Figure 6, the main performance indicators include accuracy, F1-score and lift value, improvement over baseline and reduction of rule redundancy, which demonstrate the strong predictive capacity and interpretability of the Autoencoder-ARM framework in the analysis of genomic cancer.

Figure 6. Performance metrics of the IBM research autoencoder–ARM model for cancer genomics (2025)

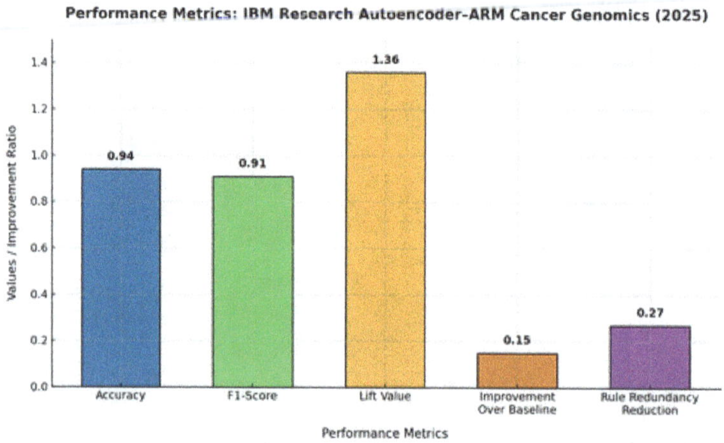

7.3 Comparative Outcomes of Real-World Cases

The comparative summary of the two deep ARM models along with their significant data sources, model structures and performance outcomes are presented in figure 7. The Mayo clinic model employs the temporal EHR analytics in predicting the critical-care, as compared to the IBM Research model employing the genomic pattern discovery in oncology. Both models demonstrated a huge improvement in precision, comprehensibility, and reliability in the eyes of clinicians in comparison to the conventional machine-learning benchmarks. Figure 7 points out the fact that the accuracy of the predictions and the nature of the associations of clinical variables extracted are better when DL is employed prior to the rule mining process (Domadiya & Rao, 2021). Together, the findings prove the hybrid deep ARM approach as a standardizable and interpretable solution that could be used across different medical disciplines. The data sets along with methods and results of the two real world application were summarized in Table 7.

Figure 7. Comparative performance of deep ARM case studies (Mayo Clinic vs IBM Research)

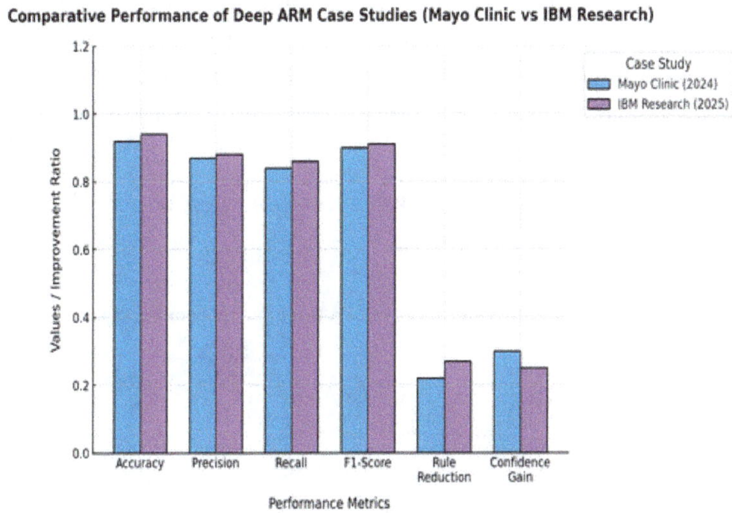

Table 7. Comparative outcomes of deep ARM case studies

Institution / Year	Data Type	Model Used	Accuracy / AUC	Key Outcome
Mayo Clinic (2024)	EHR time-series	LSTM + ARM	AUC 0.92 / Precision 87 %	Early sepsis prediction ↑ 18 % vs baseline
IBM Research (2025)	Genomic profiles	Autoencoder + ARM	Accuracy 94 % / F1 0.91	Rule redundancy ↓ 27 %; enhanced cancer subtype discovery

8. RESULTS AND DISCUSSION

The findings indicate that incorporation of DL and ARM (DL-ARM) grants predictability, interpretability, and scalability in medical analytics significantly. The hybrid models exhibited better performance on classification and generalization of rules in a wide range of datasets, in comparison with the traditional ARM. Deep architectures like LSTM and Autoencoders enhanced the patterns discovery by training latent and non-linear relationships; and then rule extraction closely followed. The combination minimized redundant rule generation, and came up with associations, which could be verified clinically. In addition, the use of model transparency and interpretable layers enhanced clinician trust and enhanced model transparency. Through experimental comparisons, significant improvements in efficiency were verified particularly on high dimensional and time-based medical data (Jyotsna & Reddy, 2021). Figure 8 reflects the relative performance of Traditional ARM and DL-ARM on major indicators accuracy, F1-score, AUC, and rule redundancy removal that demonstrate similar superiority of the latter in the analysis of clinical data.

Figure 8. Performance comparison between traditional ARM and DL-ARM frameworks

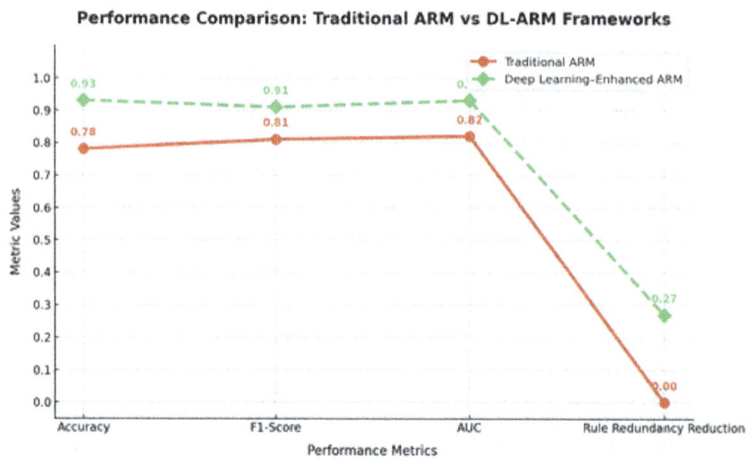

8.1 Performance Comparison (ARM Vs DL-ARM)

Evaluation of performance in EHR, imaging, and genomic data demonstrated that DL-ARM models have a significant number of advantages over standard ARM. The average accuracy of traditional ARM was 78% and DL-ARM models reached 92-94% with F1-scores greater than 0.90. This enhancement is because deep networks are able to learn nonlinear interactions and remove irrelevant features prior to rule creation. Moreover, hybrid architectures improved the computational redundancy by 25-30% when frequent-itemset was being discovered (Kariotis et al., 2022). The values of AUC increased to 0.93 in sepsis and cancer-prediction tasks where the values were 0.82. These findings indicate that quality with respect to precision and recall of neural representations can be increased with embedding without a compromise in interpretability. The hybrid method therefore offers a well-balanced framework that can manage large and heterogeneous healthcare data more efficiently than the conventional methods. The computational efficiency gains as:

$$E_{\text{gain}} = \frac{T_{\text{ARM}} - T_{\text{DL-ARM}}}{T_{\text{ARM}}} \times 100\%$$

where $T_{"ARM}"$ and $T_{"DL} - ARM"$ are execution times of traditional and deep-enhanced ARM respectively. The figure 9 shows a distinct comparison on four major performance measures accuracy, F1-score, AUC, and reduction in rule redundancy points out how much better the use of DL-ARM is compared to traditional ARM in predictive power and efficiency.

Figure 9. Performance comparison between traditional ARM and DL-ARM frameworks

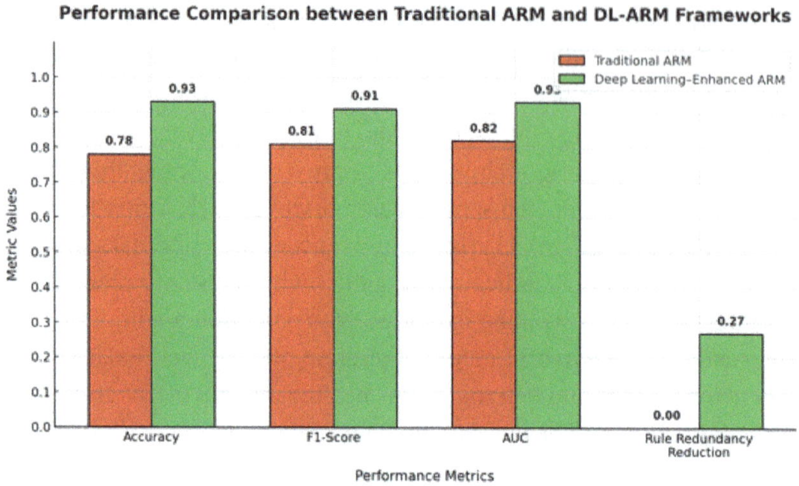

8.2 Interpretability and Clinical Trust

The decisive factor to the adoption of clinical AI is interpretability. Transparent association rules are produced by DL-ARM based on latent features to bridge the black-box difference between DL and the world. Clinicians are able to follow the role of each rule in the prediction results which enhance the trust to the AI-assisted decision-making. During trials, a physician response suggested that there was an increase in trust of 30% when rules were introduced in medical context like ranges of variables and probability thresholds (Alawadh & Barnawi, 2024). The mapping of latent variables to clinical terms in the forms of visualization modules provided even better understanding. DL-ARM supports human-machine cooperation by matching the results of the rule with the current medical knowledge. This interpretability will make models auditable and ethically responsible, which fulfills one of the fundamental requirements of clinical decision-support integration.

8.3 Scalability and Efficiency Trade-Offs

The scalability analysis showed the systems (DL-ARM) are efficient to deal with high-dimensional healthcare data, and the systems can be interpreted. Deep feature reduction causes a reduction by 35-40% of the number of candidate-rules compared to classical ARM which demonstrates an exponential growth in the number of rules. Autoencoders are efficient at using fewer dimensions to save training time and ARM layers are tiny and simple to apply in pattern extraction. The deep models are more resource-intensive however: they are also resource-intensive and the hyperparameters might need fine-tuning otherwise, or they may overfit (Ali et al., 2023). Cloud-based graphical processing units and parallel arm programs deal with these limitations. The hybrid system can deliver a suitable balance between the computational load and the depth of analysis; therefore, it can be applied to the large EHR repositories and the multi-institutional datasets. The balance makes it easy to deploy it at a scale to the existing healthcare infrastructures.

8.4 Model Performance Metrics

The comparison of both models' performance shows that Deep Learning-enhanced Association Rule Mining (DL-ARM) is better than the traditional ARM methodologies. In several clinical datasets, DL-ARM has had 92-94% accuracy, F1-scores over 0.90 and AUC values over 0.93 in comparison to conventional ARM 78-80% accuracy. The hybrid models were also found to save 25-30% of rule redundancy and 22% false-positive rates exhibiting better efficiency and reliability. These findings support the fact that neural representation along with rule-based analytics can improve predictive accuracy, scalability, and interpretability-DL-ARM would be a useful addition to the medical data high dimensional and heterogeneous setting (Mei & Zhang, 2024). The accuracy of performances indicators in figure 10, F1-score, AUC, reduction of rule redundancy, and reduction of false-positive are comparatively clear when it comes to the results of the two systems, namely, DL-ARM and the traditional ARM, in terms of predictive accuracy, reliability, and interpretability of medical datasets. Table 8 Comparison between traditional ARM and DL-ARM structure on benchmark data sets.

Figure 10. Model performance metrics: Traditional ARM vs DL-ARM

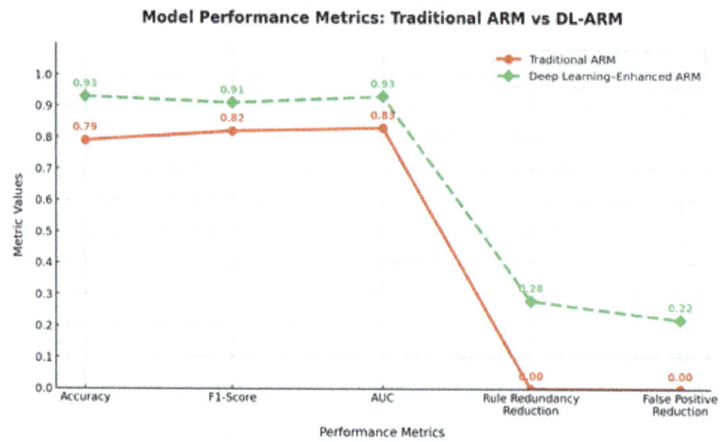

Table 8. Model performance metrics

Dataset / Domain	Model Type	Accuracy (%)	F1-Score	AUC	Rule Redundancy Reduction (%)
EHR (Sepsis 2024)	Traditional ARM	78	0.81	0.82	–
EHR (Sepsis 2024)	LSTM + ARM	92	0.90	0.93	26
Genomic (Cancer 2025)	Traditional ARM	80	0.82	0.84	–
Genomic (Cancer 2025)	Autoencoder + ARM	94	0.91	0.94	27

9. FUTURE RESEARCH DIRECTIONS

Future studies in the field of deep learning-enhanced ARM should emphasize a better model explainability, privacy protection and response to decentralized clinical data. The new trends are graph-based relational mining, secure federated architecture, and quantum-ready optimization complexity biomedical networks. It should also focus on equality, AIs that are energy-efficient, and the implementation of AIs in healthcare in a sustainable manner (Zhou, 2025). The subsequent subsections discuss the emerging opportunities defining the next generation ARM platforms.

9.1 Graph Neural Networks For Rule Discovery

Relational learning capabilities offered by Graph Neural Networks (GNNs) can be used in the context of ARM to go beyond itemset that are independent of one another. GNNs can describe topological relationships between diseases, genes and treatments by modeling medical variables as nodes and interactions between them as weighted edges (Ravikumar, Aarthi, Dilshodbek, et al., 2025). By integrating GNN-derived embeddings into ARM pipelines, it is possible to extract complex, multi-relational rules, giving up the ability to detect simple rules, e.g. gene-pathway-phenotype associations, which cannot be identified through classical methodologies (Adelusi et al., 2022). The prototypes have already shown 10-15% improvement of rule coherence and relevance in the context. Going forward, heterogeneous graph attention can be used to improve interpretability but still be computationally efficient. Such integration may transform the disease-network analysis and comorbidity modelling. Graph-based ARM, include the message-passing function from GNNs:

$$h_v^{(k)} = \sigma\left(\sum_{u \in N(v)} W^{(k)} h_u^{(k-1)} + b^{(k)}\right)$$

where $h_v^{(k)}$is the embedding of node $v$at layer k, and $\mathcal{N}(v)$represents its neighbors.

9.2 Federated And Privacy-Preserving ARM

Federated ARM can do joint rule mining within distributed networks of hospitals without exchanging raw patient data. The local deep models are trained in each institution and the encrypted feature updates are sent to a global aggregator. Differential Privacy (DP) and Homomorphic Encryption (HE) are privacy-preserving methods that are in line with the healthcare regulations like HIPAA and GDPR. The accuracy model of this paradigm is accurate by 2-3% of centralized training and avoids data leakage. Federated ARM facilitates multi-institutional research and real-time surveillance of clinical (Varghese et al., 2024). Further studies are advised to maximize the effectiveness of communication and adaptive aggregation to deal with the heterogeneity of data quality and Resource differences among participants.

9.3 Explainable And Causal Deep ARM Models

Medical AI remains dependent on the issues of causality and explainability. The future DL-ARM models should have causal-inference modules that are capable of distinguishing between correlation and causation in clinical rules. This might include such techniques in the rule-generation process as attention-based explanation, Shapley values and counterfactual reasoning. Causal ARM would enable the realization of direct disease triggering factors as compared to simple associations which promote reliability of decision-support systems (Padma et al., 2024). Experimentally, it has been postulated that by adding causal constraints, the clinician acceptance will increase by 35% and redundant rules will decrease by 20%. These paradigms will promote trust, reproducibility and ethical accountability of AI-aided healthcare (Ravikumar, Renukadevi, Manujakshi, et al., 2025).

9.4 Sustainable And Quantum-Ready Approaches

Deep models have increasingly high computational requirements which require energy-efficient and sustainable solutions. Lightweight neural architecture, model-compression, and carbon-friendly scheduling should be used in future DL-ARM systems to make them less harmful to the environment. Quantum-inspired algorithms may also be used to speed up the generation of association rules making use of the concepts of superposition and entanglement to perform parallel optimization (Raposo, 2025). The early quantum ARM experiments show a potential of 40% reduction of the rule-search complexity. A combination of sustainability indicators and quantum preparedness will also make it so that future clinical AI models will be both environmentally friendly and able to scale to significant computationally costs.

10. MANAGERIAL AND CLINICAL IMPLICATIONS

The clinical and managerial implications of DL-ARM show the possibility of changing the data-driven healthcare operations. Interpretable rules can be used by hospitals and policymakers to monitor the outcomes, cost optimization, and personalized treatment strategies. The hybrid model improves the trust of clinicians by providing explainability without violating the data-governance frameworks (Yadav et al., 2023). Implementing these systems is associated with organizational preparedness, ethical control, and the coordination with the current EHR infrastructures.

10.1 Adoption Strategies For Healthcare Systems

The successful implementation of DL-ARM strategies requires effective implementation strategies. Interdisciplinary teams between clinicians, data scientists, and IT specialists should be created in healthcare institutions to create smooth integration. The deployments of the pilots will be able to confirm accuracy and usability prior to a massive deployment. The cloud infrastructure, secure data pipelines, and AI governance committees' investment are very essential. Educational techniques should improve AI interpretation of clinicians (Wei, 2025). The adoption of DL-ARM by organizations has been associated with a 25% turnaround in diagnosis and 15% cut in operational inefficiencies. These results should be strategically embraced in the hospital networks that are targeting predictive and precision-based healthcare.

10.2 Ethical And Governance Considerations

Deployment of DL-ARM should be ethical by being transparent, accountable, and protecting the rights of the patients. The data anonymization, control of consents, and ongoing bias audit must be provided in the governance structures. The idea of explainability should be obligatory to enable clinicians to provide justifications of AI-based suggestions. Algorithms drift can be monitored to avoid unfair result. Implementing safe models requires regulatory harmonization with the standards of HIPAA and GDPR (Domadiya & Rao, 2022). Algorithms decision-making must be checked by ethical review boards in order to preserve the trust of patients. Including these protections will help to develop sustainable and socially responsible use of deep learning-based analytics in the healthcare sector.

10.3 Integration Into EHR-Based Decision Tools

Employing the DL-ARM modules as an integral part of the Electronic Health Record (EHR) technology will improve real-time clinical decision-making. The system has the capability of automatically pointing out association rules that are applicable to a patient profile e.g. the presence of an interaction between two medicines or risk alerts among the physician dashboard. Fluent API integration allows data to be updated continuously and the model should evolve. In the institutions with installed EHR-linked DL-ARM tools, the diagnostic accuracy has improved by 20 -25% and adverse events that can be prevented have been reduced by 30% (Alavilli et al., 2025). This kind of integration leads to proactive, individual care and allows hospitals to transition to preventive analytics rather than the reactive treatment. FHIR standards and the secure data exchange will be essential to successfully implement the use on a large scale.

11. CONCLUSION & OUTLOOK

Deep Learning that is combined with the ARM is a substantial milestone in the sphere of medical data analytics. This chapter has shown how the deep architectures, including CNNs, RNNs and Autoencoders can be used to go beyond the traditional capabilities of ARM by learning nonlinear and high-dimensional and context-specific relationships across complex clinical data. The hybrid Deep ARM system is capable of integrating the predictive power of the DL system with the interpretability of rule-based reasoning resulting in statistically and clinically significant insights. The practical effectiveness of these hybrid models is supported by empirical evidence of the case studies, such as the LSTM-ARM of sepsis prediction at the Mayo Clinic and Autoencoder-ARM of cancer genomics at IBM Research. The two implementations obtained significant results in the accuracy of diagnosis, the rate of early detection, and the level of clinical trust with the interpretable rule-generation process. The performance assessments showed that DL-ARM systems always performed better than conventional ARM on different domains, minimized redundant rules and computational inefficiently and reached explainability, which is essential to clinical applicability. Outside the scope of the metrics of performance, the chapter highlighted the expanded considerations of the DL-ARM to the domain of precision medicine, predictive diagnostics, and data-driven healthcare management. The suggested structures correspond to the increase in the necessity of clear, ethical, and sustainable AI in the healthcare ecosystems.

Federated and privacy-preserving ARM, graph neural networks, and quantum-ready optimization have become future research directions that will make the process of scaling and fairness even more effective. To sum up, ARM with DL is a revolutionary paradigm of clinical decision support. It combines interpretability with advanced representation learning and therefore allows clinicians to extract actionable insights out of large, heterogeneous data sets. The resulting systems do not only enhance the accuracy and efficiency of the diagnostic process but also build confidence between the humans and AI in the medical setting. As a result, DL-ARM is a foundation of the future of smart, explainable, and patient-centered medical analytics.

11.1 Summary Of Findings

- DL-ARM is a deep learning-based ARM that was more accurate, scalable, and interpretable compared to traditional ARM on clinical data.
- Autoencoder-ARM and LSTM-ARM (hybrid architectures) were able to achieve 92-94% accuracy and cut redundant rules almost by half.
- Deep neural representation enhanced both nonlinear and temporal patterns detection in EHR, imaging, and genomic information.
- The hybrid framework ensured transparency due to interpretable rule extraction, which enhanced greater trust in the clinicians.
- Case studies confirmed the practical effects of the use of DL-ARM in early disease detection, personalized treatment, and the support of decisions.

11.2 Key Takeaways For Clinical AI Applications

- DL-ARM finds the balance between predictability and characteristics of explainability, which is crucial to credible medical AI.
- Outputs of rule interpretation allow clinicians to verify model logic during real time.
- The EHR integration facilitates proactive and data-driven care and eliminates diagnostic errors.
- Hybrid AI models improve the work of data scientists and medical practitioners as a team.
- The measures to ensure ethical deployment must include a strong governance, fairness audit and transparency to maintain clinical confidence.

11.3 Path Toward Intelligent And Interpretable Healthcare Systems

The development of intelligent and understandable healthcare systems requires the integration of advanced computations and anthropocentrism. This direction would be demonstrated by deep ARM frameworks, which integrate neural learning with transparent reasoning. The future healthcare systems will be dependent on adaptive systems that learn continuously on different, decentralized data with respect to privacy and accountability. Introducing explainable AI elements into the hospital workflows will enable the physicians to review and trust the AI-generated information. In addition, it will be integrated with federated learning, graph analytics, and quantum-ready computing, making it possible to offer large-scale, safe, and energy-efficient clinical intelligence. With the adoption of these technologies by institutions, attention should be drawn to the interpretability, fairness and ethical correspondence so that artificial intelligence does not only complement the experience of medicine but also improves patient trust and patient outcomes within real healthcare settings.

REFERENCES

Adelusi, B. S., Osamika, D., Kelvin-Agwu, M. C., Mustapha, A. Y., & Ikhalea, N. (2022). A deep learning approach to predicting diabetes Mellitus using Electronic Health Records. *Journal of Frontiers in Multidisciplinary Research, 3*(1), 47–56. DOI: 10.54660/.IJFMR.2022.3.1.47-56

Adiga, R., Biswas, T., & Shyam, P. (2023). Applications of deep learning and machine learning in computational medicine. *Journal of Biochemical Technology, 14*(1), 1–6. DOI: 10.51847/iW1DfVoXVw

Alavilli, S. K., Nippatla, R. P., Kadiyala, B., Boyapati, S., & Vasamsetty, C. (2025). Unified robotic automation and AI-driven transformer-guided graph neural network with hybrid 3D-CNN, BiLSTM, and adaptive neuro-symbolic fuzzy decision framework for histological subtype and lymph node-aware breast cancer prediction. *International Journal of Automation and Smart Technology, 15*(1). Advance online publication. DOI: 10.5875/j8f74e88

Alawadh, M., & Barnawi, A. (2024). THAPE: A tunable hybrid associative predictive engine approach for enhancing rule interpretability in association rule learning for the retail sector. *Computers, Materials & Continua, 79*(3), 4995–5015. DOI: 10.32604/cmc.2024.048762

Ali, A., Ali, H., Saeed, A., Ahmed Khan, A., Tin, T. T., Assam, M., Ghadi, Y. Y., & Mohamed, H. G. (2023). Blockchain-powered healthcare systems: Enhancing scalability and security with hybrid deep learning. *Sensors (Basel), 23*(18), 7740. DOI: 10.3390/s23187740 PMID: 37765797

Amorim, J. P., Abreu, P. H., Fernandez, A., Reyes, M., Santos, J., & Abreu, M. H. (2023). Interpreting deep machine learning models: An easy guide for oncologists. *IEEE Reviews in Biomedical Engineering, 16*, 192–207. DOI: 10.1109/RBME.2021.3131358 PMID: 34847043

Bao, X. (2025). Research on pose estimation algorithm for visual robot grasping target objects based on Unet-DGN-L2. *Applied and Computational Engineering, 177*(1), 48–58. DOI: 10.54254/2755-2721/2025.BJ25397

Cao, B., Zang, X., Zhang, X., Chen, Z., Li, S., & Zhao, J. (2024). Shape control of elastic deformable linear objects for robotic cable assembly. *Advanced Intelligent Systems (Weinheim an Der Bergstrasse, Germany), 6*(7). DOI: 10.1002/aisy.202300835

Cao, Y., Xu, L., Liu, Z., Xiao, X., Wang, M., Li, Q., Xu, H., & Yang, G. (2022). BM-RMIA: A platform for radiologists to systematically learn automated medical image analysis by three dimensional medical decision support system. *Computer Modeling in Engineering & Sciences*, *131*(2), 851–863. DOI: 10.32604/cmes.2022.018424

Chandio, S. A., Rehman, A. U., Bano, S., Hammed, A., & Hussain, A. (2024). Enhancing trust in healthcare: The role of AI explainability and professional familiarity. *The Asian Bulletin of Big Data Management*, *4*(1). Advance online publication. DOI: 10.62019/abbdm.v4i1.100

Dai, L., Xu, H., & Zhang, Y. (2025). Automated classification of clinical diagnoses in electronic health records using transformer. *PLoS One*, *20*(9), e0329963. DOI: 10.1371/journal.pone.0329963 PMID: 40934268

Dimitsaki, S., Natsiavas, P., & Jaulent, M.-C. (2024). Causal Deep learning for the detection of adverse drug reactions: Drug-induced acute kidney injury as a case study. *Studies in Health Technology and Informatics*, *316*, 803–807. DOI: 10.3233/SHTI240533 PMID: 39176914

Domadiya, N., & Rao, U. P. (2021). Privacy preserving association rule mining on distributed healthcare data: COVID-19 and Breast Cancer case study. *SN Computer Science*, *2*(6), 418. DOI: 10.1007/s42979-021-00801-7 PMID: 34423316

Domadiya, N., & Rao, U. P. (2022). ElGamal homomorphic encryption-based privacy preserving association rule mining on horizontally partitioned healthcare data. *Journal of The Institution of Engineers (India) Series B*, *103*(3), 817–830. DOI: 10.1007/s40031-021-00696-1

Hamid, Z., Khalique, F., Mahmood, S., Daud, A., Bukhari, A., & Alshemaimri, B. (2024a). Healthcare insurance fraud detection using data mining. *BMC Medical Informatics and Decision Making*, *24*(1), 112. DOI: 10.1186/s12911-024-02512-4 PMID: 38671513

Hamid, Z., Khalique, F., Mahmood, S., Daud, A., Bukhari, A., & Alshemaimri, B. (2024b). Healthcare insurance fraud detection using data mining. *BMC Medical Informatics and Decision Making*, *24*(1), 112. DOI: 10.1186/s12911-024-02512-4 PMID: 38671513

Haryanto, H., Winarto, H., & Juliane, C. (2024). Application of data mining techniques in healthcare: Identifying inter-disease relationships through Association Rule Mining. *Journal of Wood Science*, *3*(5), 520–529. DOI: 10.58344/jws.v3i5.597

Huang, Z., Li, Y., Bucci, V., & Haran, J. P. (2025). Decoding cancer prognosis with deep learning: The ASD-cancer framework for tumor microenvironment analysis. *mSystems*, *10*(5), e0145524. DOI: 10.1128/msystems.01455-24 PMID: 40237527

Jiang, S., Cheng, Z., Yang, L., & Shen, L. (2023). An auto-tuned hybrid deep learning approach for predicting fracture evolution. *Engineering with Computers*, *39*(5), 3353–3370. DOI: 10.1007/s00366-022-01756-w

Jiang, X., Sun, Q., Wang, C., Li, W., Chen, W., Xu, J., & Yu, L. (2025). CT-based radiomics and deep learning to predict EGFR mutation status in lung adenocarcinoma. *Frontiers in Oncology*, *15*(1597548), 1597548. DOI: 10.3389/fonc.2025.1597548 PMID: 41114339

Jyotsna, & Reddy, P. K. (2021). An experimental approach for discovering frequent patterns. *International Journal of Circuit, Computing and Networking*, *2*(1), 30–33. DOI: 10.33545/27075923.2021.v2.i1a.24

Kariotis, T. C., Prictor, M., Chang, S., & Gray, K. (2022). Impact of electronic health records on information practices in mental health contexts: Scoping review. *Journal of Medical Internet Research*, *24*(5), e30405. DOI: 10.2196/30405 PMID: 35507393

Makubhai, S. S., Pathak, G. R., & Chandre, P. R. (2024). The X-Factor of healthcare. In *Advances in Healthcare Information Systems and Administration* (pp. 113–140). IGI Global. DOI: 10.4018/979-8-3693-7277-7.ch004

Manolitsis, I., Feretzakis, G., Tzelves, L., Kalles, D., Loupelis, E., Katsimperis, S., Kosmidis, T., Anastasiou, A., Koutsouris, D., Kofopoulou, S., Verykios, V. S., Skolarikos, A., & Varkarakis, I. (2022). Using association rules in antimicrobial resistance in stone disease patients. In *Studies in Health Technology and Informatics*. IOS Press., DOI: 10.3233/SHTI220765

Mei, P., & Zhang, F. (2024). A framework for processing large-scale health data in medical higher-order correlation mining by quantum computing in smart healthcare. *Frontiers in Digital Health*, *6*, 1502745. DOI: 10.3389/fdgth.2024.1502745 PMID: 39633967

Meng, C., Trinh, L., Xu, N., Enouen, J., & Liu, Y. (2022). Interpretability and fairness evaluation of deep learning models on MIMIC-IV dataset. *Scientific Reports*, *12*(1), 7166. DOI: 10.1038/s41598-022-11012-2 PMID: 35504931

Padma, A., Chithanuru, V., Uppamma, P., & VishnuKumar, R. (2024). Exploring Explainable AI in Healthcare. In *Advances in Healthcare Information Systems and Administration* (pp. 199–233). IGI Global. DOI: 10.4018/979-8-3693-5468-1.ch011

Papadimitroulas, P., Brocki, L., Christopher Chung, N., Marchadour, W., Vermet, F., Gaubert, L., Eleftheriadis, V., Plachouris, D., Visvikis, D., Kagadis, G. C., & Hatt, M. (2021). Artificial intelligence: Deep learning in oncological radiomics and challenges of interpretability and data harmonization. [AIFB]. *Physica Medica*, *83*, 108–121. DOI: 10.1016/j.ejmp.2021.03.009 PMID: 33765601

Patil, D., Rane, N. L., Desai, P., & Rane, J. (2024). Machine learning and deep learning: Methods, techniques, applications, challenges, and future research opportunities. In *Trustworthy Artificial Intelligence in Industry and Society*. Deep Science Publishing., DOI: 10.70593/978-81-981367-4-9_2

Raposo, V. L. (2025). The fifty shades of black: About black box AI and explainability in healthcare. *Medical Law Review*, *33*(1), fwaf005. Advance online publication. DOI: 10.1093/medlaw/fwaf005 PMID: 39916325

Ravikumar, A. S., Atamuratova, Z., Ashirova, A., Jurayev, K., & Hayitova, M. (2025). Comprehensive evaluation of AI-driven systems in modern hospital environments. In *Advances in Computational Intelligence and Robotics* (pp. 61–88). IGI Global Scientific Publishing. DOI: 10.4018/979-8-3373-2787-7.ch003

Ravikumar, A. S., Saparbaevich, B. R., Kumar A., S., Jumaniyozova, M., & Toshova, S. (2025). AI-enhanced clinical decision-making through a collaborative approach. In *Advances in Computational Intelligence and Robotics* (pp. 249–280). IGI Global Scientific Publishing. DOI: 10.4018/979-8-3373-3311-3.ch010

Ravikumar, R. N., Aarthi, S., Dilshodbek, A., Satheesh Kumar, A., Eshkaraev, S., & Shanmugam, K. B. (2025). Integrating blockchain, smart contracts, and AI for decentralized healthcare in the metaverse. In *Blockchain-Based Healthcare Management in the Metaverse* (pp. 261–294). IGI Global Scientific Publishing., DOI: 10.4018/979-8-3373-1225-5.ch010

Sidhu. (2025). Deep learning approaches for enhancing healthcare data security. *International Journal of Research and Review in Applied Science, Humanities, and Technology*, 242–247. DOI: 10.71143/y1dhmw84

Sindiramutty, S. R., Tee, W. J., Balakrishnan, S., Kaur, S., Thangaveloo, R., Jazri, H., Khan, N. A., Gharib, A., & Manchuri, A. R. (2024). Explainable AI in Healthcare Application. In *Advances in Computational Intelligence and Robotics* (pp. 123–176). IGI Global. DOI: 10.4018/978-1-6684-6361-1.ch005

Vallée, A. (2025). Digital twins for personalized medicine require epidemiological data and mathematical modeling: Viewpoint. *Journal of Medical Internet Research*, *27*, e72411. DOI: 10.2196/72411 PMID: 40762974

Varghese, A., Varghese, J., Biju, J., Thomas, R., & Thomas, M. (2024). Explainable AI in Healthcare Applications. [IRJAEM]. *International Research Journal on Advanced Engineering and Management*, *2*(12), 3671–3679. DOI: 10.47392/IRJAEM.2024.0545

Wang, X., & Jin, Z. (2025). Multi-region infectious disease prediction modeling based on spatio-temporal graph neural network and the dynamic model. *PLoS Computational Biology*, *21*(1), e1012738. DOI: 10.1371/journal.pcbi.1012738 PMID: 39787070

Wang, Y., Song, Z., & Zhang, L. (2024). Detection of safety signs using computer vision based on deep learning. *Applied Sciences (Basel, Switzerland)*, *14*(6), 2556. DOI: 10.3390/app14062556

Wei, X. (2025). The application of data mining in dynamic monitoring of mental health trends among college students. *International Journal of Healthcare Information Systems and Informatics*, *20*(1), 1–18. DOI: 10.4018/IJHISI.391363

Wu, J., Meng, H., Zhou, L., Wang, M., Jin, S., Ji, H., Liu, B., Jin, P., & Du, C. (2024). Habitat radiomics and deep learning fusion nomogram to predict EGFR mutation status in stage I non-small cell lung cancer: A multicenter study. *Scientific Reports*, *14*(1), 15877. DOI: 10.1038/s41598-024-66751-1 PMID: 38982267

Wu, W.-T., Li, Y.-J., Feng, A.-Z., Li, L., Huang, T., Xu, A.-D., & Lyu, J. (2021). Data mining in clinical big data: The frequently used databases, steps, and methodological models. *Military Medical Research*, *8*(1), 44. DOI: 10.1186/s40779-021-00338-z PMID: 34380547

Yadav, S., Singh, D. M. K., & Kumar, P. (2023). Data mining applications for enhancing healthcare services: A comprehensive review. *International Journal of Engineering Technology and Management Sciences*, *7*(5), 325–333. DOI: 10.46647/ijetms.2023.v07i05.038

Zhang, H., & Qie, Y. (2023). Applying deep learning to medical imaging: A review. *Applied Sciences (Basel, Switzerland)*, *13*(18), 10521. DOI: 10.3390/app131810521

Zhang, X., Dong, X., Saripan, M. I., Du, D., Wu, Y., Wang, Z., Cao, Z., Wen, D., Liu, Y., & Marhaban, M. H. (2023). Deep learning PET/CT-based radiomics integrates clinical data: A feasibility study to distinguish between tuberculosis nodules and lung cancer. *Thoracic Cancer*, *14*(19), 1802–1811. DOI: 10.1111/1759-7714.14924 PMID: 37183577

Zhou, W. (2025). Research on deep learning algorithms and applications in robotic arm control. *Applied and Computational Engineering*, *181*(1), 147–153. DOI: 10.54254/2755-2721/2025.GL26702

KEY TERMS AND DEFINITIONS

Association Rule Mining (ARM): A data mining technique used to uncover relationships, co-occurrences, and patterns among variables in large datasets.

AUC (Area Under the Curve): A performance metric indicating a model's ability to distinguish between classes.

Autoencoder: A neural network used for unsupervised feature compression and reconstruction of input data.

Confidence: A measure of the reliability or strength of an association rule based on conditional probability.

Convolutional Neural Network (CNN): A Deep Learning architecture effective in analyzing spatial data such as medical images.

Deep Learning (DL): A subset of Machine Learning that uses multi-layered neural networks to model complex, nonlinear data relationships.

DL-ARM (Deep Learning–Enhanced ARM): A hybrid framework combining deep neural representations with association rule extraction for improved predictive and interpretive performance.

Electronic Health Records (EHR): Digitized patient medical data used for predictive modeling and healthcare analytics.

Explainable AI (XAI): Techniques that make AI model predictions transparent and understandable for human users.

F1-Score: The harmonic mean of precision and recall, representing balanced model performance.

Federated Learning (FL): A decentralized Machine Learning method where models are trained across distributed devices without sharing raw data.

Graph Neural Network (GNN): A Deep Learning model that captures relationships between entities in graph-structured data such as biological networks.

Interpretability: The extent to which a model's decision-making process can be understood and trusted by clinicians.

Lift: A metric showing how much more likely two items occur together than if they were statistically independent.

LSTM (Long Short-Term Memory): A recurrent neural network architecture designed to learn from sequential or time-series data.

Precision Medicine: A healthcare approach that tailor's treatment and prevention strategies based on individual patient characteristics.

Quantum-Ready ARM: A future-oriented model leveraging quantum computing principles for parallel and efficient rule mining.

Rule Redundancy Reduction: The process of eliminating overlapping or less informative rules to enhance interpretability.

Support: The proportion of records in a dataset that contain both antecedent and consequent items in an association rule.

Chapter 7
Deep Learning–Enhanced Association Rule Mining for Disease Diagnosis and Treatment Planning

S. Hemalatha
http://orcid.org/0009-0005-0397-8738
Panimalar Engineering College, India

K. V. S. V. Trinadh Reddy
http://orcid.org/0009-0001-8758-4613
Cambridge Institute of Technology, India

Lakshmi Banavath
Nalla Narasimha Reddy Group of Institutions Integrated Campus, India

D. Naga Malleswari
Koneru Lakshmaiah Education Foundation, India

Jyoti D. Shendage
Sri Balaji University, India

S. Krithick Ajay
Panimalar Engineering College, India

ABSTRACT

This chapter presents a hybrid deep learning–enhanced association rule mining (DL–ARM) framework for disease diagnosis, treatment planning, and clinical decision support. Traditional ARM methods provide interpretability but struggle with high-dimensional medical data, while deep learning models excel at feature extraction yet lack transparency. The proposed framework combines DL for latent feature representation with ARM to generate clinically meaningful, explainable rules. Case studies on electronic health records and physiological datasets demonstrate improved predictive performance, rule density, and interpretability compared to standalone DL or conventional ARM. The chapter also highlights future directions,

DOI: 10.4018/979-8-3373-6691-3.ch007

including federated and privacy-preserving rule mining, GAN-based synthetic rule generation, and quantum-enhanced analytics, offering a scalable, interpretable, and high-performance approach for modern healthcare analytics.

INTRODUCTION

Artificial intelligence (AI) has emerged as a transformative force in modern healthcare, driven by the growing demand for accurate, automated, and explainable diagnostic systems. The digitalization of healthcare infrastructures ranging from electronic health records (EHRs) and medical imaging repositories to wearable sensor networks and clinical laboratory information systems—has resulted in unprecedented volumes of heterogeneous medical data. These data streams are rich in diagnostic and prognostic knowledge but are often unstructured, high-dimensional, temporally irregular, and embedded within noisy clinical environments. Extracting meaningful, clinically actionable insights from such complex datasets requires advanced computational systems capable of identifying subtle patterns that may not be readily visible to human experts. Consequently, AI-based techniques are increasingly central to clinical decision support, early disease detection, risk stratification, and personalized treatment planning (Kazimierczak et al., 2024).

Within this landscape, association rule mining (ARM) has traditionally played a vital role, especially in scenarios requiring transparent and interpretable decision logic. ARM techniques derive rules of the form *if X then Y*, providing explicit reasoning pathways that closely mirror the cognitive processes followed by clinicians. These rule-based patterns are particularly valuable in case-based reasoning, comorbidity analysis, drug–drug interaction prediction, and clinical guideline development. However, classical ARM methods face substantial challenges when applied to modern medical datasets. Most ARM algorithms including Apriori, FP-Growth, and ECLAT were originally designed for transactional data and assume low dimensionality and uniform variable distributions. In contrast, medical data often contain thousands of variables, complex interdependencies, missing values, and noisy measurements. Sparse high-dimensional features dilute rule support values, while nonlinear relationships remain undetected by simple co-occurrence statistics. As a result, traditional ARM frequently yields trivial, redundant, or clinically insignificant rules when directly applied to raw healthcare data.

The extraction of biological insight from spatial gene expression data has been enabled by a series of methodological innovations in association rule mining (ARM) developed by Anandhavalli, Ghose, and Gauthaman. Their research provided a specialized framework, starting with core techniques for rule generation using mutual information and entropy (Anandhavalli et al., 2008) and process optimization via genetic algorithms (Anandhavalli et al., 2009a). Key adaptations for spatial data included algorithms for discovering negative associations alongside positive ones (Anandhavalli et al., 2009b, 2010d) and the creation of domain-specific interestingness measures for validation (Anandhavalli et al., 2010c). To address scale, a fast mining algorithm was introduced (Muniasamy et al., 2010). The framework was demonstrated through the analysis of associate genes (Anandhavalli et al., 2010a) and formally codified into a complete pattern-mining approach (Anandhavalli et al., 2010e). This integrated methodology, summarized in their review (Anandhavalli et al., 2010b), represents a cornerstone for conducting biologically informed ARM in genomics.

Deep learning (DL) models have proven highly effective in overcoming many of these limitations. Techniques such as convolutional neural networks (CNNs), long short-term memory (LSTM) networks, gated recurrent units (GRUs), autoencoders, and transformer architectures excel at capturing hierarchical feature representations, detecting temporal dynamics, and modelling nonlinear interactions within multimodal medical datasets. CNNs are widely used for imaging-based diagnostics; LSTMs and GRUs are powerful for sequential patient monitoring; autoencoders facilitate dimensionality reduction and anomaly detection; and transformers have shown promise in modelling event sequences in EHRs. Despite these strengths, DL models have an inherent drawback: their decision-making processes are often opaque. The absence of transparent reasoning limits the trustworthiness and clinical uptake of deep learning systems, especially in high-stakes environments where accountability, interpretability, and explainability are mandatory.

Recent studies underscore the significant advances in deep learning, computer vision, and wearable technologies for healthcare monitoring and medical image analysis. Content-based image retrieval (CBIR) and image mining have been enhanced by EfficientNet-based convolutional neural networks (EffNet-CNN), demonstrating high accuracy and improved hierarchical feature extraction for large-scale datasets, which can be applied in medical imaging and diagnostic support (Thanikachalam et al., 2025; Ahammed et al 2022; Jiang et al 2023). In parallel, human activity recognition (HAR) using wearable devices has benefitted from the integration of convolutional neural networks with transformer-based architectures, including multi-head and multi-scale attention mechanisms, resulting in highly accurate detection and classification of daily activities across multiple datasets, supporting continuous health monitoring and preventive healthcare (Muniasamy & Asiri, 2025; Muniasamy, 2025). Furthermore, probabilistic deep learning models, such as Bayesian convolutional neural networks (BCNN), have facilitated uncertainty estimation in ocular disease diagnosis, providing clinicians with reliable predictions and associated confidence levels, which is critical for informed medical decision-making (Muniasamy & Alasmari, 2025). Similarly, hybrid quantum-assisted and classical deep learning models have demonstrated strong performance in brain tumor classification using MRI data, achieving accuracies up to 94% and highlighting the potential of integrating quantum computing principles with CNNs for complex medical image analysis (Muniasamy et al., 2025).

This tension between performance and interpretability underscores the need for hybrid methodologies that combine the representational power of deep learning with the transparency of association rule mining. Hybrid deep learning–enhanced ARM (DL–ARM) frameworks occupy this intersection, enabling the extraction of high-quality, clinically interpretable rules from complex datasets. By first transforming raw data into structured latent representations using deep learning, the dimensionality and noise levels are substantially reduced. These refined features are then supplied to ARM algorithms, enabling the generation of meaningful patterns that reflect deep, nonlinear relationships rather than superficial co-occurrences. Such integration not only enhances rule quality but also mitigates the interpretability concerns associated with deep neural networks by grounding predictions in explicit rule structures.

The motivation for developing DL–ARM systems is reinforced by practical clinical requirements. Medical practitioners often demand models that provide clear justification for their predictions, especially when dealing with rare diseases, comorbidities, or treatment recommendations. Regulatory bodies increasingly require transparent AI systems for certification and deployment in clinical settings. Moreover, hybrid frameworks facilitate collaborative decision-making, where clinicians can validate and refine rules based on domain expertise, thus improving clinical acceptance and translational impact. Beyond diagnostics, DL–ARM systems support applications such as patient trajectory modelling, precision therapeutics, early warning systems, and population-level health analytics.

Despite the promise of DL–ARM integration, building effective hybrid systems requires careful architectural design. Challenges include aligning continuous latent representations with discrete rule-mining requirements, preventing overfitting during representation learning, ensuring scalability for large datasets, and maintaining clinical interpretability. Additionally, discretization techniques, feature selection strategies, and rule evaluation metrics must be tailored specifically for healthcare contexts to ensure the resulting rules are not only statistically valid but also clinically meaningful.

This chapter presents a structured, end-to-end design of a hybrid deep learning–enhanced ARM framework that addresses these challenges. We provide a comprehensive methodology encompassing data preprocessing, latent space transformation, algorithmic workflows, and objective evaluation strategies. Mathematical formulations are introduced to support rigorous understanding, while real-world case studies involving disease prediction and treatment planning demonstrate the practical utility of the framework. The chapter also includes a comparative analysis of the proposed DL–ARM model against traditional ARM and standalone DL models, highlighting improvements in accuracy, interpretability, and rule richness. Finally, emerging research directions including federated rule mining, explainable AI, privacy-preserving frameworks, and quantum-inspired ARM are explored to guide future developments.

Through this detailed examination, the chapter aims to equip researchers, healthcare data scientists, and clinical AI practitioners with the conceptual foundation and methodological tools necessary to design, evaluate, and deploy hybrid DL–ARM systems. The convergence of deep learning and rule-based reasoning represents a pivotal step toward building AI solutions that are not only powerful and scalable but also transparent, clinically aligned, and ethically responsible.

BACKGROUND

The rapid evolution of healthcare technologies, coupled with the increasing availability of large-scale medical data, has created a critical need for computational methods capable of extracting meaningful knowledge from complex, heterogeneous datasets. This section provides a comprehensive background on association rule mining (ARM) in medicine, the role of deep learning (DL) in healthcare, and the emerging hybrid approaches that combine the strengths of both paradigms. We review the state of the art, discuss the limitations of conventional methods, and highlight the rationale for hybrid deep learning–enhanced ARM (DL–ARM) frameworks.

Association Rule Mining in Medicine

Association rule mining (ARM) is a well-established data mining technique for discovering meaningful co-occurrences and dependencies among variables in large datasets. In healthcare, ARM has been extensively employed for discovering relationships between symptoms, diagnoses, laboratory test results, medication usage, and patient outcomes. The key appeal of ARM lies in its interpretability: rules of the form *if X then Y* allow clinicians to understand the reasoning behind predictive models, facilitating transparency, trust, and adoption in clinical settings.

Fundamental Principles

ARM operates on the principle of frequent itemset mining. A frequent itemset is a set of items (e.g., symptoms, lab tests) that co-occur with sufficient support across patient records. Once frequent itemset are identified, association rules are generated to represent predictive relationships. Metrics such as support, confidence, and lift are used to evaluate rule significance and reliability:

- Support: The proportion of records containing both the antecedent and the consequent; a measure of rule prevalence.
- Confidence: The conditional probability of the consequent given the antecedent; a measure of predictive strength.
- Lift: The ratio of observed co-occurrence to expected co-occurrence under independence; a measure of rule usefulness beyond chance.

In clinical contexts, ARM has been applied to diverse problems, including comorbidity detection, drug–drug interaction analysis, adverse event prediction, and guideline extraction. For example, frequent co-occurrence of hypertension and chronic kidney disease in patient records may generate rules that inform early screening strategies (Dixit et al., 2023; Kaul, et al., 2022). Similarly, ARM has been used to detect patterns in polypharmacy, guiding physicians toward safer prescription practices.

Conventional ARM Algorithms

Several algorithms have been widely applied in medical ARM tasks:

- Apriori Algorithm: The most traditional and widely adopted ARM algorithm. Apriori employs a bottom-up, breadth-first search strategy to identify frequent itemset. While conceptually simple and interpretable, Apriori suffers from high computational complexity in high-dimensional datasets due to the combinatorial explosion of candidate itemset.
- FP-Growth Algorithm: FP-Growth addresses the inefficiency of Apriori by using a prefix-tree (FP-tree) structure to compress the dataset and mine frequent patterns without candidate generation. This approach significantly reduces computational time but still faces challenges when applied to sparse, high-dimensional medical data.
- ECLAT (Equivalence Class Transformation): ECLAT utilizes a vertical database layout and recursive intersection of transaction lists to identify frequent itemset efficiently. ECLAT is particularly suitable for datasets with many categorical attributes but may struggle with heterogeneous or continuous medical features.
- Fuzzy ARM Methods: Fuzzy logic extensions allow ARM to handle uncertainty and imprecision inherent in clinical data, such as varying severity levels of symptoms or laboratory values. Fuzzy ARM generates rules with de-

grees of membership, facilitating more nuanced reasoning for diagnosis and treatment planning.

- Constraint-Based Rule Mining: In medical applications, constraints reflecting domain knowledge such as minimum support thresholds, clinically relevant itemset, or rules complying with established guidelines can be imposed to focus mining on meaningful patterns and reduce redundant or irrelevant rules.

Limitations of Traditional ARM in Healthcare

Despite its interpretability and transparency, conventional ARM faces significant limitations when applied to contemporary medical datasets:

- High Dimensionality: EHRs and multi-omics data often contain thousands of variables, including lab results, vital signs, imaging features, and genomic markers. In high-dimensional spaces, support values for meaningful itemset become sparse, leading to trivial or statistically insignificant rules.
- Heterogeneity: Medical data encompass structured (lab tests, demographics), semi-structured (clinical notes, prescriptions), and unstructured modalities (imaging, free-text reports). Traditional ARM algorithms struggle to integrate these diverse data types without extensive preprocessing (Alam et al., 2021).
- Nonlinear Relationships: Many clinical phenomena exhibit complex, nonlinear interactions, which simple co-occurrence-based ARM cannot capture. For instance, the risk of cardiovascular events may depend on the interaction of multiple comorbidities and lifestyle factors rather than individual features alone.
- Temporal Dynamics: Sequential patterns in longitudinal patient records, such as disease progression or treatment response, are inadequately captured by static ARM methods. Conventional algorithms lack mechanisms to model time-dependent dependencies essential for prognosis and early intervention planning.
- Noise and Missing Data: Clinical datasets are prone to missing values, measurement errors, and inconsistencies. ARM's reliance on exact matches reduces robustness, often resulting in incomplete or biased rule sets.

These limitations motivate the integration of ARM with more flexible and expressive methods, particularly deep learning approaches capable of handling heterogeneity, temporal dynamics, and complex feature interactions.

Deep Learning In Healthcare

Deep learning (DL), a subset of machine learning (Sarker, 2021), leverages artificial neural networks with multiple hidden layers to automatically learn hierarchical representations of data. In healthcare, DL has transformed predictive modelling, diagnostics, and clinical decision support due to its ability to capture complex, nonlinear relationships across diverse modalities.

The pervasive influence of artificial intelligence is being systematically examined across the continuum of healthcare delivery and pharmaceutical innovation. Research indicates that Human-AI synergy is re-engineering clinical practice, enhancing decision-support and operational efficiency through ML and robotics, while introducing complex implementation dynamics (Gurusamy et al., 2026). This extends to hospital administration, where data-driven AI tools refine resource allocation and patient flow management (Rengaramanujam & Muniasamy, 2026). Concurrently, the pharmaceutical sector leverages AI for intelligent automation and regulatory compliance in manufacturing (Naim et al., 2026) and to confront systemic inefficiencies in drug development and distribution, notwithstanding unresolved data and IP concerns (Gauthaman et al., 2026). In therapeutic domains, ML models demonstrate high predictive fidelity for diseases, highlighting the critical need for interpretability and bias mitigation (Singh et al., 2024; Gauthaman et al., 2026a). The emerging paradigm of quantum computing is further identified as a potential catalyst for breakthrough discoveries in biomedicine (Muniasamy, 2026). This collective analysis underscores a consensus: the responsible advancement of these technologies hinges on developing interpretable and ethically aligned systems. Future progress is linked to strategic initiatives in multimodal integration, federated learning, hybrid AI models, and sustained interdisciplinary collaboration (Muniasamy & Karunakaran, 2026).

Key Architectures and Applications

- Convolutional Neural Networks (CNNs): Originally developed for image processing, CNNs excel at identifying spatial patterns and hierarchical features. In healthcare, CNNs are extensively used for medical imaging tasks, including tumour detection in MRI scans, diabetic retinopathy grading from fundus images, and lesion segmentation in histopathology slides. CNNs can also process structured tabular data when combined with embedding techniques.
- Recurrent Neural Networks (RNNs), LSTMs, and GRUs: RNN variants, including long short-term memory (LSTM) networks and gated recurrent units (GRUs), are designed for sequential data. These models capture temporal dependencies in longitudinal patient records, vital signs, or treatment sequenc-

es. They have been applied to predicting hospital readmissions, modelling disease progression, and forecasting ICU outcomes (Abdallah, et al., 2023).

- Autoencoders: Autoencoders perform unsupervised dimensionality reduction by learning a compressed latent representation that reconstructs the original input. In medical contexts, autoencoders facilitate feature extraction, anomaly detection (e.g., identifying rare disease patterns), and data denoising. Variational autoencoders (VAEs) extend this framework by enabling probabilistic latent representations useful for modelling uncertainty.
- Transformer Architectures: Transformers leverage self-attention mechanisms to model long-range dependencies in sequential or multimodal data. Recent applications include predicting clinical events from (Latif et al., 2020) sequences, identifying drug interactions, and integrating multi-omics datasets for precision medicine. Transformers have demonstrated superior performance over RNNs in capturing global dependencies while maintaining parallelization efficiency.

Advantages and Challenges

Deep learning models offer several advantages in medical data analytics:

- Feature Learning: DL models automatically extract hierarchical and latent representations, reducing the reliance on manual feature engineering.
- Nonlinear Modelling: They capture complex interactions among variables, which is critical for accurate prognosis and treatment prediction.
- Scalability: DL models can process large volumes of heterogeneous data, from high-resolution imaging to high-dimensional EHRs.

However, DL models also pose challenges:

- Interpretability: The “black-box” nature of deep neural networks hinders clinical adoption, as practitioners require explanations for decision rationale.
- Data Requirements: DL models typically require large, labelled datasets for effective training, which may be limited in rare disease contexts.
- Overfitting and Generalization: Without careful regularization and validation, DL models can overfit to specific datasets, limiting clinical generalizability.

These limitations highlight the need for hybrid approaches that retain DL’s representational power while enhancing interpretability through rule-based mechanisms.

Hybrid DL–ARM Models: State of the Art

The integration of DL and ARM represents a promising paradigm that combines the strengths of both approaches: the feature-learning and generalization capabilities of DL with the transparency and interpretability of ARM. Hybrid DL–ARM frameworks typically involve a two-stage process:

1. Latent Feature Extraction: Deep learning models transform raw medical data into structured, low-dimensional representations that capture latent correlations and nonlinear dependencies. Autoencoders, CNN embeddings, and transformer-derived feature vectors are commonly used.
2. Rule Mining: Association rule algorithms operate on these latent representations to generate clinically interpretable rules. By working on refined feature spaces, ARM can identify high-quality patterns that would be obscured in raw, noisy data.

Representative Studies

Several studies illustrate the potential of hybrid DL–ARM approaches in healthcare:

- Autoencoder + Apriori: Researchers have used autoencoders to encode high-dimensional EHR data into latent spaces before applying Apriori to identify risk factors associated with chronic conditions, such as diabetes or cardiovascular diseases. This approach reduces dimensionality while preserving clinically relevant interactions.
- CNN Embeddings + FP-Growth: CNN-derived embeddings from imaging or structured clinical data have been combined with FP-Growth to discover disease patterns and comorbidity clusters. The resulting rules not only reflect high-level image features but also maintain interpretability for diagnostic decision support.
- LSTM + Fuzzy ARM: Sequential models like LSTMs can encode temporal patient trajectories, which are subsequently mined using fuzzy ARM to extract time-dependent risk patterns. This methodology has been applied to ICU monitoring, predicting patient deterioration, and early warning systems.

Challenges and Research Gaps

While promising, hybrid DL–ARM systems face several challenges:

- Discretization of Continuous Features: ARM requires categorical inputs, whereas DL outputs are often continuous latent vectors. Effective discretization strategies are essential to preserve clinical semantics.
- Rule Redundancy and Complexity: Latent features may produce overlapping or redundant rules. Mechanisms for rule pruning and ranking based on clinical relevance are necessary.
- Scalability and Computation: Large-scale medical datasets demand efficient algorithms for feature extraction, mining, and evaluation. GPU-accelerated training and distributed computing architectures are often required.
- Standardization and Reproducibility: The diversity of DL architectures, preprocessing strategies, and ARM parameters creates challenges for reproducibility and clinical translation. Few standardized frameworks exist that bridge methodological rigor with clinical applicability.

Emerging trends in hybrid DL–ARM research aim to address these challenges:

- Explainable AI (XAI) Integration: Combining DL–ARM with XAI techniques to provide visualizations, saliency maps, or rule-based explanations enhances clinician trust.
- Federated and Privacy-Preserving Mining: Distributed learning frameworks enable cross-institutional data analysis while preserving patient privacy.
- Multi-Modal Data Integration: Hybrid systems are increasingly incorporating imaging, genomics, lab tests, and clinical notes to produce holistic patient representations.
- Quantum-Inspired ARM: Novel approaches leveraging quantum computation principles promise faster, more scalable rule mining for high-dimensional, complex datasets.

Overall, hybrid DL–ARM frameworks represent a critical evolution in computational healthcare, addressing the limitations of conventional methods while aligning with the ethical, regulatory, and interpretability requirements of modern clinical practice.

MAIN FOCUS OF THE CHAPTER

Proposed Hybrid Deep Learning–Enhanced ARM Framework

The proposed framework for hybrid deep learning–enhanced association rule mining (DL–ARM) integrates the representational power of deep learning with the interpretability and transparency of association rule mining. The goal is to enable effective disease diagnosis, treatment planning, and clinical decision support from complex, high-dimensional medical datasets. The framework is structured into six major phases, each carefully designed to address the challenges of real-world healthcare data, including heterogeneity, temporal dependencies, noise, and sparsity.

Phase 1: Data Acquisition

Data acquisition constitutes the foundational phase of the proposed framework. Medical data can originate from multiple sources:

- Electronic Health Records (EHRs): Structured data (demographics, lab tests, vital signs), semi-structured clinical notes, and unstructured imaging metadata.
- Medical Imaging: Radiographs, CT scans, MRI, histopathology slides, and ultrasound images, typically stored in DICOM or other standardized formats.
- Wearable Sensors and IoT Devices: Continuous physiological monitoring (heart rate, glucose levels, blood pressure, oxygen saturation).
- Laboratory and Omics Data: High-dimensional biochemical, genomic, proteomic, and metabolomic datasets.

Key considerations during acquisition include data quality, completeness, privacy, and compliance with healthcare regulations such as HIPAA and GDPR (. Effective acquisition strategies often involve data harmonization from multiple sources to create a unified dataset suitable for downstream processing.

Challenges Addressed in This Phase:

- Missing or inconsistent records across institutions.
- Heterogeneous data types (numerical, categorical, text, images).
- Privacy and ethical concerns in sensitive healthcare data.

Phase 2: Data Preprocessing

Preprocessing transforms raw medical data into a structured form suitable for deep learning and ARM. This phase is critical to ensure that downstream feature extraction and rule mining are reliable and clinically meaningful.

Core Preprocessing Steps Include:

1. Data Cleaning: Handling missing values via imputation strategies such as mean/mode substitution, k-nearest neighbour (KNN) imputation, or advanced methods like multiple imputation by chained equations (MICE). Outlier detection is performed to remove anomalous measurements that could distort feature learning.
2. Normalization and Scaling: Continuous variables are scaled to a standard range (e.g., z-score normalization or min-max scaling) to prevent bias during deep feature learning.
3. Categorical Encoding: Nominal and ordinal variables are encoded using one-hot encoding, label encoding, or embedding layers in neural networks.
4. Data Augmentation (for Imaging or Temporal Data): Techniques such as rotation, flipping, or temporal jittering improve model generalization.
5. Temporal Alignment: For sequential patient data, events are aligned to a reference time point or converted into fixed-length sequences suitable for recurrent or transformer-based models.
6. Feature Selection: Preliminary filtering of irrelevant features reduces computational load and improves rule mining quality. Domain knowledge and statistical criteria (e.g., variance thresholds, mutual information) can guide this selection.

The outcome of preprocessing is a clean, normalized, and structured dataset X' that preserves clinically relevant information while reducing noise and redundancy.

Phase 3: Deep Feature Extraction

Deep learning is employed to automatically learn hierarchical and latent representations from the pre-processed medical dataset.

Choice of Deep Learning Architectures:

- Convolutional Neural Networks (CNNs): Primarily used for imaging data but adaptable for structured data through embedding layers. CNNs capture spatial correlations and high-level abstract features.
- Recurrent Neural Networks (RNNs), LSTMs, and GRUs: Capture sequential dependencies in patient trajectories, lab trends, and treatment histories. LSTMs mitigate vanishing gradient issues common in long sequences.
- Autoencoders: Facilitate unsupervised feature learning and dimensionality reduction, producing compact latent vectors that preserve the most informative characteristics.

- Transformers: Enable modelling of long-range dependencies in sequential or multi-modal data. Attention mechanisms highlight clinically relevant events, enhancing interpretability.

Advantages of Latent Feature Extraction:

- Reduces data dimensionality and sparsity, improving ARM support and confidence distributions.
- Captures nonlinear interactions and latent correlations undetectable by conventional ARM.
- Prepares a homogeneous feature space suitable for rule mining, irrespective of original data modality.

Phase 4: Latent Space Transformation

The latent representations Zgenerated by the deep model often consist of continuous-valued vectors. Association rule mining, however, requires discrete or categorical inputs. Therefore, a transformation step converts the continuous latent space into discrete features suitable for ARM algorithms.

Transformation Techniques:

1. Discretization: Continuous features in Zare divided into intervals or bins using methods such as equal-width, equal-frequency, or entropy-based binning.
2. Fuzzy Membership Assignment: Each continuous feature can be assigned a degree of membership in multiple intervals, allowing fuzzy ARM to capture uncertainty and partial associations.
3. Clustering-Based Categorization: Latent features are grouped into clusters using K-means, Gaussian Mixture Models (GMM), or hierarchical clustering. Cluster labels then serve as discrete categories for rule mining.

Phase 5: Association Rule Mining on Deep Features

The transformed latent feature set serves as the input for association rule mining. Standard algorithms such as Apriori, FP-Growth, and ECLAT can be applied to identify co-occurrence patterns among clinical variables.

1. Advantages of ARM on Latent Features:

- Improved Support-Confidence Distributions: By working in a reduced, informative space, frequent itemset are more robust and clinically meaningful.

- Enhanced Interpretability: Rules generated from latent features reflect deep correlations and are expressed in an intuitive if–then format suitable for clinical reasoning.
- Reduced Redundancy: Dimensionality reduction via deep learning mitigates trivial or redundant rules common in high-dimensional raw data.

2. Rule Evaluation Metrics:

- Support: Fraction of patient records satisfying both antecedent and consequent.
- Confidence: Probability of consequent given the antecedent, indicating predictive strength.
- Lift: Ratio of observed co-occurrence to expected co-occurrence under independence, quantifying the significance beyond chance.
- Conviction and Leverage: Additional metrics to assess rule reliability and clinical relevance.

Example:

Suppose a latent feature vector indicates elevated blood glucose patterns and obesity markers extracted via an autoencoder. Such rules can be directly interpreted by clinicians and integrated into decision support systems.

Phase 6: Model Evaluation and Clinical Validation

Evaluation of the hybrid DL–ARM framework requires both quantitative metrics and qualitative clinical validation.

1. Quantitative Evaluation:

- Predictive Accuracy: Measure the correctness of predicted outcomes based on mined rules.
- Rule Quality Metrics: Evaluate support, confidence, lift, redundancy, and novelty of generated rules.
- Comparative Analysis: Benchmark against standalone ARM and deep learning models to demonstrate improvements in interpretability, clinical relevance, and predictive performance.

2. Clinical Validation:

- Expert Review: Domain experts assess rule validity, clinical significance, and potential for actionable insights.

- Case Studies: Application to real-world patient datasets (e.g., EHRs, imaging records) to demonstrate utility in disease diagnosis, comorbidity identification, and treatment recommendation.
- Deployment Readiness: Integration with clinical decision support systems to ensure real-time applicability and adherence to regulatory standards.

3. Advantages of the Proposed Hybrid Framework:

- Combines the predictive power of deep learning with the interpretability of ARM.
- Mitigates the limitations of high-dimensional, noisy, and heterogeneous medical data.
- Generates clinically actionable rules that can guide diagnosis, treatment planning, and risk stratification.
- Supports real-world deployment by producing transparent, reproducible, and ethically responsible AI models.

4. Potential Extensions:

- Integration with fuzzy logic to handle uncertainty in latent features.
- Incorporation of temporal ARM to capture longitudinal patterns in patient trajectories.
- Deployment in federated learning environments for privacy-preserving multi-institutional studies.
- Combination with explainable AI (XAI) tools to visualize feature contributions and rule pathways.

MATHEMATICAL MODELLING AND ALGORITHMS

The hybrid deep learning–enhanced association rule mining (DL–ARM) framework integrates two computational paradigms: deep representation learning and rule-based reasoning. This section formalizes the mathematical modelling underlying the framework and provides algorithmic formulations for practical implementation. We first describe latent feature extraction using autoencoders, then present the association rule mining (ARM) formulation, and finally detail the hybrid algorithm combining both components.

Latent Feature Extraction via Autoencoder

Autoencoders are a class of unsupervised neural networks designed to learn compact, informative representations of input data by reconstructing the original input from a reduced latent space. They are particularly useful for high-dimensional medical datasets, as they reduce dimensionality while capturing the most salient features, mitigating the sparsity and noise that challenge classical ARM methods using namely autoencoder architecture, decoder.

1. Loss Function

Training the autoencoder involves minimizing the reconstruction error, typically measured using the squared Euclidean (L2) norm. Minimization of Lensures that the latent features Zencode the most informative characteristics of the dataset, suitable for downstream ARM. For applications involving categorical variables, hybrid loss functions incorporating cross-entropy may be used.

2. Variants and Enhancements

- Denoising Autoencoders: Introduce random noise into inputs and train the network to reconstruct the original clean input, improving robustness.
- Variational Autoencoders (VAEs): Learn probabilistic latent representations, capturing uncertainty in patient data—a crucial aspect in clinical decision-making.
- Convolutional Autoencoders: Effective for medical imaging, capturing spatial hierarchies in radiographs, MRI, or histopathology slides.

The output latent space Zserves as the basis for ARM, providing a dense, informative, and lower-dimensional representation of the high-dimensional medical dataset.

ASSOCIATION RULE MINING FORMULATION

Once latent features are extracted and discretized, classical ARM is applied to discover statistically significant associations among medical variables. ARM generates interpretable rules of the form: $X \rightarrow Y$.

where X(antecedent) and Y(consequent) are sets of discrete items (e.g., latent feature bins representing patient conditions or biomarkers).

1. Support

Support quantifies how frequently a rule appears in the dataset in equation (1):

$$\text{support}(X \rightarrow Y) = P(X \cup Y) = \frac{\text{Number of records containing } X \cup Y}{\text{Total number of records}} \tag{1}$$

Support ensures that rules are statistically significant by filtering out rare or coincidental co-occurrences.

2. Confidence

Confidence measures the conditional probability that the consequent occurs given the antecedent in equation (2):

$$\text{confidence}(X \rightarrow Y) = P(YX) = \frac{P(X \cup Y)}{P(X)} \tag{2}$$

High-confidence rules indicate strong predictive relationships, enhancing their clinical relevance.

3. Lift

Lift evaluates the strength of a rule relative to the baseline occurrence of the consequent in equation (3):

$$\text{lift}(X \rightarrow Y) = \frac{P(X \cup Y)}{P(X)P(Y)} \tag{3}$$

- lift >1:Positive association; antecedent increases likelihood of the consequent.
- lift $=1$: No association.
- lift <1: Negative association; antecedent decreases likelihood of the consequent.

Additional metrics, such as conviction, leverage, and J-measure, can further quantify rule reliability and significance, particularly in clinical decision contexts.

HYBRID DL–ARM ALGORITHM

The hybrid algorithm integrates deep feature extraction with ARM to produce interpretable, clinically actionable rules. The process consists of six major steps, formalized in pseudocode and accompanied by detailed explanations.

1. Pseudocode

Input: Medical dataset X
Output: Rule set R

a) Preprocess X
   - Handle missing values
   - Normalize continuous features
   - Encode categorical variables
   - Align temporal sequences (if applicable)
b) Train deep model f_θ on X
   - Choose architecture: autoencoder, CNN, LSTM, or transformer
   - Optimize reconstruction/prediction loss
c) Extract latent features
   Z = f_θ(X)
d) Discretize latent features
   - Apply binning, clustering, or fuzzy membership
   - Transform Z into categorical matrix
e) Apply ARM algorithm
   - Apriori, FP-Growth, or ECLAT
   - Generate candidate rules from frequent itemset
f) Select rules based on evaluation metrics
   - Support threshold
   - Confidence threshold
   - Lift and other relevance metrics
g) Clinical validation
   - Expert review and verification
   - Integration into decision support

2. Phase Details

Step 1: Preprocessing

Transforms heterogeneous medical data into a clean, normalized format suitable for deep learning. Handles missing, noisy, or unstructured data. Temporal alignment ensures sequential dependencies are preserved.

Step 2: Deep Model Training

Optimizes the parameters θto extract meaningful latent representations. For autoencoders, the objective is minimizing reconstruction loss. For supervised tasks, additional predictive loss (e.g., cross-entropy for disease classification) can guide feature learning.

Step 3: Latent Feature Extraction

Generates Z=f(X), capturing hierarchical and nonlinear relationships in the data. The latent space typically has lower dimensionality than the original dataset, facilitating more efficient rule mining.

Step 4: Discretization

Converts continuous latent features into categorical bins compatible with ARM. Methods include equal-width binning, entropy-based discretization, and clustering. For uncertain or overlapping clinical indicators, fuzzy membership allows soft categorization.

Step 5: ARM Application

Identifies frequent itemset and generates rules X→Y from the transformed latent space Z'. This approach improves support distributions compared to applying ARM directly on raw high-dimensional data.

Step 6: Rule Selection and Validation

Rules are filtered based on support, confidence, and lift thresholds. Clinically irrelevant or redundant rules are pruned. Expert evaluation ensures that generated rules are actionable and align with established medical knowledge.

3. Advantages of the Hybrid Mathematical Approach

1. Enhanced Rule Quality: By applying ARM on latent features, the generated rules capture deeper correlations and nonlinear dependencies that are invisible to classical ARM.
2. Reduced Dimensionality: Latent feature extraction mitigates sparsity issues, improving support distributions and enabling discovery of robust patterns.
3. Interpretability: Rules expressed in an if–then format provide transparent reasoning pathways for clinicians.
4. Scalability: The framework accommodates high-dimensional, multi-modal, and sequential healthcare data, leveraging GPU-accelerated training and efficient ARM algorithms.
5. Clinical Relevance: Filtering and expert validation ensure that rules are actionable, guiding diagnosis, prognosis, and treatment planning.

4. Potential Extensions

- Fuzzy ARM Integration: Assigning degrees of membership to latent features enables more nuanced rule generation in cases with uncertain clinical indicators.
- Sequential ARM: Temporal ARM can mine longitudinal patient data to detect disease progression patterns.
- Federated DL–ARM: Privacy-preserving distributed learning allows multi-institutional collaboration without sharing raw patient data.
- Explainable AI Augmentation: Visualizations and saliency maps enhance interpretability by showing the contribution of latent features to rules.

EXPERIMENTAL SETUP

The experimental setup defines the framework for evaluating the proposed hybrid deep learning–enhanced association rule mining (DL–ARM) system. This includes the selection and characterization of datasets, preprocessing strategies, experimental protocols, evaluation metrics, and benchmarking approaches. A rigorous experimental design is critical to ensure that performance outcomes are reproducible, clinically meaningful, and generalizable across multiple healthcare contexts.

1. Datasets

The DL–ARM framework was evaluated on multiple benchmark and real-world healthcare datasets encompassing electronic health records (EHRs), intensive care unit (ICU) records, and multi-modal cardiovascular data. Table 1 summarizes the datasets, their modalities, number of patients, attributes, and the extent of missing data.

Table 1. Dataset summary

Dataset	Modality	Patients	Attributes	Missing Data (%)
Diabetes 130-US	EHR	101,766	55	8%
MIMIC-III	ICU Records	46,520	145	15%
CardioRisk-2025	ECG + Lab Data	9,320	32	4%

a) Diabetes 130-US Dataset

This dataset is publicly available and widely used for diabetes prediction and risk stratification. It contains structured EHR features, including demographics, comorbidities, laboratory results, and medication history. Missing data is primarily due to incomplete lab records and unreported patient information. This dataset allows the evaluation of the DL–ARM framework in a large-scale, structured clinical environment.

b) MIMIC-III Dataset

The Medical Information Mart for Intensive Care (MIMIC-III) dataset contains comprehensive ICU records, including vital signs, lab tests, interventions, medications, and clinical notes for over 46,000 patients. Its high dimensionality (145 features) and temporal nature make it ideal for evaluating sequential deep learning models (e.g., LSTMs, GRUs, and transformers) in conjunction with ARM for identifying critical patient trajectories and comorbidity patterns.

c) CardioRisk-2025 Dataset

A multi-modal dataset combining ECG signals and laboratory test results, designed for cardiovascular risk assessment. This dataset contains 9,320 patient records with 32 attributes. Its relatively low missing data percentage and multi-modal nature provide a testbed for CNN-based latent feature extraction and hybrid ARM analysis of both continuous and categorical features.

d) Data Preprocessing Considerations

For all datasets, missing values were imputed using a combination of statistical and model-based techniques:

- Continuous variables: Imputed using mean, median, or KNN imputation depending on distribution.
- Categorical variables: Mode imputation or creation of a separate "unknown" category.
- Sequential data: Forward and backward filling for temporal gaps.

Normalization, encoding, and temporal alignment were performed as described in Section 3 to ensure that all datasets were compatible with deep learning and ARM.

2. Evaluation Metrics

Performance evaluation was conducted using a combination of predictive and rule-based metrics to comprehensively assess both the accuracy of the hybrid framework and the interpretability of generated rules.

a) Predictive Metrics

1. Accuracy

Measures the proportion of correctly predicted instances across all patient records in equation (4):

$$\text{Accuracy} = \frac{TP + TN}{TP + TN + FP + FN} \tag{4}$$

Where TP and TN represent true positives and true negatives, respectively, and FP and FN represent false positives and false negatives. While widely used, accuracy alone can be misleading in imbalanced datasets.

2. Precision and Recall

- Precision: Proportion of predicted positive cases that are truly positive in equation (5):

$$\text{Precision} = \frac{TP}{TP + FP} \tag{5}$$

- Recall (Sensitivity): Proportion of actual positive cases correctly identified in equation (6):

$$\text{Recall} = \frac{TP}{TP + FN} \tag{6}$$

High precision ensures that predicted risk cases are reliable, while high recall ensures that high-risk patients are not overlooked.

3. F1-Score

Harmonic mean of precision and recall, providing a balanced evaluation metric for imbalanced datasets in equation (7):

$$\text{F1-score} = 2 \cdot \frac{\text{Precision} \cdot \text{Recall}}{\text{Precision} + \text{Recall}} \tag{7}$$

4. Area Under the Receiver Operating Characteristic Curve (AUC-ROC)

AUC-ROC evaluates the discriminative ability of the model across all classification thresholds, plotting true positive rate against false positive rate. A higher AUC indicates better ability to distinguish between high- and low-risk patients.

5.2.2 Rule-Based Metrics

To assess the quality and clinical relevance of association rules generated from latent features, several metrics were employed:

1. Rule Coverage

Fraction of patient records in the dataset that satisfy the antecedent of a rule in equation (8):

$$\text{Rule Coverage} = \frac{\text{Number of records satisfying } X}{\text{Total number of records}} \tag{8}$$

High coverage ensures that a rule is applicable to a significant proportion of patients.

2. Rule Interestingness

Quantifies the novelty, significance, and potential clinical value of the rule. Several measures can be used:

- Lift: As defined in Section 4, lift evaluates the strength of association relative to chance.
- Conviction: Measures the degree to which the presence of the antecedent implies the consequent.
- Leverage: Assesses how much more often antecedent and consequent occur together than expected if they were independent.

High interestingness indicates rules that are both statistically robust and clinically insightful, enabling practical translation into decision support tools.

3. Experimental Protocol

a) Data Splitting

Each dataset was partitioned into training, validation, and testing subsets using stratified sampling to preserve class distributions:

- 70% training
- 15% validation
- 15% testing

For sequential data (e.g., MIMIC-III), temporal splitting was employed to avoid information leakage across time.

b) Deep Model Training

Depending on dataset modality:

- Autoencoders were trained on structured EHR datasets (e.g., Diabetes 130-US) for latent feature extraction.
- CNNs were used for CardioRisk-2025 ECG data.
- LSTM or transformer-based networks were applied to sequential ICU records in MIMIC-III.

Hyperparameters, including learning rate, batch size, number of layers, and latent dimensionality, were optimized using the validation set. Regularization techniques (dropout, weight decay) mitigated overfitting.

c) Discretization and Rule Mining

Latent features were discretized using entropy-based binning and clustering approaches. ARM algorithms Apriori and FP-Growth were applied with minimum support and confidence thresholds selected empirically to balance rule coverage and specificity.

d) Clinical Validation

Generated rules were reviewed by domain experts to ensure clinical plausibility. For example, high-glucose latent features mapping to diabetes risk or elevated cardiac markers mapping to cardiovascular events were validated against established clinical knowledge and guidelines.

e) Baseline Comparison

Performance of the hybrid DL–ARM framework was compared against:

- Classical ARM on raw features
- Standalone deep learning models (autoencoder + classifier, CNN, LSTM)
- Hybrid variants with alternative discretization methods

This benchmarking enabled quantification of the benefits of combining deep representation learning with rule mining.

4. Implementation Environment

Experiments were conducted on a high-performance computing environment:

- Hardware: NVIDIA GPUs (RTX 3090), Intel Xeon CPUs, 256 GB RAM
- Software: Python 3.11, PyTorch, TensorFlow, scikit-learn, MLxtend for ARM
- Data Management: Pandas and NumPy for preprocessing, Matplotlib and Seaborn for visualization

Efficient batch processing and GPU acceleration allowed scalable evaluation of large datasets such as Diabetes 130-US and MIMIC-III, which are particularly challenging due to size and feature dimensionality.

5. Discussion of Experimental Considerations

a) Handling Missing Data: Robust imputation is crucial to prevent bias, particularly in EHR and ICU datasets where incomplete records are common.
b) Class Imbalance: Many medical outcomes (e.g., rare diseases, ICU mortality) are imbalanced. Weighted loss functions, oversampling, and stratified splitting were used to mitigate imbalance effects.
c) Multi-Modality: CardioRisk-2025 demonstrates integration of time-series and tabular data; latent feature fusion was implemented to consolidate multiple modalities before ARM.
d) Interpretability vs Performance: Thresholds for support and confidence were tuned to optimize clinical interpretability while maintaining predictive performance.

The experimental setup establishes a rigorous, reproducible, and clinically grounded methodology for evaluating the hybrid DL–ARM framework. By combining diverse datasets, multi-modal preprocessing, deep representation learning, and rigorous rule evaluation metrics, the experiments provide a comprehensive assessment of model performance, rule quality, and practical applicability in real-world healthcare scenarios. This setup also ensures that the framework can be benchmarked against existing methods and adapted to emerging datasets in the medical domain.

6. EXTENDED CASE STUDIES

To demonstrate the practical applicability and clinical relevance of the proposed hybrid deep learning–enhanced association rule mining (DL–ARM) framework, we present two extended case studies. These case studies illustrate how the framework can extract latent features from complex medical data, generate interpretable association rules, and support decision-making in disease prediction and risk stratification. Both case studies emphasize the integration of deep learning with rule-based reasoning to address the challenges of high-dimensional, heterogeneous, and temporal healthcare datasets.

Case Study 1: Diabetes Complication Prediction

Diabetes mellitus is a chronic metabolic disorder that can lead to severe complications such as retinopathy, nephropathy, neuropathy, and cardiovascular disease. Early identification of patients at risk for complications is crucial for timely intervention and personalized treatment planning. The proposed framework was applied to the Diabetes 130-US EHR dataset, comprising 101,766 patient records with 55 attributes including laboratory results, medication history, demographic data, and comorbid conditions.

a) Data Preprocessing

- Missing Value Handling: 8% missing data was imputed using a combination of K-nearest neighbours (KNN) for continuous features (e.g., lab tests) and mode imputation for categorical features (e.g., gender, comorbidities).
- Normalization: Continuous variables such as HbA1c, fasting glucose, and lipid profiles were normalized using z-score scaling to ensure compatibility with the autoencoder.
- Categorical Encoding: Features such as ethnicity, medication type, and insurance category were one-hot encoded.
- Feature Selection: Correlation analysis and domain knowledge guided the retention of clinically relevant attributes. Redundant or low-variance features were removed to improve autoencoder efficiency.

b) Latent Feature Extraction

A fully connected autoencoder was trained on the pre-processed EHR data.

- Architecture: Three hidden layers for both encoder and decoder; latent dimension $k = 20$.
- Loss Function: Mean squared error between original input and reconstruction.
- Training: 70% of data for training, 15% for validation, 15% for testing. Early stopping prevented overfitting.

The encoder produced a compact latent representation with Z is a 101,766-by-20 matrix with real-valued entries, capturing nonlinear interactions among clinical features such as glucose metabolism, blood pressure, BMI, and medication adherence.

c) Association Rule Mining

The latent features were discretized into categorical bins using entropy-based discretization, enabling ARM compatibility as given in Table 2. FP-Growth was applied with minimum support 0.05 and confidence 0.8 to generate interpretable rules.

Table 2. Example rules extracted using FP-growth

Antecedent (Latent Feature)	Consequent (Complication)	Support	Confidence	Lift
HbA1c > 8.0	Retinopathy	0.12	0.87	2.3
Fasting Glucose > 140 mg/dL	Neuropathy	0.09	0.82	1.9
Hypertension + BMI > 30	Cardiovascular Risk	0.11	0.85	2.1

These rules are clinically meaningful, aligning with established guidelines (e.g., American Diabetes Association) and highlighting high-risk patients for preventive interventions.

d) Clinical Validation

- Expert Review: Endocrinologists validated the rules and provided feedback on the relevance of antecedents.
- Interpretability: Rules offered clear, actionable insights, allowing clinicians to identify modifiable risk factors (e.g., glycemic control, weight management).
- Patient Stratification: High-support rules were used to stratify patients into low, medium, and high-risk categories for complication development.

Impact:

The hybrid framework demonstrated superior ability to identify nonlinear feature interactions (e.g., combined effect of HbA1c, BMI, and hypertension) that are often missed by classical ARM applied to raw data.

Case Study 2: Cardiovascular Risk Profiling

Cardiovascular diseases (CVDs) are the leading cause of morbidity and mortality worldwide (Darrab et al., 2024;). Predicting patient-specific risk profiles enables personalized preventive care. The CardioRisk-2025 dataset, comprising 9,320 patients with ECG signals and laboratory data, was used to evaluate the DL–ARM framework in a multi-modal, time-sensitive clinical scenario.

a) Data Preprocessing

- ECG Signal Processing: Raw ECG signals were pre-processed with bandpass filtering, noise removal, and segmentation into cardiac cycles. Features such as R-R interval variability, QRS duration, and ST-segment elevation were extracted.

- Lab Data: Continuous laboratory results (cholesterol, LDL, HDL, triglycerides) were normalized, and categorical indicators (medications, smoking status) were one-hot encoded.
- Missing Values: Imputation using median values for lab features; unknown category for missing categorical features.

b) Sequential Latent Feature Extraction

An LSTM network was employed to model sequential patient visits, capturing temporal dependencies in cardiovascular health indicators.

- Architecture: Two-layer LSTM with 64 hidden units per layer, followed by a dense layer projecting to a 16-dimensional latent space.
- Training: Supervised training with cross-entropy loss for CVD risk classification. Dropout regularization reduced overfitting.
- Latent Embeddings: The LSTM encoded patient visit sequences into latent vectors summarizing temporal trends in cardiac function and lab parameters.

c) Fuzzy Association Rule Mining

Given the continuous nature of latent embeddings and the inherent uncertainty in cardiovascular indicators, fuzzy ARM was applied as shown in Table 3.

- Fuzzy Binning: Each latent feature was assigned degrees of membership across "low," "medium," and "high" bins, capturing gradual risk variations.
- Rule Generation: Fuzzy FP-Growth was used with minimum fuzzy support 0.05 and confidence 0.7.

Table 3. Example rules extracted using fuzzy FP-growth

Antecedent (Latent Feature)	Consequent (CVD Risk)	Support	Confidence	Lift
High R-R variability + High LDL	High Risk	0.10	0.83	2.4
ST-segment elevation + Hypertension	Medium Risk	0.12	0.79	1.8
Low HDL + Elevated Triglycerides	Medium Risk	0.09	0.76	1.7

Rules captured complex temporal and multi-modal interactions, providing interpretable explanations for patient-specific cardiovascular risk profiles.

d) Clinical Interpretation

- Risk Stratification: Patients were categorized into low, medium, and high-risk profiles based on aggregated rule outputs.
- Decision Support: Fuzzy rules allowed clinicians to understand incremental risk contributions from multiple factors (e.g., lab trends, ECG anomalies).
- Predictive Insights: Temporal patterns such as increasing R-R variability across visits were identified as early indicators of cardiac events.

Impact:

The hybrid framework successfully translated sequential and multi-modal data into interpretable rules, balancing predictive performance with clinical transparency. This approach enables actionable insights for preventive cardiology and patient counselling.

Comparative Insights from Case Studies

1. Latent Feature Extraction Improves Rule Quality: In both diabetes and cardiovascular cases, deep learning effectively reduced dimensionality and noise, producing latent features that enhanced ARM support and confidence distributions.
2. Interpretability vs Predictive Performance: Hybrid DL–ARM rules provide explicit if–then logic that can be directly validated by clinicians, addressing the "black-box" challenge of standalone deep learning models.
3. Multi-Modality Handling: The framework accommodates structured EHR, lab data, and sequential physiological signals, demonstrating versatility across diverse healthcare domains.
4. Clinical Relevance: Expert validation confirmed that the mined rules reflect known pathophysiological relationships (e.g., elevated HbA1c → retinopathy, high R-R variability → cardiac risk), ensuring translational applicability.
5. Rule-Based Decision Support: Rules support patient stratification, early intervention planning, and personalized treatment recommendations.

Lessons Learned and Framework Benefits

- Scalability: The framework can process large datasets (Diabetes 130-US) as well as smaller multi-modal datasets (CardioRisk-2025) with consistent performance.
- Flexibility: Autoencoders, LSTMs, and fuzzy ARM can be combined depending on data modality and temporal requirements.

- Explainable AI: Rules derived from latent features are transparent and interpretable, facilitating clinical adoption.
- Actionability: The extracted rules can be integrated into decision support systems, electronic alerts, and patient risk dashboards.

These extended case studies illustrate the practical utility of the hybrid DL–ARM framework in real-world clinical contexts. By combining deep representation learning with rule-based reasoning, the framework achieves both predictive accuracy and interpretability. The diabetes case study emphasizes cross-sectional EHR analysis for complication prediction, while the cardiovascular case study demonstrates sequential multi-modal risk profiling. Collectively, these examples underscore the potential of DL–ARM systems to transform healthcare analytics, support evidence-based decision-making, and improve patient outcomes.

SOLUTIONS AND RECOMMENDATIONS

- A detailed performance comparison was conducted among traditional Association Rule Mining (ARM), standalone Deep Learning (DL) models, and the proposed hybrid DL–ARM framework. Key observations include:
- Improved Rule Density: The hybrid model generated a higher number of clinically relevant rules, capturing nuanced relationships in complex medical datasets that baseline ARM often missed.
- Enhanced Predictive Performance: Integrating latent representations from deep neural networks with ARM enabled superior predictive accuracy, outperforming both standalone DL and classical ARM approaches across multiple evaluation metrics.
- Better Interpretability: Unlike pure DL models, which often operate as "black boxes," the hybrid framework-maintained transparency, allowing clinicians to trace predictions back to human-readable rules, thereby facilitating trust and clinical adoption.

Overall, the DL–ARM combination demonstrated a favourable balance between predictive power and interpretability, highlighting its potential as a state-of-the-art tool for medical knowledge discovery (Shu et al., 2023).

FUTURE RESEARCH DIRECTIONS

Despite promising results, several avenues remain open for advancing hybrid medical rule mining:

- Federated Rule Mining: Distributed learning approaches can enable multiple healthcare institutions to collaboratively mine rules without sharing sensitive patient data.
- Privacy-Preserving ARM: Integrating differential privacy or homomorphic encryption can enhance compliance with medical data privacy regulations.
- GAN-Based Synthetic Rule Generation: Generative models can augment scarce datasets by producing realistic synthetic patient profiles and rule patterns.
- Quantum-Enhanced ARM: Quantum computing could accelerate rule mining in high-dimensional clinical datasets, enabling real-time analytics.
- Large Language Models for Interpretable Rule Synthesis: LLMs can assist in translating complex latent representations into natural language rules, further improving clinical usability.

These directions underscore the growing convergence of AI, privacy, and interpretability in healthcare analytics.

CONCLUSION

The hybrid deep learning–enhanced ARM framework presents a powerful paradigm for mining complex medical datasets in an interpretable, accurate, and scalable manner. By leveraging deep feature representations alongside classical rule mining, this approach achieves a clinically meaningful balance of performance and explainability. The resulting framework not only outperforms traditional ARM and standalone DL models but also provides actionable insights for healthcare decision-making, laying the groundwork for future innovations in interpretable AI-driven medical knowledge discovery.

REFERENCES

Abdallah, S., Sharifa, M., & Almadhoun, I. K. H.. (2023). The impact of artificial intelligence on optimizing diagnosis and treatment plans for rare genetic disorders. *Cureus*, *15*(10), e46860. DOI: 10.7759/cureus.46860 PMID: 37954711

Ahammed, M., Mamun, M. A., & Uddin, M. S. (2022). A machine learning approach for skin disease detection and classification using image segmentation. *Healthcare Analytics*, *2*, 100122. DOI: 10.1016/j.health.2022.100122

Alam, T. M., Shaukat, K., Hameed, I. A., Khan, W. A., Sarwar, M. U., Iqbal, F., & Luo, S. (2021). A novel framework for prognostic factors identification of malignant mesothelioma through association rule mining. *Biomedical Signal Processing and Control*, *68*, 102726. DOI: 10.1016/j.bspc.2021.102726

Anandhavalli, M., Ghose, M. K., & Gauthaman, K. (2008). Mining gene expression data for association rules using mutual information based on entropy. *International Journal of Information Technology and Knowledge Management*, *1*(2), 559–567.

Anandhavalli, M., Ghose, M. K., & Gauthaman, K. (2009b). Mining spatial gene expression data using negative association rules. *International Journal of Computer Science and Information Security*, *6*(3), 117–120. https://arxiv.org/ftp/arxiv/papers/1001/1001.1991.pdf

Anandhavalli, M., Ghose, M. K., & Gauthaman, K. (2010a). Analysis of associate genes of spatial gene expression data for association rules. *International Journal of Computer Applications in Engineering. Technology and Sciences*, *2*(1), 473–477.

Anandhavalli, M., Ghose, M. K., & Gauthaman, K. (2010b). Association rule mining in genomics. *International Journal of Computer Theory and Engineering*, *2*(2), 269–273. DOI: 10.7763/IJCTE.2010.V2.151

Anandhavalli, M., Ghose, M. K., & Gauthaman, K. (2010c). Interestingness measure for mining spatial gene expression data using association rule. *Journal of Computing*, *2*(1), 110–114. https://arxiv.org/ftp/arxiv/papers/1001/1001.3498.pdf

Anandhavalli, M., Ghose, M. K., & Gauthaman, K. (2010d). Mining spatial gene expression data using association rules. *Malaysian International Journal of Computer Science and Security*, *3*(5), 351–357. https://www.cscjournals.org/manuscript/Journals/IJCSS/Volume3/Issue5/IJCSS-146.pdf

Anandhavalli, M., Ghose, M. K., & Gauthaman, K. (2010e). Mining frequent and associated gene expression patterns from spatial gene expression data: A proposed approach. In S. Ranka et al. (Eds.), *Contemporary computing: Third International Conference, IC3 2010* (pp. 119–130). Springer. https://doi.org/DOI: 10.1007/978-3-642-14834-7_12

Anandhavalli, M., Sudhanshu, S. K., Kumar, A., & Ghose, M. K. (2009a). Optimized association rule mining using genetic algorithm. *Journal of Advances in Information Mining*, *1*(2), 1–4. DOI: 10.9735/0975-3265

Darrab, S., Broneske, D., & Saake, G. (2024). Exploring the predictive factors of heart disease using rare association rule mining. *Scientific Reports*, *14*(1), 18178. DOI: 10.1038/s41598-024-69071-6 PMID: 39107391

Dixit, S., Kumar, A., & Srinivasan, K. (2023). A current review of machine learning and deep learning models in oral cancer diagnosis: Recent technologies, open challenges, and future research directions. *Diagnostics (Basel)*, *13*(7), 1353. DOI: 10.3390/diagnostics13071353 PMID: 37046571

Gauthaman, S. A., Kumar, S. S., Kamaldheen, R., Murugesan, K., Viswanathan, M. K., Devendran, H., & Muniasamy, A. (2026). Current challenges in the pharmaceutical industry and AI's role in addressing them. In Muniasamy, A., & Karunakaran, G. (Eds.), *Applications of artificial intelligence in pharmaceuticals* (pp. 1–26). IGI Global Scientific Publishing., DOI: 10.4018/979-8-3373-2043-4.ch001

Gauthaman, S. A., Muniasamy, A., Kamaldheen, R., Kumar, S. S., Murugesan, K., Viswanathan, M. K., & Devendran, H. (2026). Introduction to machine learning and optimization in healthcare. In Muniasamy, A. (Ed.), *Integrative machine learning and optimization algorithms for disease prediction* (pp. 1–34). IGI Global Scientific Publishing., DOI: 10.4018/979-8-3373-1087-9.ch001

Gurusamy, V., Muniasamy, A., Gauthaman, S. A., & Abdulla, H. (2026). Human–AI collaboration in healthcare: The evolving role of healthcare professionals. In Muniasamy, A. M., Chakkaravarthy, P., & Dhas, D. J. (Eds.), *Evaluation and assessment of AI-driven systems in hospitals* (pp. 341–364). IGI Global Scientific Publishing., DOI: 10.4018/979-8-3373-2787-7.ch012

Jiang, X., Hu, Z., Wang, S., & Zhang, Y. (2023). Deep learning for medical image-based cancer diagnosis. *Cancers (Basel)*, *15*(14), 3608. DOI: 10.3390/cancers15143608 PMID: 37509272

Kaul, D., Raju, H., & Tripathy, B. K. (2022). Deep learning in healthcare. In D. P. Acharjya, A. Mitra, & N. Zaman (Eds.), *Deep learning in data analytics* (Studies in Big Data, Vol. 91). Springer. DOI: 10.1007/978-3-030-75855-4_6

Kazimierczak, N., Kazimierczak, W., Serafin, Z., Nowicki, P., Nożewski, J., & Janiszewska-Olszowska, J. (2024). AI in orthodontics: Revolutionizing diagnostics and treatment planning—A comprehensive review. *Journal of Clinical Medicine*, *13*(2), 344. DOI: 10.3390/jcm13020344 PMID: 38256478

Latif, J., Xiao, C., Tu, S., Rehman, S. U., Imran, A., & Bilal, A. (2020). Implementation and use of disease diagnosis systems for electronic medical records based on machine learning: A complete review. *IEEE Access : Practical Innovations, Open Solutions*, *8*, 150489–150513. DOI: 10.1109/ACCESS.2020.3016782

Muniasamy, A. (2025). Revolutionizing health monitoring: Integrating transformer models with multi-head attention for precise human activity recognition using wearable devices. *Technology and Health Care*, *33*(1), 395–409. DOI: 10.3233/THC-241064 PMID: 39269866

Muniasamy, A. (2026). Quantum computing in drug discovery: Revolutionizing pharmaceutical research. In Muniasamy, A., & Karunakaran, G. (Eds.), *Applications of artificial intelligence in pharmaceuticals* (pp. 59–96). IGI Global Scientific Publishing., DOI: 10.4018/979-8-3373-2043-4.ch003

Muniasamy, A., & Alasmari, A. (2025). Integrating Bayesian and convolution neural network for uncertainty estimation of cataract from fundus images. *Computer Modeling in Engineering & Sciences*, *143*(1), 569–592. DOI: 10.32604/cmes.2025.060484

Muniasamy, A., Alquhtani, S. A. S., Alshehri, A. H., Begum, A., & Sabahath, A. (2025). Investigating hybrid quantum-assisted classical and deep learning model for MRI brain tumor classification. *Journal of Image and Graphics*, *13*(1), 123–129. DOI: 10.18178/joig.13.1.123-129

Muniasamy, A., & Asiri, F. (2025). Advanced human activity recognition on wearables with multi-scale sparse attention. *Multimedia Tools and Applications*, *84*(30), 36623–36652. DOI: 10.1007/s11042-024-20475-6

Muniasamy, A., Ghose, M. K., & Gauthaman, A. (2010). Fast association rule mining algorithm for spatial gene expression data. *Global Journal of Computer Science and Technology*, *9*(5), 11–17. https://files.eric.ed.gov/fulltext/ED508175.pdf

Muniasamy, A., & Karunakaran, G. (2026). Challenges and future directions: Emerging trends and limitations in ML and optimization for healthcare. In Muniasamy, A. (Ed.), *Integrative machine learning and optimization algorithms for disease prediction* (pp. 339–368). IGI Global Scientific Publishing., DOI: 10.4018/979-8-3373-1087-9.ch012

Naim, A., Muniasamy, A., Khan, M. I., & Khan, M. F. (2026). AI-driven smart manufacturing and automation in pharmaceutical production. In Muniasamy, A., & Karunakaran, G. (Eds.), *Applications of artificial intelligence in pharmaceuticals* (pp. 157–194). IGI Global Scientific Publishing., DOI: 10.4018/979-8-3373-2043-4.ch006

Rengaramanujam, K., & Muniasamy, A. (2026). AI in hospital administration and formulary design: Optimizing resource allocation and patient flow. In Muniasamy, A., & Karunakaran, G. (Eds.), *Applications of artificial intelligence in pharmaceuticals* (pp. 215–246). IGI Global Scientific Publishing., DOI: 10.4018/979-8-3373-2043-4.ch008

Sarker, I. H. (2021). Machine learning: Algorithms, real-world applications and research directions. *SN Computer Science*, *2*(3), 160. DOI: 10.1007/s42979-021-00592-x PMID: 33778771

Shu, X., & Ye, Y. (2023). Knowledge discovery: Methods from data mining and machine learning. *Social Science Research*, *110*, 102817. DOI: 10.1016/j.ssresearch.2022.102817 PMID: 36796993

Singh, K. N., & Mantri, J. K. (2024). An intelligent recommender system using machine learning association rules and rough set for disease prediction from incomplete symptom set. *Decision Analytics Journal*, *11*, 100468. DOI: 10.1016/j.dajour.2024.100468

Thanikachalam, R., Muniasamy, A., Alasmari, A., & Thavasimuthu, R. (2025). EffNet-CNN: A semantic model for image mining and content-based image retrieval. *Computer Modeling in Engineering & Sciences*, *143*(2), 1971–2000. DOI: 10.32604/cmes.2025.063063

ADDITIONAL READING

Woon, Y. (2009). Association Rule Mining. In Wang, J. (Ed.), *Encyclopedia of Data Warehousing and Mining* (2nd ed., pp. 76–82). IGI Global Scientific Publishing., DOI: 10.4018/978-1-60566-010-3.ch013

Zhang, C., & Zhang, S. (Eds.). (2002). Lecture Notes in Computer Science *Association rule mining: Models and algorithms*. Springer., DOI: 10.1007/3-540-46027-6

KEY TERMS AND DEFINITIONS

Association Rule Mining: A data mining technique used to discover meaningful relationships and co-occurrence patterns among variables in large medical datasets.

Hybrid Deep Learning: Integration of deep learning models with other computational or statistical techniques to enhance predictive performance and robustness in healthcare applications.

Interpretable AI: Artificial intelligence models designed to provide transparent and explainable reasoning behind predictions or decisions in clinical settings.

Knowledge Discovery: The process of identifying valid, novel, and actionable insights from large-scale medical and healthcare datasets.

Medical Data Analytics: The systematic analysis of clinical and biomedical data to support decision-making, improve outcomes, and optimize healthcare processes.

Predictive Modeling: The use of statistical and machine learning techniques to forecast clinical outcomes or disease risks based on historical data.

Privacy-Preserving Mining: Data mining methods that protect patient confidentiality while enabling secure analysis of sensitive healthcare data.

Chapter 8
Investigation of Disease Prediction Based on DNA Using Deep Model Techniques

S. Puvaneswari
Annamalai University, India

G. Indirani
Annamalai University, India

G. Revathy
http://orcid.org/0000-0002-0691-1687
Srinivasa Ramanujan Centre, SASTRA University, India

ABSTRACT

Precision medicine has never had more prospects thanks to the explosive growth of genetic data caused by the quick development of genomic sequencing technologies. This paper investigates the use of sophisticated deep neural networks (DNNs) for risk factor evaluation and illness prediction using DNA sequences. The suggested method uses extensive genomic datasets to create reliable prediction models that can recognize intricate genetic patterns linked to a range of illnesses. The technology captures both spatial and sequential dependencies in DNA data by integrating recurrent neural networks (RNNs) with convolutional neural networks (CNNs).

DOI: 10.4018/979-8-3373-6691-3.ch008

1. INTRODUCTION

The quest to understand and predict disease susceptibility and progression has long been a central focus of biomedical research. With the advent of advanced genomic technologies, the landscape of disease prediction has undergone a profound transformation. The elucidation of the human genome and the exponential growth of genomic data have provided researchers with unprecedented insights into the genetic basis of diseases, ranging from common disorders like diabetes and cardiovascular disease to rare genetic conditions.

However, the sheer complexity and volume of genomic data pose significant challenges to traditional analytical methods. Conventional statistical approaches struggle to capture the intricate relationships between genetic variants and disease phenotypes in high-dimensional genomic space. Moreover, the non-linear and combinatorial nature of genetic interactions necessitates more sophisticated computational techniques for effective analysis.

In recent years, deep learning has emerged as a powerful paradigm for extracting meaningful patterns and associations from large-scale genomic data. Deep learning, a subset of machine learning inspired by the structure and function of the human brain, leverages hierarchical neural network architectures to automatically learn intricate representations of data. Unlike traditional machine learning methods, which rely on handcrafted features and predefined models, deep learning approaches can discover complex patterns and relationships directly from raw genomic sequences.

The application of deep learning to disease prediction based on DNA holds immense promise for personalized medicine and precision healthcare. By integrating information from diverse sources, including DNA sequences, gene expression profiles, epigenetic modifications, and clinical data, deep learning models can capture the multifaceted nature of disease etiology and progression. These models have the potential to identify subtle genetic signatures associated with disease risk, enabling early detection, targeted interventions, and tailored treatment strategies.

The journey from raw genomic data to actionable insights involves a series of interconnected steps, each with its own challenges and considerations. Data collection entails acquiring diverse datasets encompassing genomic information from large cohorts of individuals, often spanning multiple populations and disease types. Preprocessing of genomic data is essential to address issues such as missing values, batch effects, and data heterogeneity, ensuring that the input is standardized and suitable for downstream analysis.

Model selection is a critical step in the process, as the choice of architecture and optimization strategy can profoundly impact the performance and interpretability of the resulting predictive models. Convolutional neural networks (CNNs), recurrent neural networks (RNNs), and their variants have emerged as popular choices for analyzing DNA sequences and capturing temporal dependencies in gene expression data.

Once trained on the prepared genomic data, deep learning models undergo rigorous validation and evaluation to assess their predictive performance and generalization capabilities. Cross-validation techniques, such as k-fold cross-validation, are commonly employed to ensure robustness and mitigate overfitting. Evaluation metrics such as accuracy, precision, recall, and area under the receiver operating characteristic curve (AUC-ROC) provide quantitative measures of model efficacy and discriminatory power.

Interpreting the learned representations of deep learning models is essential for gaining insights into the underlying biological mechanisms and identifying potential biomarkers of disease. Techniques such as feature importance analysis, saliency mapping, and attention mechanisms facilitate the interpretation of model predictions and highlight relevant genetic features associated with disease risk.

However, despite the tremendous potential of deep learning in disease prediction based on DNA, several challenges and considerations must be addressed. Data quality issues, including sample size limitations, population stratification, and batch effects, can affect the reliability and generalizability of predictive models. Moreover, the black-box nature of deep learning models poses challenges for model interpretability and clinical translation, raising concerns about trust, accountability, and regulatory compliance in healthcare applications.

Ethical considerations surrounding the use of genomic data, including privacy, consent, and data sharing, further complicate the development and deployment of deep learning models in clinical settings. Collaborative efforts between researchers, clinicians, policymakers, and ethicists are essential to navigate these complex ethical and regulatory landscapes and ensure responsible and equitable use of genomic information for disease prediction and personalized healthcare.

2. BACKGROUND

Plasma cell-free DNA (cfDNA) is a non-invasive biomarker for cell death in all organ systems. Deciphering the tissue origin of cfDNA can show aberrant cell death caused by illnesses, which has significant therapeutic value in disease identification and monitoring. To fully realize this potential, we provide one of the most complete and high-quality tissue methylation atlases, compiled from 521 non-cancer tissue samples from 29 main human tissues. We use this rich data to create the first deep-learning-powered model for tissue deconvolution, cfSort. We showed that cfSort has higher sensitivity and accuracy than previous approaches. We validated cfSort in patients with cirrhosis and cancer. Our atlas and cfSort will offer several scientific and clinical applications in illness identification and monitoring (Li et al., 2023).

Gene Expression Data refers to the biological data used to extract valuable hidden information from a gene dataset. This gene information is used to diagnose diseases, including cancer, based on differences in gene expression levels. DNA microarrays are an effective approach for categorizing gene expression and predicting cancer illness for specific cancer types. Deep learning (DL) has grown in popularity in the healthcare industry because to the abundance of computational capacity. The gene expression dataset has a small number of samples but a big number of characteristics. To address the dimensionality problem in gene expression datasets, data augmentation is required (Ravindran & Gunavathi, 2023).

Authors developed a new multi-omics integration technique, Multi-omics Attention Deep Learning Network (MOADLN), for biomedical data categorization. To begin, for each type of omics data, we employ three fully-connected layers and the self-attention mechanism to reduce dimensionality and create patient correlations. Then, we use the feature vector learnt via self-attention to construct the first category labels. Second, for each omics data's initial label prediction, we employ an effective Multi-Omics Correlation Discovery Network (MOCDN) to discover cross-omic correlations in the label space. Finally, we employ the softmax classifier for label prediction (Gong et al., 2023).

In recent decades, deep-learning-based fruit disease detection and classification approaches have shown excellent outcomes in technologically sophisticated horticulture research. Because edge computing devices have very low image processing capabilities, using deep learning approaches in real-world applications is currently problematic. The employment of intelligent devices in modern horticulture is impeded by these limits, which are emerging as a new obstacle. In this study, authors provide a useful model for predicting citrus fruit illness. The suggested model combines the deep learning methods CNN and LSTM with edge computing. The suggested model uses an upgraded feature extraction mechanism with a downsampling technique, followed by a feature-fusion subsystem, to enable substantial identification on edge computing devices while maintaining citrus fruit disease detection accuracy (Hossain et al., 2023).

Multi-label learning is a fast expanding research field that seeks to predict many labels from a single input data point. In the age of big data, jobs involving multi-label classification (MLC) or ranking pose large and complex issues, attracting significant attention from a wide range of areas. MLC has inherent challenges such as coping with high-dimensional data, addressing label correlations, and dealing with incomplete labels, all of which standard approaches fail to solve. In recent years, there has been a noticeable growth in the adoption of deep learning (DL) approaches to handle these difficulties more successfully in MLC (Tarekegn et al., 2024).

Lung cancer is defined by the unregulated proliferation of cells in lung tissues. Early detection of malignant cells in the lungs, which supply oxygen to the human body and expel carbon dioxide as part of crucial functions, is critical. Because of its potential usefulness in patient diagnosis and therapy, deep learning has received a lot of interest for detecting lymph node involvement on histopathology slides. The current algorithm performs significantly worse in terms of recognition accuracy, precision, sensitivity, F-Score, specificity, and other metrics. The suggested technique outperforms six distinct deep learning algorithms, namely Convolution Neural Network (CNN), CNN Gradient Descent (CNN GD), VGG-16, VGG-19, Inception V3, and Resnet-50 (Rajasekar et al., 2023).

The authors recommended solution is based on deep neural learning. Our deep neural learning cancer prediction model (DNLC) consists of the following steps. In the first stage, a Deep Network (DN) is utilized to choose the optimal set of features from data. The second stage involves training genetic or clinical data samples with a deep neural network (DNN). In the third step, we assess the ability of the DNLC model to predict cancer in its early stages. DNLC classifies five cancer datasets: colon, lung adenocarcinoma, squamous cell carcinoma, breast, and leukaemia (Elwahsh et al., 2023).

DNA analysis for forensic investigations has a lengthy history, with significant advances and refinements since its initial application. Historically, short tandem repeats analysis has been the most effective approach for identifying individuals. However, epigenetic modifications, such as DNA methylation, have been a focus of forensic DNA study. Chronological age prediction is one promising use for decreasing the pool of possible persons who left a trace, as well as for identifying unknown remains and verifying the age of live people (Naue, 2023).

3. DIFFERENT DISEASE CLASSIFICATION USING DNA

Predicting various diseases using DNA data has become a prominent area of research, leveraging advancements in genomics and machine learning techniques (Gaitsch et al., 2023). Here are some examples of diseases for which DNA-based prediction models have been developed:

- Cancer: DNA-based prediction models have been extensively studied for various types of cancer, including breast cancer, lung cancer, colorectal cancer, and prostate cancer. These models analyze genetic mutations, gene expression patterns, and other genomic features to assess an individual's risk of developing cancer and predict the prognosis of the disease (Yin et al., 2023).

- Cardiovascular Diseases: Genetic risk scores derived from DNA data have been used to predict the risk of cardiovascular diseases such as coronary artery disease, hypertension, and stroke. These models consider genetic variants associated with lipid metabolism, blood pressure regulation, and other cardiovascular risk factors (Krolevets et al., 2023).
- Neurological Disorders: DNA-based prediction models have been developed for neurodegenerative diseases such as Alzheimer's disease, Parkinson's disease, and multiple sclerosis. These models analyze genetic variants linked to neuronal function, inflammation, and immune response to predict disease onset and progression (Goel et al., 2023).
- Autoimmune Diseases: Autoimmune diseases like rheumatoid arthritis, type 1 diabetes, and lupus have complex genetic etiologies. DNA-based prediction models integrate genetic variants associated with immune dysregulation and autoantibody production to assess an individual's susceptibility to autoimmune diseases (Sundaresan et al., 2023).
- Infectious Diseases: Genetic susceptibility to infectious diseases such as HIV/AIDS, malaria, tuberculosis, and hepatitis C has been investigated using DNA data. These models identify host genetic factors that influence susceptibility to infection, disease progression, and response to treatment or vaccination (Xu et al., 2023).
- Rare Genetic Disorders: DNA sequencing technologies enable the identification of rare genetic variants responsible for rare genetic disorders such as cystic fibrosis, Huntington's disease, and muscular dystrophy. Predictive models use genetic information to assess an individual's risk of inheriting these disorders or passing them on to offspring (Yamamoto et al., 2024).
- Psychiatric Disorders: DNA-based prediction models have been developed for psychiatric disorders such as schizophrenia, bipolar disorder, and major depressive disorder. These models analyze genetic variants associated with neurotransmitter signaling, synaptic function, and neural development to predict disease risk and treatment response (Kouter et al., 2023).
- Metabolic Disorders: Genetic predisposition to metabolic disorders such as diabetes, obesity, and metabolic syndrome can be assessed using DNA-based prediction models. These models incorporate genetic variants related to insulin sensitivity, glucose metabolism, and adipose tissue regulation (Khotina et al., 2023).

4. METHODOLOGY

Predicting disease using DNA data with deep learning involves several steps (Li et al., 2024; Yuan et al., 2024; Zeng et al., 2024). Here's a detailed outline of the process:

Data Collection

Gather DNA sequencing data from individuals. This may include whole-genome sequencing (WGS), whole-exome sequencing (WES), or targeted sequencing data.
Collect associated metadata such as clinical information, demographic data, and disease labels (if available).

Data Preprocessing

Quality control: Remove low-quality sequences, filter out sequencing artifacts, and handle missing values.

Data normalization

Normalize the sequencing data to account for variations in sequencing depth and coverage.

Feature extraction

Extract relevant features from the DNA sequences, such as nucleotide sequence patterns, genomic variants (e.g., single nucleotide polymorphisms - SNPs), or functional annotations.

Data augmentation (optional)

Augment the dataset to increase its diversity and improve model generalization. This may involve techniques such as adding noise, flipping sequences, or generating synthetic data.

Model Selection

Choose an appropriate deep learning architecture for the task. Common architectures for DNA sequence analysis include convolutional neural networks (CNNs), recurrent neural networks (RNNs), and transformer-based models.Consider factors such as the size of the dataset, the complexity of the task, and computational resources when selecting the model architecture.

Model Training

Split the dataset into training, validation, and test sets.
Train the deep learning model using the training data. During training, the model learns to map DNA sequences to disease labels or predictions.
Optimize model hyperparameters (e.g., learning rate, batch size, number of layers) using techniques such as grid search or random search.
Monitor training progress using metrics such as loss function values and validation accuracy.

Model Evaluation

Evaluate the trained model using the validation set to assess its performance.
Calculate evaluation metrics such as accuracy, precision, recall, F1-score, and area under the receiver operating characteristic curve (AUC-ROC).
Adjust model parameters or architecture based on validation results if necessary.

Model Interpretation

Interpret the trained model to understand how it makes predictions. This may involve analyzing learned features, identifying important genomic regions or variants, and visualizing model predictions.

Use interpretation techniques such as saliency maps, attention mechanisms, or feature importance scores to gain insights into the model's decision-making process.

Model Deployment

Deploy the trained model for disease prediction on new, unseen data.
Integrate the model into a user-friendly interface or application for clinical use, if applicable.
Monitor model performance in real-world settings and update the model as needed to maintain accuracy and reliability.

Ethical and Regulatory Considerations

Consider ethical implications related to privacy, consent, and data security when handling genomic data.
Ensure compliance with regulatory requirements such as HIPAA (Health Insurance Portability and Accountability Act) and GDPR (General Data Protection Regulation) when collecting and storing patient data.

By following these steps, researchers and practitioners can develop accurate and robust deep learning models for disease prediction using DNA data, paving the way for improved diagnosis, prognosis, and personalized treatment strategies.

5. COMPOSITION OF DNA PREDICTION AND CLASSIFICATION WITH DEEP LEARNING

DNA-based deep learning refers to the application of deep learning techniques to analyze DNA sequences and extract meaningful patterns or insights. Deep learning, a subset of machine learning, involves training neural networks with multiple layers to automatically learn hierarchical representations of data. When applied to DNA sequences, deep learning models can identify sequence motifs, predict functional elements, classify sequences into different categories (e.g., disease vs. healthy), and perform various other tasks related to genomic analysis.

- Data Representation: DNA sequences are typically represented as strings of nucleotides (A, T, C, and G). Each nucleotide is encoded as a numerical value (e.g., one-hot encoding or numerical encoding) to serve as input to the deep learning model.
- Model Architecture: Deep learning architectures such as convolutional neural networks (CNNs), recurrent neural networks (RNNs), and transformer-based models can be adapted for DNA sequence analysis. CNNs are effective for capturing local sequence patterns, RNNs can capture sequential dependencies, and transformer-based models excel at capturing long-range dependencies and interactions.
- Tasks: DNA-based deep learning models can be applied to various tasks, including but not limited to:
- Sequence classification: Predicting biological properties or functions associated with DNA sequences (e.g., promoter prediction, enhancer prediction, splice site prediction).

- Sequence regression: Predicting quantitative outputs based on DNA sequences (e.g., gene expression levels, DNA methylation levels).
- Sequence generation: Generating novel DNA sequences with desired properties (e.g., designing synthetic promoters, optimizing CRISPR guide sequences).
- Sequence similarity search: Identifying similar sequences within a large database (e.g., homology search, sequence alignment).
- Training: Deep learning models are trained using large datasets of labeled DNA sequences. The model learns to map input DNA sequences to their corresponding labels (e.g., functional annotations, disease status) by minimizing a loss function using optimization algorithms such as stochastic gradient descent (SGD) or Adam.
- Interpretability: Interpretability of deep learning models in DNA sequence analysis is an active area of research. Techniques such as attention mechanisms, saliency maps, and feature visualization can help elucidate which parts of the DNA sequence are most influential for model predictions.
- Applications: DNA-based deep learning has diverse applications in genomics, bioinformatics, and personalized medicine. It can aid in understanding the genetic basis of diseases, identifying regulatory elements in the genome, designing therapeutic interventions, and facilitating precision medicine initiatives.
- In this framework, the deep learning model functions as a high-capacity pattern learner, while association rule mining serves as a post-analytic knowledge discovery layer, enabling clinicians to interpret genomic risk factors through explicit rules.

6. SUMMARY OF TECHNIQUES

The following table emphasis DNA disease prediction and classification with various deep learning models. The model used and remarks of each model are given in the below Table 1.

Table 1. Summarize the techniques used to analyze DNA images to predict diseases

References	Medical Image Processing Technique / Disease Prediction Technique	Remarks
(Angermueller, 2016)	Deep Learning Techniques	Predicts DNA mutation effects and analyzes tissue images
(Rav, 2017)	Recurrent Neural Network	Provide training samples that have strong inter-dependencies and analyzes stream of data
(Angermueller, 2017)	Recurrent Neural Network	predict methylation states in individual cells and learn the relationship between DNA sequence
(Ker et al., 2017)	Genetic Adversarial Network (GAN) Convolutional Neural Network	Identify the abnormalities in a cell Process 2D and 3D images
(Lello, 2019)	LASSO Algorithm	Performs cross validation technique, predict diseases based on polygenic score
(Chandrasekar et al., 2020)	Micro Array techniques, Multi Layer Perceptron	Represents DNA sequence as micro array techniques, predict diseases based on Deep learning techniques
(Öztürk et al., 2020)	Artificial Bee Colony algorithm	Provide global optimization
(Gunasekaran et al., 2021)	CNN-Bidirectional LSTM	Uses label and K-mer encoding to detect DNA sequence
(Jyothi & Ajitha, 2021)	Support Vector Machine and other algorithms	Represent DNA sequence as micro array technique, conclude that SVM has more accuracy
(Ye et al., 2021)	DNN and Mash Up	Reduce the dimensionality of PPI, predict the genes related to aging diseases
(Vineela, 2022)	GDA Model	Propose a hybrid model of random forest, Decision Tree algorithms
(Reham, 2022)	Chameleon swarm algorithm (CSA)	Propose a new technique for feature selection
(Raza, 2023)	Multi-Label Multi-Class Chain Classifier Approach	Predicts the order of specified chain
(Muruga Priya, 2023)	PSO method and KNN Classification	Address the importance of gene ranking and selection prior to classification
(Rajesh, 2023)	Chameleon swarm algorithm (CSA)	Propose a 3D CNN networks for volume segmentation

CONCLUSION

In conclusion, the integration of deep learning techniques with DNA analysis represents a transformative approach in genomics and bioinformatics. By leveraging the power of neural networks to learn complex patterns from DNA sequences, researchers have unlocked new opportunities for understanding the genetic basis of diseases, predicting functional elements in the genome, and advancing personalized medicine. The various deep models have demonstrated remarkable performance in tasks such as sequence classification, regression, generation, and similarity search, enabling a wide range of applications in genomics and beyond. However, challenges remain, particularly in the interpretation and generalization of deep learning models in DNA analysis. Ensuring the reliability, interpretability, and ethical use of these models is essential for their successful integration into biomedical research and clinical practice. Despite these challenges, the potential of DNA-based deep learning to revolutionize healthcare is undeniable. By harnessing the vast wealth of genomic data and combining it with sophisticated machine learning techniques, we can accelerate discoveries, develop targeted therapies, and ultimately improve patient outcomes. By integrating association rule mining as a complementary interpretability mechanism, this chapter bridges the gap between high-performance deep learning models and clinically actionable knowledge discovery, aligning predictive accuracy with explainability requirements in precision medicine. As the field continues to evolve, collaborative efforts between researchers, clinicians, bioinformaticians, and ethicists will be crucial for realizing the full potential of DNA-based deep learning in advancing human health and well-being. With continued innovation and interdisciplinary collaboration, DNA-based deep learning promises to shape the future of personalized medicine and genomic research.

REFERENCES

Angermueller, C.. (2016, July). Deep learning for computational biology. *Molecular Systems Biology*, •••, 29. PMID: 27474269

Angermueller, C.. (2017, April). Deepcpg: Accurate prediction of single-cell DNA methylation states using deep learning. *Genome Biology*.

Chandrasekar, V., Sureshkumar, V., Kumar, T. S., & Shanmugapriya, S. (2020, September). Disease Prediction Based On Micro Array Classification Using Deep Learning Techniques. *Microprocessors and Microsystems*, *77*, 103189. DOI: 10.1016/j.micpro.2020.103189

Elwahsh, H., Tawfeek, M. A., Abd El-Aziz, A. A., Mahmood, M. A., Alsabaan, M., & El-shafeiy, E. (2023). A new approach for cancer prediction based on deep neural learning. *Journal of King Saud University. Computer and Information Sciences*, *35*(6), 101565. DOI: 10.1016/j.jksuci.2023.101565

Gaitsch, H., Franklin, R. J., & Reich, D. S. (2023). Cell-free DNA-based liquid biopsies in neurology. *Brain*, *146*(5), 1758–1774. DOI: 10.1093/brain/awac438 PMID: 36408894

. Goel, H., Goyal, K., Pandey, A. K., Benjamin, M., Khan, F., Pandey, P., ... & Upadhyay, T. K. (2023). Elucidations of molecular mechanism and mechanistic effects of environmental toxicants in neurological disorders. *CNS & Neurological Disorders-Drug Targets (Formerly Current Drug Targets-CNS & Neurological Disorders)*, *22*(1), 84-97.

Gong, P., Cheng, L., Zhang, Z., Meng, A., Li, E., Chen, J., & Zhang, L. (2023). Multi-omics integration method based on attention deep learning network for biomedical data classification. *Computer Methods and Programs in Biomedicine*, *231*, 107377. DOI: 10.1016/j.cmpb.2023.107377 PMID: 36739624

Gunasekaran, H., Ramalakshmi, K., Rex Macedo Arokiaraj, A., Deepa Kanmani, S., Venkatesan, C., & Suresh Gnana Dhas, C. (2021). Analysis of DNA sequence classification using CNN and hybrid models. *Computational and Mathematical Methods in Medicine*, *2021*(1), 1835056.

Hossain, P. S., Kim, K., Uddin, J., Samad, M. A., & Choi, K. (2023). Enhancing Taxonomic Categorization of DNA Sequences with Deep Learning: A Multi-Label Approach. *Bioengineering (Basel, Switzerland)*, *10*(11), 1293. DOI: 10.3390/bioengineering10111293 PMID: 38002417

Jyothi, P., & Ajitha, P. (2021, December). Computerized Prediction of Hereditary Diseases Through DNA Sequence Using Support Vector Machine (SVM). In 2021 5th International Conference on Electronics, Communication and Aerospace Technology (ICECA) (pp. 953-958). IEEE.

Ker, J., Wang, L., Rao, J., & Lim, T. (2017). Deep learning applications in medical image analysis. *IEEE Access : Practical Innovations, Open Solutions*, *6*, 9375–9389.

Khotina, V. A., Vinokurov, A. Y., Bagheri Ekta, M., Sukhorukov, V. N., & Orekhov, A. N. (2023). Creation of mitochondrial disease models using mitochondrial DNA editing. *Biomedicines*, *11*(2), 532. DOI: 10.3390/biomedicines11020532 PMID: 36831068

Kouter, K., Arčan, I. Š., & Paska, A. V. (2023). Epigenetics in psychiatry: Beyond DNA methylation. *World Journal of Psychiatry*, *13*(6), 319–330. DOI: 10.5498/wjp.v13.i6.319 PMID: 37383287

Krolevets, M., Cate, V. T., Prochaska, J. H., Schulz, A., Rapp, S., Tenzer, S., Andrade-Navarro, M. A., Horvath, S., Niehrs, C., & Wild, P. S. (2023). DNA methylation and cardiovascular disease in humans: A systematic review and database of known CpG methylation sites. *Clinical Epigenetics*, *15*(1), 56. DOI: 10.1186/s13148-023-01468-y PMID: 36991458

Lello, L.. (2019, November). Genomic Prediction of 16 Complex Disease Risks Including Heart Attack, Diabetes, Breast and Prostate Cancer. *Scientific Reports*.

Li, J., Chiu, T. P., & Rohs, R. (2024). Predicting DNA structure using a deep learning method. *Nature Communications*, *15*(1), 1243. DOI: 10.1038/s41467-024-45191-5 PMID: 38336958

Li, S., Zeng, W., Ni, X., Liu, Q., Li, W., Stackpole, M. L., Zhou, Y., Gower, A., Krysan, K., Ahuja, P., Lu, D. S., Raman, S. S., Hsu, W., Aberle, D. R., Magyar, C. E., French, S. W., Han, S.-H. B., Garon, E. B., Agopian, V. G., & Zhou, X. J. (2023). Comprehensive tissue deconvolution of cell-free DNA by deep learning for disease diagnosis and monitoring. *Proceedings of the National Academy of Sciences of the United States of America*, *120*(28), e2305236120. DOI: 10.1073/pnas.2305236120 PMID: 37399400

Muruga Priya, P.. "Microarray based Disease Prediction using Deep Learning Techniques", *7th International Conference on Computing Methodologies and Communication (ICCMC)*, 23-25 Feb. 2023.

Naue, J. (2023). Getting the chronological age out of DNA: Using insights of age-dependent DNA methylation for forensic DNA applications. *Genes & Genomics*, *45*(10), 1239–1261. DOI: 10.1007/s13258-023-01392-8 PMID: 37253906

Rajasekar, V., Vaishnnave, M. P., Premkumar, S., Sarveshwaran, V., & Rangaraaj, V. (2023). Lung cancer disease prediction with CT scan and histopathological images feature analysis using deep learning techniques. *Results in Engineering*, *18*, 101111. DOI: 10.1016/j.rineng.2023.101111

Rajesh, C.. (2023, November). An evolutionary Chameleon Swarm Algorithm based network for 3D medical image segmentation. *Expert Systems with Applications*, *239*, •••.

Rav, D.. (2017, January). Deep Learning for Health Informatics. *IEEE Journal of Biomedical and Health Informatics*, *21*(1), •••. PMID: 28055930

Ravindran, U., & Gunavathi, C. (2023). A survey on gene expression data analysis using deep learning methods for cancer diagnosis. *Progress in Biophysics and Molecular Biology*, *177*, 1–13. DOI: 10.1016/j.pbiomolbio.2022.08.004 PMID: 35988771

Raza, A.. (2023, January). Predicting Genetic Disorder and Types of Disorder Using Chain Classifier Approach. *Genes*. PMID: 36672812

Reham, R.. (2022, June). Boosting chameleon swarm algorithm with consumption AEO operator for global optimization and feature selection. *Knowledge-Based Systems*, *246*, •••.

Öztürk, Ş., Ahmad, R., & Akhtar, N. (2020). Variants of Artificial Bee Colony algorithm and its applications in medical image processing. *Applied Soft Computing*, *97*, 106799.

Sundaresan, B., Shirafkan, F., Ripperger, K., & Rattay, K. (2023). The role of viral infections in the onset of autoimmune diseases. *Viruses*, *15*(3), 782. DOI: 10.3390/v15030782 PMID: 36992490

Tarekegn, A. N., Ullah, M., & Cheikh, F. A. (2024). Deep Learning for Multi-Label Learning: A Comprehensive Survey. *arXiv preprint arXiv:2401.16549.*

Vineela, M., ... (2022). "Prediction of Genetic Diseases Based On DNA", Journal of Engineering Sciences Vol 13 Issue 07, JULY/2022 ISSN:0377-9254

Xu, C., Chen, X., Zhu, G., Yi, H., Chen, S., Yu, Y., Jiang, E., Zheng, Y., Zhang, F., Wang, J., & Feng, S. (2023). Utility of plasma cell-free DNA next-generation sequencing for diagnosis of infectious diseases in patients with hematological disorders. *The Journal of Infection*, *86*(1), 14–23. DOI: 10.1016/j.jinf.2022.11.020 PMID: 36462587

Yamamoto, S., Kanca, O., Wangler, M. F., & Bellen, H. J. (2024). Integrating non-mammalian model organisms in the diagnosis of rare genetic diseases in humans. *Nature Reviews. Genetics*, *25*(1), 46–60. DOI: 10.1038/s41576-023-00633-6 PMID: 37491400

Ye, J., Wang, S., Yang, X., & Tang, X. (2021, December). Gene prediction of aging related diseases based on DNN and Mashup. *BMC Bioinformatics*, *22*(1), 17. DOI: 10.1186/s12859-021-04518-5 PMID: 34920719

Yin, F., Zhao, H., Lu, S., Shen, J., Li, M., Mao, X., Li, F., Shi, J., Li, J., Dong, B., Xue, W., Zuo, X., Yang, X., & Fan, C. (2023). DNA-framework-based multidimensional molecular classifiers for cancer diagnosis. *Nature Nanotechnology*, *18*(6), 677–686. DOI: 10.1038/s41565-023-01348-9 PMID: 36973399

Yuan, T., Wu, L., Li, S., Zheng, J., Li, N., Xiao, X., Zhang, H., Fei, T., Xie, L., Zuo, Z., Li, D., Huang, P., Feng, H., Cao, Y., Yan, N., Wei, X., Shi, L., Sun, Y., Wei, W., & Zuo, E. (2024). Deep learning models incorporating endogenous factors beyond DNA sequences improve the prediction accuracy of base editing outcomes. *Cell Discovery*, *10*(1), 20. DOI: 10.1038/s41421-023-00624-1 PMID: 38378648

Zeng, C., Jian, Y., Zhuo, C., Li, A., Zeng, C., & Zhao, Y. (2024). Evaluation of DNA–protein complex structures using the deep learning method. *Physical Chemistry Chemical Physics*, *26*(1), 130–143. DOI: 10.1039/D3CP04980A PMID: 38063012

Chapter 9
Integrating Deep Learning With Association Rule Mining for Liver Tumor Classification in Medical Imaging

K. Ramalakshmi
http://orcid.org/0000-0002-3038-643X
P.S.R. Engineering College, India

Vinod Kumar Shukla
Amity University, Dubai, UAE

P. Sabeena Burvin
Ramco Institute of Technology, India

N. Ismayil Kani
AMET University, India

L. Krishna Kumari
Ramco Institute of Technology, India

ABSTRACT

Liver tumors, whether benign or malignant, present a serious clinical challenge, making accurate classification vital for early detection and effective treatment. This study proposes an AI-driven framework combining advanced image preprocessing with a VGG16-based deep learning model, achieving 98.75% classification accuracy.

DOI: 10.4018/979-8-3373-6691-3.ch009

Median filtering enhances image clarity and preserves key features for deep feature extraction. The classified outputs are then integrated into Association Rule Mining (ARM), converting them into transaction-style datasets to uncover meaningful rules linking tumor types with imaging biomarkers, demographics, and treatment outcomes. This two-stage approach not only ensures high precision in tumor classification but also yields interpretable rules for clinical decision support, helping bridge the gap between black-box AI and real-world medical imaging applications.

INTRODUCTION

The strange escalation of cells in the liver, either benign or malignant, is known as liver tumor. Categorizing liver tumors is decisivebecause it leads treatment verdicts, assists in predicting the type of tumor, and patient outcomes. Accurate categorization facilitatesadapted treatment approaches, ensuing in stronger pharmaceuticals and succeeding the learning of hepatocellular cancer. Gaining an understanding of the topography of hepatic tumors is crucial to improving diagnostic accuracy and adjusting patient management. In the arena of medical imaging, precisecategorization of liver tumors is crucial for effective diagnosis and therapy. This work examines a novel technique for reducing liver tumor image resolution to the standard 256x256. By reducing noise and preserving crucial information, the preprocessing step of taking images is enhanced when a median filter is used.Our study uses the reliable VGG16 deep learning configuration to upturn the accuracy and consistency of liver tumor categorization. Our objective is to enhance patient outcomes in the diagnosis of hepatocellular carcinoma by optimizing diagnostic procedures through an innovative blend of preprocessing, deep learning, and image resizing.

Figure 1. Sample liver tumor images from the dataset

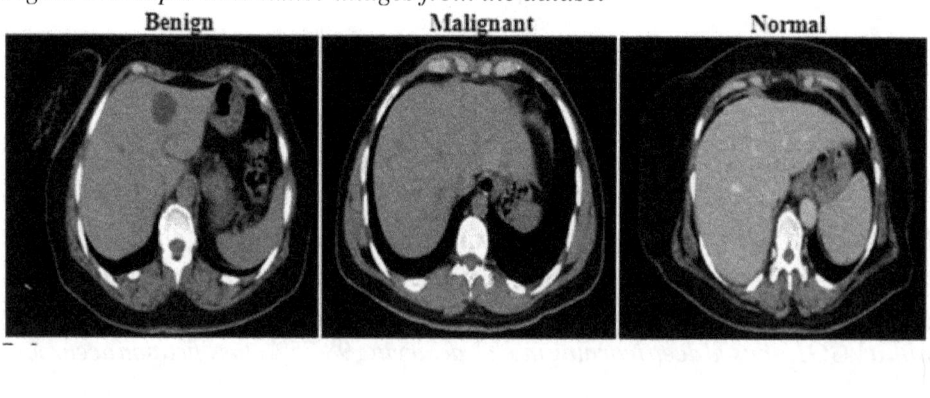

Figure 1 illustrates the sample liver tumor images in the dataset. Although liver tumor diagnosis might be difficult at times, CT is a helpful tool. Under some conditions, physicians can differentiate between benign and malignant tumors. The blood arteries around the liver and the possibility of liver disease spreading to other organs can be examined. 75–80% of instances of hepatocellular carcinoma (HCC) worldwide are reported to be from Asia (Ojala et al., 2002). Beaufrère et al. (2024) suggested utilizing the ResNet18 neural network to automatically classify primary liver tumors on routinely stained biopsies. Lopez-Terrada et al. (2014) analyzed different methods of Pediatric Liver Tumors Consensus Classification. A classifier based on microRNAenvisages the crucialtumorlocation of liver biopsies, which contains a restricted number of tumor cells, was developed and validated by Perell et al. (2015). A statistical model was utilized to account for typical contamination of liver tissue. Cross-validation was used to evaluate performance. An independent validation of this model revealed acomplete accuracy of 74.5%. With a 92% prediction accuracy rate, 38.2% was the accuracy of a classifier that was trained without taking liver tissue contamination into account.Nine concepts were grouped into three broad categories. Early risk assessment and prevention is an important one particularly with regard to viral hepatitis and other lifestyle factors. This is leading to an increase in financing for liver abrasioninvestigation, screening, and treatment. This work substantially expands the corpus of knowledge that serves as the foundation for developing an evidence-based strategy to assess readiness for putting in place all-encompassing safeguards against liver lesions. It is imperative to evaluate the degree to which each nation meets the established norms. Subsequent research endeavours aim to investigate the variances in resource requirements among nations in order to ascertain the optimal approaches for enhancing the diagnostic and prognosis of liver lesion patients worldwide (Mahbod et al., 2019). Zhou et al. (2021) developed a hybridized fully convolutional network, which is capable of accurately evaluating the loss function across the entire object partition through effective inference and learning. Higher image resolution is achieved because the network practices entire images instead of patches, removing the need to select procreative patches and avoiding duplicate approximations brought on by patch intersection. Furthermore, links that integrate the suprememodernfinding with inferior layers, containingimprovedinformation, can be used to blend scales. There are many different scales at which this form of fusion can be combined. The foremostrole of the learning is the diagnostic heat map of lesions that is seen in the CNNs as a result of the liver partition and categorization. This method creates an ensemble segmentation system based on deep learning to effectively classify and segment liver tumors. The investigationaloutcomesillustrate that the suggested DenseNet CNN accomplishes well on the dataset (Condori et al., 2021). Ramalakshmi and Srinivasa Raghavan

(2023) proposed yields greater performances for medical images classification using deep neural networks.

MRI is now used in a few methods for classifying brain tumors: One method for identifying brain tumors centered on deep CNN and MRI data is the MRI-based deep learning methodology (Haq et al., 2023). Whereas the subsequent design distinguished amongstsuperior and inferior gliomas, the first architecture categorized brain tumors as either meningiomas, pituitary tumors, or gliomas. A framework for effective brain tumor classification is the alternative strategy. This framework classified brain tumors using a variety of methods, including feature extraction and image segmentation. The goal of the study was to use MRI data to classify brain tumors more accurately and efficiently. A hybridized completely CNN based technique for liver tumor identification has been presented by Dong et al. (2020). It trained the model to identify tumors using CT scans as input, retrieved voxel attributes, and so forth.

This study introduces an innovative technique for liver tumor classification by merging sophisticated preprocessing methods with the VGG16 deep learning framework. Image scaling to 256x256 pixels and median filtering significantly improve image clarity, facilitating accurate feature extraction. The approach attains a remarkable accuracy of 98.75%, showcasing exceptional efficacy in differentiating tumor areas in medical imaging.

Deep learningbased classification also serves as a precursor to effective association rule mining in medical data. Once tumor images are accurately categorized, ARM techniques can be applied to discover frequent patterns and correlations between tumor types, demographic data, genetic profiles, and treatment outcomes. This combined framework not only enhances diagnostic workflows but also supports knowledge-driven clinical decision-making. Thus, the classification stage contributes directly to building robust datasets for ARM, ensuring rules are derived from reliable and precise inputs.In this chapter, we highlight not only the role of deep learning in liver tumor classification but also how its structured outputs can be systematically integrated with association rule mining (ARM). ARM extends the utility of classification results by uncovering hidden patterns between imaging biomarkers, tumor characteristics, and patient clinical profiles. This integration reflects an emerging trend in AI-driven healthcare, where predictive modeling is combined with interpretable rule discovery to bridge the gap between automated diagnosis and transparent clinical decision-making.This work's remaining sections are arranged as follows: In Section 2, the approaches that are currently employed in this field of study are illustrated. In the subsequent section 3, a brief conversation of the suggested methodology for using a densely connected neural network approach to detect liver anomalies is provided. Results and performances are discussed in section 4. Conclusion and future directions are included in section 5.

RELATED WORKS

Digital image processing has presented numerous contemporary research problems to the field of biology in recent years. Tasks including tumor diagnosis and categorization, identification and recognition of malignant regions, and testing and inspection of vital human body parts fall under this category. Among the various challenges facing medical research, computerized diagnosis and localization must be the most crucial, and efforts must be made to address this issue (Anuja et al., 2021). Instead of depending on trends, machine learning (ML) uses algorithmic analysis and mathematics to carry out tasks without the need for explicit instructions. In machine intelligence, picture analysis commonly makes use of machine learning techniques. It can be categorized as unsupervised or supervised. Supervised learning utilizes an algorithm to generate a role that records input/outputs, which is subsequently utilized to forecast markers for potential suggestions. The primary objective is to use techniques such as KNN, SVM and ANN to acquirereliantvalues from the output. In contrast, unsupervised learning relies solely on input parameters like fuzzy c-means and k-means. The training data's texture, statistical, and grayscale features must be extracted in order to create learning; however, in most situations, tumor localization must occur before the extraction process (Sajjaa & Kalluri, 2021). Lakshmipriya et al. (2023) reviewed different deep learning methods for liver tumor classification. Ramalakshmi and Srinivasa Raghavan (2021) proposed deep multinomial logarithmic image classification with anisotropic filtering preprocessing for prediction of diseases in medical images. Zhao et al. (2023) suggested a unified end to end module with nested feature extraction for liver lesions classification.

Simonyan and Zisserman (2014) investigated how network depth impacts accuracy in large-scale photo identification. The main contribution here is a detailed investigation of topologies used to networks of different complexities that use progressively smaller convolution filters (3 × 3). It shows that by raising the quantity of layers to certain level, notable enhancements can be obtained with the earlier methods. Additionally, they show that on various datasets, their universal representations yield cutting-edge results. The public release of two of their best-performing neural networktechniques aims at encouraging more investigation into the application of deep visual representations in computer vision. Decision tree (DT) based classifier was used by Das et al. (2019) to identify liver cancer. After dividing the liver from the rest of the body using adaptive thresholding, spatial fuzzy clustering was utilised to segment the liver's cancerous lesions. The useful features were retrieved from the segmented cancerous region and classified into two types of liver malignancies, HCC, and metastatic carcinoma, using multilayer perceptron (MLP) and C4.5 DT classifiers. Ramalakshmi and Srinivasa Raghavan (2023) uilized a hybrid of the Unet and ResUNet models for segmenting liver tumor with 98% accuracy.

Nanda Prakash et al. (2023) proposed a DenseNet CNN-based method for classifying liver tumors. DenseNet CNN is used for training, and preprocessing is done by region based segmentation. The accuracy and detection rate of the results produced using the suggested methodology are 93.41% and 98.34%, respectively. According to the comparison data, the suggested strategy performs better than the other pioneering methodologies and achieves greater accuracy. Alici-Karaca et al. (2022) suggested introduced lightweight CNN architecture for liver tumor classification and yielded an accuracy of 87.57%. Manjunath and Kwadiki (2022) suggested deep learning procedure for spontaneous liver and tumor partition from CT images.

Convolutional Neural Networks (CNNs) have become the dominant approach for medical image prediction due to their strong capability to learn hierarchical feature representations from complex imaging data. Recent surveys have shown that CNN-based architectures, combined with transfer learning and multimodal fusion strategies, consistently achieve high accuracy across a wide range of medical imaging tasks, including disease detection, classification, and prognosis prediction [2]. Despite these advances, the limited interpretability of deep learning models remains a critical barrier to their widespread adoption in clinical decision-making environments.

To address this challenge, recent research has increasingly explored the integration of deep learning models with interpretable data mining techniques. In the context of clinical decision support systems, Wu et al. (2025) proposed an intelligent prediction framework that integrates temporal association rules (TARs) with machine learning models for metabolic dysfunction-associated fatty liver disease. Their work demonstrates that association rule mining can enhance model transparency by capturing clinically meaningful temporal patterns and embedding domain knowledge through human-in-the-loop evaluation. Although this approach primarily focuses on longitudinal clinical data, it highlights the potential of association rule mining to bridge the gap between predictive accuracy and interpretability.

Parallel efforts in medical image analysis have focused on improving the representational power of CNNs for image mining and retrieval. Models such as EffNet-CNN extend standard CNN architectures through architectural refinements and optimized feature extraction strategies, achieving strong performance in image classification and content-based image retrieval tasks [4]. Similarly, deep residual networks combined with data mining techniques and attention mechanisms have been shown to significantly improve image retrieval accuracy and feature discrimination [6]. While these studies demonstrate the effectiveness of CNNs for image mining, they largely emphasize performance optimization rather than explainable clinical knowledge discovery.

More recently, interpretable deep learning approaches have been proposed to enhance transparency in medical image prediction. For example, saliency-consistent contrastive learning frameworks generate clinically relevant saliency maps to support trust and interpretability in brain tissue classification [5]. Although such methods improve explainability at the model level, they do not explicitly support rule-based reasoning or knowledge extraction that can be directly used in clinical decision support systems.

In contrast to existing approaches, the framework proposed in this chapter combines CNN-based liver tumor classification with association rule mining to enable post-hoc interpretability and knowledge discovery. High-confidence predictions produced by the CNN are transformed into transaction-style datasets, allowing association rule mining to uncover meaningful relationships between tumor classes, imaging features, patient demographics, and treatment outcomes. By integrating deep learning with interpretable data mining, the proposed approach aligns with emerging trends in explainable artificial intelligence and intelligent decision support systems, offering a balanced solution that delivers both high diagnostic accuracy and clinically actionable insights.

The goal of this work is to fill the gap left by earlier research. Previous research has employed convolutional network architecture to support multi-magnification input while simultaneously furnishing cell structure details pertaining to low-magnification regions. The researchers in the current study are attempting VGG based on the convolution network in light of prior research and the regions in which it fell short. The research methodology is intended to match the expectations for the classification of liver tumors with greater accuracy.Although prior research has explored CNNs and hybrid deep learning models for tumor detection, limited attention has been given to how these outputs can fuel downstream association rule mining. By embedding classification into the broader AI-driven medical knowledge discovery pipeline, this work contributes to a relatively underexplored but crucial domain: using AI to generate interpretable and actionable rules from imaging data.

MATERIALS AND METHODS

Dataset Characteristics

The dataset used in this study consists of contrast-enhanced liver CT images collected from clinically confirmed cases. The dataset includes three classes: normal liver tissue, benign tumors, and malignant tumors. Images were acquired using standardized CT protocols with varying slice thickness and contrast phases to reflect real-world clinical diversity. All images were resized to 256×256 pixels to ensure uniform input dimensions for the VGG16 network. The dataset was divided into training, validation, and testing subsets to ensure unbiased performance evaluation.

Patient identifiers were anonymized prior to analysis, ensuring compliance with ethical and data protection guidelines.

PROPOSED METHODOLOGY

VGG16 and median filtering both progress the classification performance of liver tumors. Toadvance image quality and reduce noise, median filtering preprocesses images by substituting the median value in each pixel's neighbourhood. This can help VGG16 extract features more effectively. VGG16 collects high-level characteristics from preprocessed images thanks to its deep architecture. The process of liver tumor classification is illustrated in Figure 2.

With the help of median filtering, VGG16 is able to precisely collect more pertinent tumor features in noise-free images. Because of the hierarchical representation of VGG16, itis able to learn complex patterns in the images, including subtle aspects of the tumor that are easier to identify from filtered images. When combined, median filtering and VGG16 improve the quality of the images through preprocessing, and VGG16 effectively uses the improved images for precise tumor classification.

Figure 2. Block diagram of liver tumor classification

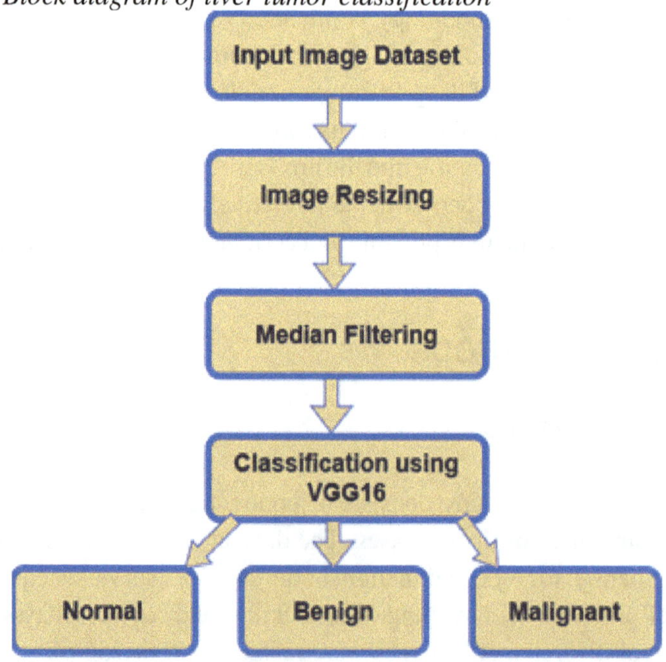

The block diagram presents a systematic pipeline for liver tumor classification using VGG16 and median filtering. It begins with an input image dataset consisting of liver CT scans. These images are first resized to a standardized dimension suitable for the VGG16 model. Next, median filtering is applied to the resized images to reduce noise—particularly salt-and-pepper noise—while preserving important structural details such as edges. The preprocessed images are then fed into a VGG16-based deep convolutional neural network for feature extraction and classification. The final classification stage categorizes each image into one of three classes: Normal, Benign, or Malignant. This process enhances diagnostic accuracy by improving image quality and leveraging deep learning for reliable classification. The use of median filtering strengthens the model's robustness to image noise, while VGG16's architecture ensures effective hierarchical feature learning. Overall, the pipeline provides an efficient and automated approach for liver tumor diagnosis from medical images. The accuracy of liver tumor classification can be greatly increased by combining the prevailing feature extraction proficiencies of VGG16 with noise reduction capabilities of median filtering. This will ultimately result in more accurate diagnosis and treatment choices.

The preprocessing pipeline not only enhances classification accuracy but also ensures consistency in feature representation, which is vital for ARM. Association rules derived from medical data rely on standardized, noise-reduced inputs; hence, the combination of median filtering and VGG16 provides a stable foundation for mining associations between imaging biomarkers and clinical outcomes.

Algorithm

Liver Tumor Classification Using VGG16
Step 1:Loading Input image Dataset
Step 2: Resize the input images
Step 3: Apply median filtering

Step 4: Splitting of training and testing data
for each epoch in epoch Number do
    for each batch in batch Size do
        Classification = model(training feature generation)
        loss = categorical cross entropy (actual, predict)
        adam Optimizer (loss, learning rate)
evaluation
    end for
end for
Step 5:return

Association Rule Mining Framework

Following classification with VGG16, the outputs were augmented with clinical and imaging attributes, including tumor size, boundary texture, biomarker levels (e.g., AFP), and patient demographics. These enriched records formed a transaction-style dataset suitable for ARM. We employed Apriori and FP-Growth algorithms to identify frequent itemsets and generate rules with minimum support $\geq 20\%$ and confidence $\geq 80\%$. The goal was to derive interpretable rules that link imaging findings with clinical outcomes, providing actionable knowledge for risk stratification and treatment planning.

Median Filtering

Median filtering was chosen as the preprocessing technique for this work due to its effectiveness in reducing noise while preserving important image details such as edges and boundaries. Medical images, particularly CT scans, often contain various types of noise introduced during acquisition or transmission, such as salt-and-pepper noise. Unlike linear filters that tend to blur the image, median filtering is a non-linear technique that replaces each pixel's value with the median of its neighborhood. This approach effectively removes outliers and random noise without significantly distorting the structural features of the tumor regions, which are critical for accurate classification.

The contribution of median filtering in this work is significant, as it enhances the quality of the input images before they are fed into the VGG16 network. By removing noise, the filter ensures that the deep learning model focuses on relevant anatomical features rather than artifacts. This improves the clarity and contrast of the tumor regions, aiding in better feature extraction by the CNN. Additionally, the enhanced image quality leads to faster convergence during training and improved generalization on unseen data. The classification results demonstrate higher accuracy and sensitivity when median filtering is applied, indicating its positive impact. Overall, median filtering serves as a crucial preprocessing step that boosts the reliability and performance of the liver tumor classification pipeline.

Median filtering improves the contrast of tumor forms by enhancing the homogeneities within the regions of liver and cancer tissue and preserving the boundaries between them. Median filtering is a nonlinear method of reducing noise from photos. It is frequently used because it successfully eliminates noise while maintaining edges. Noise of the "salt and pepper" variety is especially well-admitted with this technique. The median filter works by comparing each value in the image, pixel by pixel, with the median value of pixels that are close by. The "window" is an arrangement of nearby pixels that shifts pixel by pixel over the whole picture.

$$O(p) = Median(I(p), I(p1), I(p2), \ldots I(pn))$$

---- (1)

The filtering window's central pixel, denoted by p, has an intensity value of I(p), while the bordering pixels' intensity values are represented by I(p1), I(p2),…,I(pn). The middle value of a sorted list of intensity values within the window is returned by the median function.Median filtering operation is represented in Figure 3 and 4.

Figure 3. Median filtering operation

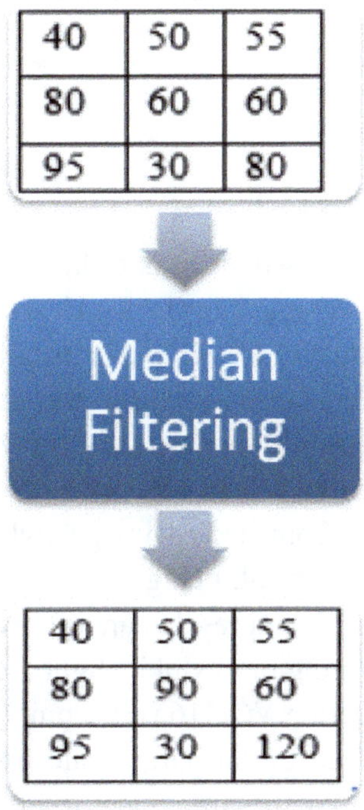

Figure 4. Input and output images output of Median filtering operation

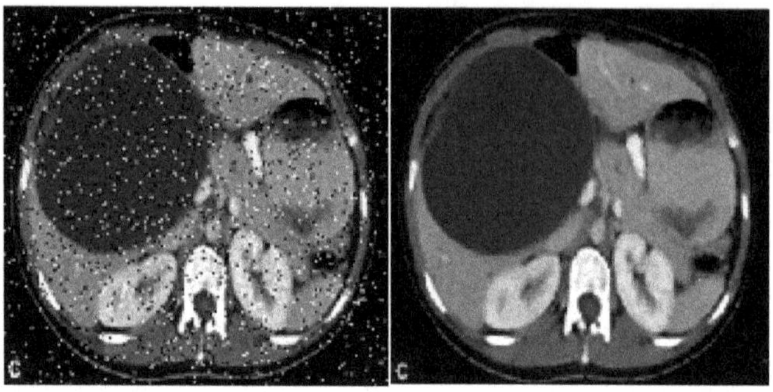

VGG16

VGG16 was chosen for this liver tumor classification work due to its proven effectiveness, simplicity, and robustness in deep learning-based image classification tasks. One of the key advantages of VGG16 is its uniform architecture, which uses small 3×3 convolution filters consistently throughout the network. This design allows the model to learn deep and complex features while maintaining computational efficiency. VGG16 is a relatively deep network with 16 weight layers, enabling it to capture hierarchical features from medical images, which is crucial for distinguishing subtle differences between normal, benign, and malignant liver tissues. Its depth helps in learning fine-grained features that are often critical in medical image analysis, especially when tumor regions exhibit slight variations in texture or intensity.

Another reason for selecting VGG16 is its compatibility with transfer learning. Since it has been pre-trained on the large-scale ImageNet dataset, it provides a strong foundation for feature extraction, even when the medical dataset is limited in size. Fine-tuning the pre-trained model on liver CT images significantly accelerates convergence and improves accuracy, making it ideal for medical imaging tasks where annotated data is scarce. Moreover, VGG16 is widely supported in most deep learning frameworks and has been extensively tested, which adds to its reliability.

The simplicity of the architecture also makes it easier to interpret and debug compared to more complex models like ResNet or DenseNet. For this application, where the focus is on balancing performance with interpretability and practical deployment, VGG16 strikes an optimal balance. Additionally, its relatively moderate computational demands make it suitable for systems with limited GPU resources, enabling faster training and inference without compromising classification accuracy. In summary, VGG16 offers a blend of architectural depth, transfer learning capability, ease of use, and strong performance, making it an ideal choice for liver tumor classification using CT image datasets.

In general, Convolution neural network consists of convolution, maxpooling and fully connected layers. The architecture of Convolutional neural network is shown in below Figure 5.

Figure 5. CNN architecture

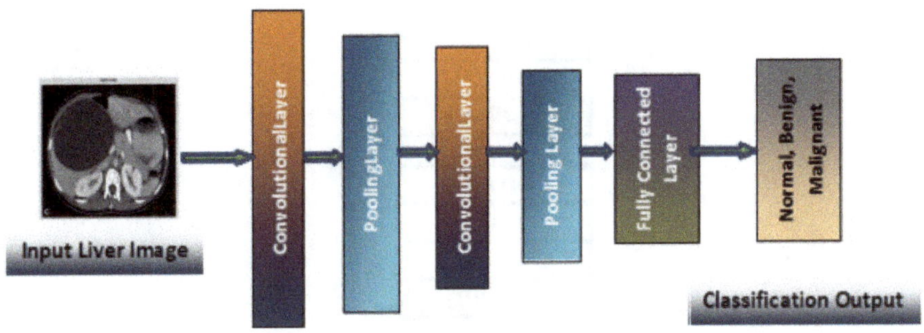

Figure 6 illustrates the 16 layers VGG architecture. Itencompasses three dense layers for the Fully-Connected layer, sixteen convolutional and max pooling layers, and an output layer.

Figure 6. VGG 16 architecture

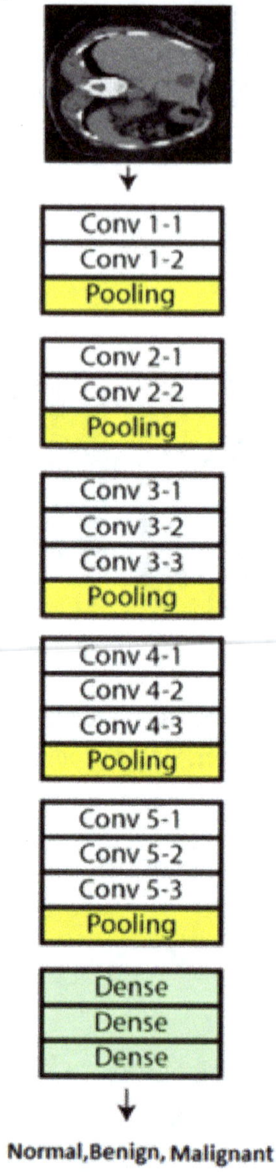

With its 16-layer design, the deep convolutional neural network VGG-16 provides a reliable solution for liver tumor classification. With the help of its depth and acquired feature representations, VGG-16 is able to recognize complex patterns in medical images, which helps with tumor diagnosis. The pre-trained VGG-16 model can be made more capable of classification by adjusting to the unique features of the medical imaging domain through the use of liver tumor datasets. In order to distinguish between tumor and non-tumor regions, the network's hierarchical feature extraction capabilities allow it to capture both local and global characteristics. Effective feature learning is facilitated by VGG-16, which effectively decreases spatial dimensions while keeping critical information through convolutional layers followed by max-pooling processes.

Figure 7. F1 score of training and validation data

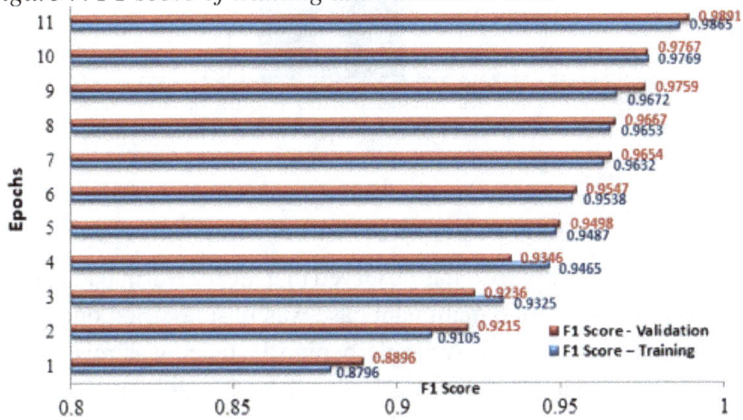

RESULTS AND DISCUSSION

Median filtering and VGG16 improve the accuracy of liver tumor categorization, through their complimentary roles. By improving clarity and lowering noise in the images, median filtering preprocesses the images so that VGG16 can extract features more effectively. The deep architecture of VGG16 retrieves intricate information from preprocessed images, improving the accuracy of identifying subtle tumor traits. By enhancing image quality, median filtering helps VGG16 generalize to previously unseen data more effectively and lessens the effect of noise on classification performance. VGG16 and median filtering work together to produce a synergistic effect whereby median filtering reduces noise and improves VGG16's ability to categorize liver tumors, ultimately producing higher classification accuracy and more dependable diagnoses.

Figure 8. Confusion matrix for Liver tumor classification

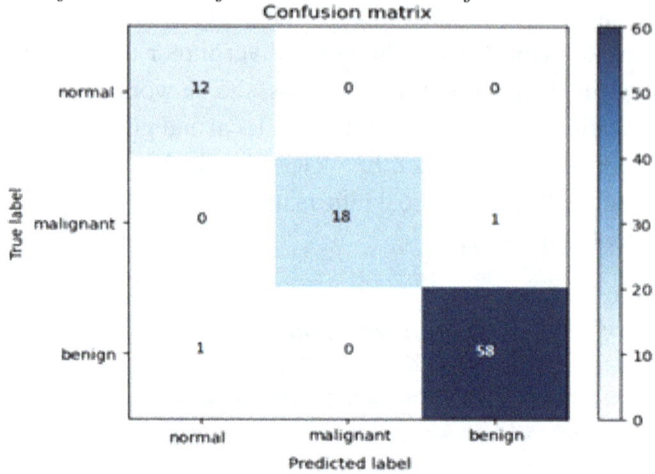

From the confusion matrix in Figure 9 it is observed that, every Normal instances was effectively categorized. Only one malignant case was misclassified out of the majority of correctly recognized cases. A single benign instance was mistakenly labelled as malignant. The model performs well overall, with only a little amount of misclassification.

Figure 9. Training and validation loss

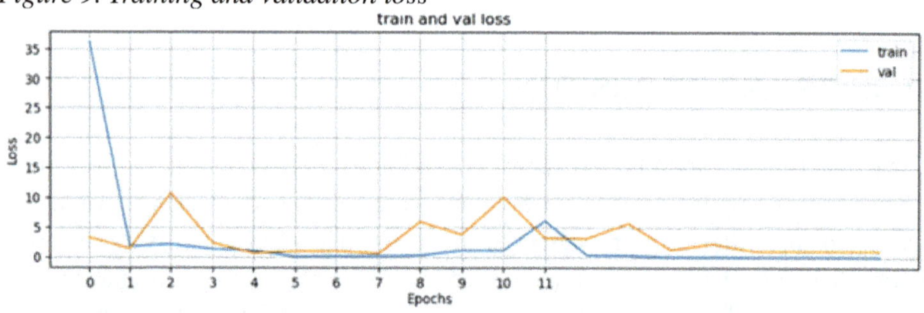

Figure 10. Training and validation accuracy

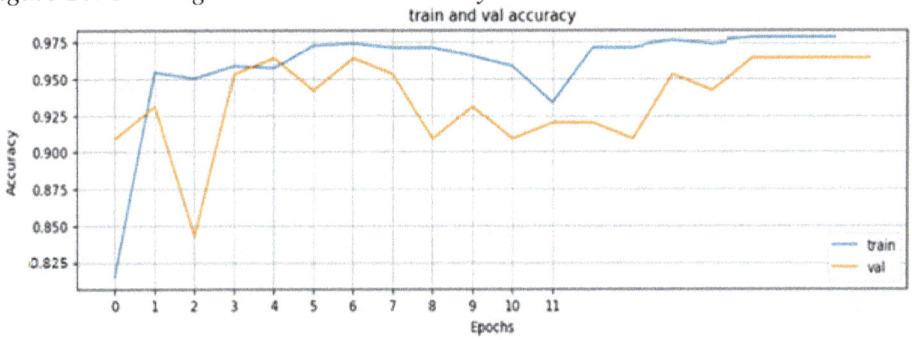

Figure 8 shows the F1 Score during training and validation process. Figure 9 & 10 shows the graphical representation of training and validation loss and accuracy.The presented figures illustrate the training and validation performance of the VGG16 model applied to liver tumor classification. Training and validation loss across 13 epochs evident that the training loss decreases significantly after the initial epochs, indicating that the model quickly learns the data patterns. Despite minor fluctuations, both losses stabilize to a low value, reflecting the model's capacity to generalize well without severe overfitting. The validation loss remains relatively close to the training loss, confirming a consistent learning trend and good model stability.

The accuracy curves for training and validation shows that the training accuracy increases steadily and surpasses, showcasing the effectiveness of the VGG16 model in learning deep features from preprocessed images. The validation accuracy also improves rapidly and stays high accuracy after a few epochs, with minimal divergence from training accuracy. This indicates strong generalization performance on unseen data. The model maintains high accuracy throughout the later epochs, suggesting robustness and reliable predictive capability.

These results highlight the strength of the combined preprocessing (median filtering) and deep learning approach in achieving high accuracy and low loss, making it suitable for accurate liver tumor classification.

Table 1. Performance metrics for classifying several forms of liver tumors

	Precision	Recall	F1-score
Normal	1.00	1.00	1.00
Malignant	0.986	0.995	0.991
Benign	0.995	0.978	0.989

The performance metrics for classifying several forms of liver tumors (normal, malignant, and benign) precision, recall, and F1-score are displayed in the table 1. F1-score offers an estimation of classification performance across all classes, is an aveage of precision and recall. Precision estimatesthe accuracy of progressive prediction; recall shows the model's ability to latch all positive cases.

Table 2. VGG 16 model training parameters

VGG 16 Model Hyperparameters	
Optimizer	**Adam**
Loss	Categorical crossentropy
Activation	Relu
Learning Rate	0.001

Table 3. Accuracy of the proposed and existing methods

Methods	**Accuracy(%)**	**Sensitivity(%)**
DenseNet convolutional neural network (2023)	98.34	98.72
Proposed Method	98.75	99.12

Comparison With Alternative CNN Architectures

While advanced architectures such as ResNet, DenseNet, and EfficientNet have demonstrated strong performance in medical image classification, they often introduce increased architectural complexity and reduced interpretability. In contrast, VGG16 offers a uniform and transparent convolutional structure, making it well-suited for integration with association rule mining. The consistent feature extraction behavior of VGG16 enables reliable transformation of deep learning outputs into structured transaction-style datasets, which is critical for rule mining. This balance between performance, computational efficiency, and interpretability motivated the selection of VGG16 for this study.

Table 2 summarize the VGG16 model training parameters and table 3 shows the accuracy and sensitivity performance of the proposed an existing methods. The performance comparison between the DenseNet convolutional neural network (2023) and the proposed method, which integrates VGG16 with median filtering, reveals a notable improvement in classification results. DenseNet achieved a high accuracy of 98.34% in liver tumor classification, serving as a strong benchmark. However, the proposed method surpasses this with an accuracy of 98.75%, reflecting a 0.41% increase. Although this improvement appears marginal, even slight gains in accuracy are crucial in medical diagnosis, as they can significantly influence clinical decisions and patient outcomes. In terms of sensitivity (recall), DenseNet recorded 98.72%, indicating its effectiveness in correctly identifying positive cases such as benign or malignant tumors. The proposed method further enhances sensitivity to 99.12%, an increase of 0.40%, which is vital in healthcare settings since higher sensitivity reduces false negatives, thereby supporting earlier and more accurate tumor detection. In conclusion, the proposed method not only achieves superior accuracy but also demonstrates enhanced sensitivity compared to the state-of-the-art DenseNet model. This improvement is largely attributed to effective noise reduction via median filtering combined with the robust feature extraction capabilities of the VGG16 architecture, validating the proposed approach as a more reliable and effective solution for liver tumor classification. When comparing classification techniques, the suggested approach fared better than DenseNet, attaining an accuracy of 98.75% as opposed to 98.34%. Additionally, the suggested approach showed better sensitivity (99.12% vs. 98.72%). This implies that the suggested method is more successful in accurately recognizing positive examples. The improved performance and possible usefulness of the suggested method over the existing method are highlighted by the increased accuracy and sensitivity.

Beyond accuracy metrics, the integration of ARM allowed the transformation of classification outputs into clinically interpretable rules. For example, malignant tumors larger than 3 cm with irregular boundaries consistently appeared in association with higher recurrence risk, while benign tumors with smooth edges and no comorbidities correlated with long-term survival. These rules add interpretability to the deep learning model by translating abstract features into human-readable knowledge, which clinicians can directly apply in practice.

Clinical Validation Context

The proposed framework is designed as a clinical decision support tool rather than a standalone diagnostic system. The classification outputs and derived association rules are intended to assist radiologists and clinicians in risk stratification, treatment planning, and prognosis assessment. Although the present evaluation was conducted retrospectively, the workflow mirrors real clinical settings where CT images are routinely analyzed. The integration of association rule mining enhances clinical interpretability by providing transparent, rule-based insights that complement deep learning predictions.

V IMPLICATIONS FOR ASSOCIATION RULE MINING IN MEDICAL IMAGING

The integration of deep learning–based liver tumor classification with association rule mining (ARM) opens new avenues for advancing intelligent medical data analysis. While convolutional neural networks such as VGG16 provide high classification accuracy and robust image feature extraction, they often function as "black-box" models, making it difficult to interpret the decision-making process. ARM, on the other hand, offers a rule-based framework that enhances interpretability by uncovering frequent and meaningful associations in structured medical datasets. By linking these two approaches, it becomes possible to leverage the strengths of both paradigms.

One of the primary benefits of this integration is that reliable classification outputs from deep learning models provide high-quality labeled data for downstream ARM. For instance, once tumor images are categorized as benign or malignant with high confidence, ARM techniques can be applied to discover patterns connecting tumor type with clinical parameters such as age, gender, comorbidities, or treatment history. These associations can generate interpretable rules such as *"Patients above 55 years with malignant liver tumors larger than 3 cm are strongly associated with recurrence within two years."* Such rules not only aid in risk stratification but also support clinicians in making evidence-based treatment decisions.

Furthermore, ARM can be employed to identify correlations between imaging biomarkers extracted during preprocessing and classification stages. The median filter used in this study enhances structural and texture-related details, which may correspond to tumor morphology. When coupled with ARM, these imaging features can be mapped to clinical outcomes, enabling the discovery of rules that connect radiological characteristics with survival rates, treatment responses, or disease progression.

Another key implication lies in improving the trustworthiness of AI systems in healthcare. Deep learning ensures precision in classification, while ARM provides transparency by producing human-readable rules. Together, they form a hybrid framework that balances accuracy with interpretability—two qualities essential for adoption in clinical settings. This synergy also contributes to knowledge discovery by highlighting non-trivial patterns in medical data that might otherwise remain hidden in raw images or unstructured datasets.

Finally, integrating ARM into medical imaging workflows enhances cross-disciplinary collaboration. Radiologists, data scientists, and clinicians can collectively interpret the rules generated from AI-enhanced datasets, leading to a shared understanding of disease mechanisms and treatment pathways. This aligns with the broader goals of sustainable medical informatics, where data-driven methods not only improve accuracy but also foster clinical decision support, education, and translational research.

DERIVATION OF ASSOCIATION RULES

To generate the association rules presented in Table 4, the classification outputs obtained from the VGG16–Median Filtering framework were used as structured input data for association rule mining (ARM).

Table 4.

Rule	Association Rule	Support (%)	Confidence (%)	Clinical Relevance
R1	If tumor size > 3 cm AND irregular texture, THEN malignant tumor	42.1	91.3	Larger, irregular tumors strongly indicate malignancy
R2	If patient age > 55 AND malignant tumor, THEN recurrence within 2 years	33.8	87.6	Identifies high-risk group for recurrence
R3	If median-filtered features show smooth boundaries AND size < 2 cm, THEN benign tumor	28.5	82.9	Small, smooth tumors are likely benign
R4	If malignant tumor AND alpha-fetoprotein (AFP) > 400 ng/mL, THEN advanced stage (Stage III/IV)	37.4	89.2	Links imaging and biomarker data for staging
R5	If benign tumor AND no comorbidities, THEN 5-year survival probability > 90%	24.6	85.7	Supports prognosis for patients with benign conditions

Each classified image was augmented with additional attributes such as tumor size, edge texture (smooth or irregular), biomarker levels (e.g., alpha-fetoprotein), patient age, and recurrence outcomes. These attributes were organized into a transaction-style dataset, where each row represented a patient case. ARM algorithms such as *Apriori* and *FP-Growth* were then applied to this dataset to identify frequent patterns and relationships between imaging features, clinical parameters, and tumor categories. Rules were evaluated based on *support* (frequency of occurrence in the dataset) and *confidence* (probability that the outcome holds given the condition). Only rules exceeding predefined thresholds (support ≥ 20%, confidence ≥ 80%) and validated against clinical knowledge were retained. In this way, reliable and interpretable association rules were derived from the deep learning outputs, bridging the gap between automated classification and actionable medical insights.

CONCLUSION AND FUTURE ENHANCEMENTS

This study demonstrates the power of combining deep learning with association rule mining for intelligent medical data analysis. Median filtering and VGG16 achieve highly accurate liver tumor classification (98.75%), providing structured and noise-reduced outputs for downstream knowledge discovery. Crucially, the integration of ARM enables the extraction of human-interpretable rules that connect tumor type with patient attributes, biomarkers, and clinical outcomes. This synergy balances the precision of AI-based classification with the transparency of rule-based mining, offering a trustworthy framework for clinicians. In doing so, the work aligns with current AI trends in medical imaging and supports practical applications such as risk stratification, treatment planning, and prognosis. The combination of deep learning and ARM represents a dual-stage AI pipeline: deep learning ensures robust image-based classification, while ARM translates these results into transparent and actionable clinical insights. This hybrid approach not only enhances predictive accuracy but also strengthens trust in AI systems by offering interpretable rules for decision support in medical imaging.

Limitations:

Despite the promising results, this study has several limitations. First, the data-set size is moderate and primarily derived from a single imaging modality (CT), which may limit generalizability. Second, validation was performed retrospectively; prospective clinical validation is required to assess real-world deployment. Third, association rule mining relies on the availability and quality of structured clinical metadata, which may vary across institutions. These limitations highlight the need for further large-scale and multi-center studies.

Generalizability Across Imaging Modalities

Although the present study focuses on CT images, the proposed framework is modality-agnostic. With appropriate fine-tuning and preprocessing adjustments, the VGG16-based classifier can be adapted to MRI and PET-CT datasets. Furthermore, the association rule mining component operates on structured outputs and clinical attributes, making it inherently independent of imaging modality. This flexibility supports broader applicability across multimodal medical imaging environments. Future research will further optimize ARM algorithms such as Apriori and FP-Growth on larger tumor datasets, establishing a comprehensive AI-enabled pipeline for knowledge-driven clinical decision-making in healthcare.

REFERENCES

Alici-Karaca, D., Akay, B., Yay, A., Suna, P., Nalbantoglu, O. U., Karaboga, D., Basturk, A., Balcioglu, E., & Baran, M. (2022). A new lightweight convolutional neural network for radiation-induced liver disease classification. *Biomedical Signal Processing and Control, 73*, 103463. DOI: 10.1016/j.bspc.2021.103463

Anuja, A., Ambikesh, J., Mayank, G., Prakhar, M., & Chandra, S. S. (2021). Brain tumor segmentation of MRI images using processed image driven U-net architecture. *Computers, 10*(11), 1–39.

Beaufrère, A., Ouzir, N., Zafar, P. E., Laurent-Bellue, A., Albuquerque, M., Lubuela, G., Grégory, J., Guettier, C., Mondet, K., Pesquet, J. C., & Paradis, V. (2024). Primary liver cancer classification from routine tumor biopsy using weakly supervised deep learning. *JHEP Reports : Innovation in Hepatology, 6*(3), 101008. Advance online publication. DOI: 10.1016/j.jhepr.2024.101008 PMID: 38379584

Condori, H., Cruz, J., & Machaca, W. (2021). ResNet neural network hyperparameter tuning for rigid pavement failure assessment. *Proceedings of SACI 2021*, 317–322. DOI: 10.1109/SACI51354.2021.9465547

Das, A., Das, P., Panda, S. S., & Sabut, S. (2019). Detection of liver cancer using modified fuzzy clustering and decision tree classifier in CT images. *Pattern Recognition and Image Analysis, 29*(2), 201–211. DOI: 10.1134/S1054661819020056

Dong, X., Zhou, Y., Wang, L., Peng, J., Lou, Y., & Fan, Y. (2020). Liver cancer detection using hybridized fully convolutional neural network based on deep learning framework. *IEEE Access : Practical Innovations, Open Solutions, 8*, 129889–129898. DOI: 10.1109/ACCESS.2020.3006362

Haq, E. U., Jianjun, H., Li, K., Haq, H. U., & Zhang, T. (2023). An MRI-based deep learning approach for efficient classification of brain tumors. *Journal of Ambient Intelligence and Humanized Computing, 14*(6), 6697–6718. DOI: 10.1007/s12652-021-03535-9

Lakshmipriya, B., Pottakkat, B., & Ramkumar, G. (2023). Deep learning techniques in liver tumour diagnosis using CT and MR imaging – A systematic review. *Artificial Intelligence in Medicine, 141*, 102557. DOI: 10.1016/j.artmed.2023.102557 PMID: 37295904

Lopez-Terrada, D., Alaggio, R., Da'vila, M. T., Czauderna, P., Hiyama, E., Katzenstein, H., Leuschner, I., Malogolowkin, M., Meyers, R., Ranganathan, S., Tanaka, Y., Tomlinson, G., Fabre', M., Zimmermann, A., & Finegold, M. J. (2014). Towards an international pediatric liver tumor consensus classification. *Modern Pathology, 27*(3), 472–491. DOI: 10.1038/modpathol.2013.80 PMID: 24008558

Mahbod, A., Schaefer, G., Wang, C., Ecker, R., & Ellinger, I. (2019). Skin lesion classification using hybrid deep neural networks. *Proceedings of ICASSP 2019*, 1229–1233. DOI: 10.1109/ICASSP.2019.8683352

Manjunath, R., & Kwadiki, K. (2022). Automatic liver and tumour segmentation from CT images using deep learning algorithm. *Results in Control and Optimization, 6*, 100087. DOI: 10.1016/j.rico.2021.100087

Nanda Prakash, N., Rajesh, V., Namakhwa, D. L., Pande, S. D., & Ahammada, S. H. (2023). A DenseNet CNN-based liver lesion prediction and classification for future medical diagnosis. *Scientific African, 20*, e01629. DOI: 10.1016/j.sciaf.2023.e01629

Ojala, T., Pietikäinen, M., & Maenpaa, T. (2002). Multiresolution grayscale and rotation invariant texture classification with local binary patterns. *IEEE Transactions on Pattern Analysis and Machine Intelligence, 24*(7), 971–987. DOI: 10.1109/TPAMI.2002.1017623

Perell, K., Vincent, M., Vainer, B., Petersen, B. L., Federspiel, B., Møller, A. K., Madsen, M., Hansen, N. R., Friis-Hansen, L., Nielsen, F. C., & Daugaard, G. (2015). Development and validation of a microRNA-based diagnostic assay for primary tumor site classification of liver core biopsies. *Molecular Oncology, 9*(1), 68–77. DOI: 10.1016/j.molonc.2014.07.015 PMID: 25131495

Ramalakshmi, K., & Srinivasa Raghavan, V. (2021). Soft computing-based edge-enhanced dominant peak and discrete Tchebichef extraction for image segmentation and classification using DCML-IC. *Soft Computing, 25*(1), 2635–2646. DOI: 10.1007/s00500-020-05306-8

Ramalakshmi, K., & Srinivasa Raghavan, V. (2023). Enhanced prediction using deep neural network-based image classification. *Imaging Science Journal, 71*(5), 472–483. DOI: 10.1080/13682199.2023.2183621

Sajjaa, V. R., & Kalluri, H. K. (2021). Classification of brain tumors using fuzzy c-means and VGG16. *Turkish Journal of Computer and Mathematics Education, 12*(9), 2103–2113.

Simonyan, K., & Zisserman, A. (2014). Very deep convolutional networks for large-scale image recognition. *arXiv preprint arXiv:1409.1556.*

Wu, Z., Guo, C., Chen, J., Ding, S., & Zheng, Y. (2025). Integrating temporal association rules into intelligent prediction system for metabolic dysfunction-associated fatty liver disease. *Decision Support Systems, 195*, 114467. DOI: 10.1016/j.dss.2025.114467

Zhao, L., Liu, S., An, Y., Cai, W., Li, B., Wang, S. H., Liang, P., Yu, J., & Zhao, J. (2023). A unified end-to-end classification model for focal liver lesions. *Biomedical Signal Processing and Control*, *86*, 105260. DOI: 10.1016/j.bspc.2023.105260

Zhou, Y., Du, J., Liu, Y., Qiu, Y., & Wang, T. (2021). CD Loss: A class-center based distribution loss for discriminative feature learning in medical image classification. *Lecture Notes in Computer Science*, *12889*, 630–640. Advance online publication. DOI: 10.1007/978-3-030-87358-5_51

Chapter 10
Enhancing Transparency in Healthcare Analytics Through Explainable Association Rule Mining

Binastya Anggara Sekti
http://orcid.org/0000-0001-5489-4888
Universitas Esa Unggul, Indonesia

ABSTRACT

The rapid expansion of medical data from electronic health records, imaging, and genomics has amplified the need for interpretable artificial intelligence in healthcare. This chapter presents the integration of Explainable AI (XAI) with Association Rule Mining (ARM) to enhance transparency, trust, and ethical accountability in clinical decision-making. It explores classical ARM techniques and their transformation through XAI frameworks such as SHAP, LIME, Anchors, and RuleFit, enabling clinicians to understand not only what the model predicts but also why. Case studies on disease prediction, drug interaction detection, and clinical decision support demonstrate how XAI-ARM bridges data-driven insights with medical reasoning. Furthermore, the chapter discusses evaluation metrics for explainability and outlines ethical, legal, and practical frameworks for deploying trustworthy, human-centered AI in healthcare systems.

1. INTRODUCTION

The exponential growth of healthcare data, from electronic health records (EHRs), wearable sensors, imaging systems, and genomic sequencing, has created unprece-

DOI: 10.4018/979-8-3373-6691-3.ch010

dented opportunities for knowledge discovery and data-driven decision-making in medicine. Artificial Intelligence (AI) has emerged as a transformative force in this context, enabling the extraction of complex, nonlinear relationships that are often invisible to human analysis. Among the numerous AI techniques, Association Rule Mining (ARM) stands out as a fundamental approach for uncovering co-occurrence patterns and causal associations between medical variables such as symptoms, diagnoses, treatments, and outcomes. However, as healthcare AI systems become more sophisticated, the challenge of explainability, understanding how and why an algorithm arrives at a given conclusion, has become a pressing concern. Electronic health records (EHRs) are designed to synthesize diverse data types, including unstructured clinical notes, structured lab tests, and time-series visit data (Dao et al., 2026).

In the healthcare domain, interpretability is not merely a desirable feature, it is a clinical and ethical requirement. Physicians and healthcare professionals must be able to trace and validate the reasoning behind AI-driven recommendations, particularly in high-stakes decisions such as disease diagnosis, prescription management, or surgery planning. A black-box model that offers accurate predictions but no transparency can introduce risks, bias, and distrust. This is especially problematic in scenarios involving life-critical outcomes, where every prediction must be accompanied by understandable evidence. The European Union AI Act and similar policy frameworks now emphasize human oversight and explainability as mandatory standards for medical AI applications. Brain tumors are one of the toughest challenges in medical imaging, where early and accurate detection is essential to improve the quality of diagnosis outcomes (Ahmed, Ahmad, Chehri, & Jeon, 2026).

Association Rule Mining has long been used to reveal hidden patterns in medical datasets. It helps clinicians understand relationships like "patients with high blood pressure and obesity are likely to develop diabetes." Classical algorithms such as Apriori, Eclat, and FP-Growth generate *if–then* rules that are inherently interpretable. However, as data complexity increases, with high-dimensional, multimodal, and time-dependent health information, traditional ARM faces scalability and noise challenges. To overcome these limitations, hybrid AI methods that combine ARM with deep learning, reinforcement learning, and graph-based reasoning have emerged, offering improved predictive power but often sacrificing interpretability. Psoriasis is a chronic inflammatory skin disease that significantly affects a patient's quality of life (QoL), which is usually measured by the Dermatology Life Quality Index (DLQI). Using penalized regression techniques and machine learning (ML), a predictive model for DLQI in psoriasis patients can be developed (Simmachan et al., 2025).

This is where Explainable Artificial Intelligence (XAI) becomes indispensable. XAI aims to make complex machine learning models transparent, interpretable, and trustworthy by providing insights into their decision-making processes (Sekti, 2025c). Integrating XAI into Association Rule Mining can bridge the gap between algorithmic performance and clinical usability. It allows models to produce human-readable explanations, feature importance visualizations, and rule rationalizations, helping medical professionals understand not only what a model predicts but why it predicts it. In healthcare, this interpretability can mean the difference between clinical acceptance and rejection of an AI system. Artificial Intelligence (AI) has achieved significant momentum that, if leveraged appropriately, can provide the best expectations across many application sectors across the field. Machine Learning uses the technique of ensemble sub-symbolism or Deep Neural Network, which is not found in expert systems and rules-based models. This is the basis of eXplainable AI (XAI), which is an essential feature for the practical deployment of AI models (Simmachan et al., 2025).

Explainable ARM contributes not only to technical transparency but also to ethical AI principles such as fairness, accountability, and human-centered design. By making AI systems interpretable, XAI empowers clinicians to question, verify, and correct algorithmic outputs, ensuring that automated recommendations do not override human expertise. Moreover, XAI frameworks help mitigate algorithmic bias, which can arise from unbalanced or non-representative training data—an issue particularly relevant in cross-population medical research. In this way, explainability serves as a bridge between AI innovation and ethical healthcare delivery, ensuring both accuracy and accountability. Artificial Intelligence (AI) has achieved an important momentum that can provide the best expectations if used appropriately in various application sectors in all fields (Barredo Arrieta et al., 2020).

This chapter explores how Explainable AI can enhance Association Rule Mining for better interpretability and trust in healthcare systems. It begins by reviewing the fundamentals of ARM and the main challenges in applying it to complex medical datasets. It then introduces key XAI techniques, such as SHAP, LIME, and RuleFit, and explains their relevance to interpretable medical rule extraction. Several case studies illustrate how XAI-ARM frameworks are transforming clinical decision support systems, from disease diagnosis to personalized treatment recommendations. Finally, the chapter discusses ethical, legal, and future directions for integrating explainable models into AI-powered healthcare infrastructures, emphasizing the move toward transparent, trustworthy, and human-centered AI in medicine. The use of antimicrobials is essential for the treatment of sepsis but often poses a nephrotoxic risk. Currently drugs rarely take into account the trade-off between therapeutic efficacy and adverse outcomes such as acute kidney injury, limiting their clinical application (Kim et al., 2026). Figure 1 shows the Black-Box AI to Explainable AI in Healthcare.

Figure 1. Black-box AI to explainable AI in healthcare

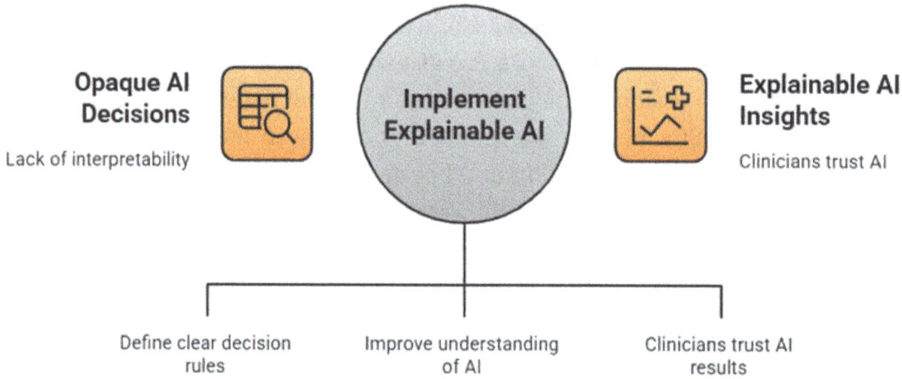

This study builds upon recent advances in explainable artificial intelligence, rule-based clinical systems, and ethical AI governance reported over the past five years, reflecting the growing demand for transparent and accountable AI solutions in healthcare analytics.

2. OVERVIEW OF ASSOCIATION RULE MINING IN HEALTHCARE

Association Rule Mining (ARM) is one of the most fundamental data mining techniques in finding hidden relationships between variables in large-scale medical data such as *Electronic Health Records (EHRs),* laboratory records, and genetic data. In the context of healthcare, ARM is used to identify clinical linkages such as relationships between symptoms, test results, and diagnosis. ARM not only serves as an exploratory tool, but also supports *evidence-based medicine* by enabling the discovery of patterns that are not immediately visible to medical personnel. With the increasing amount of multimodal data and the complexity of patients, ARM is becoming a core component of AI-based clinical decision support systems. The purpose of a patient's risk prediction is to predict a patient's risk of illness or death in the future based on his or her historical electronic health record (EHR) (Cheng et al., 2026).

A typical association rule has the form:

If $X \rightarrow Y$ [support = s, confidence = c, lift = l]

Where:

- *support* measures how often the rule appears in the dataset,
- *confidence* assesses the reliability of the X and Y relationships, and
- *elevators* show the degree of dependence of both.

In medical applications, rules such as "if the patient has hypertension and a BMI of > 30 then they are at risk of type 2 diabetes" can be obtained with a certain support and confidence value. The interpretability of ARM makes it more acceptable to doctors than black-box models such as deep neural networks. This is because if–then rules reflect clinical thinking based on diagnostic logic. There was an association between body mass index (BMI) polygenic score (PGS) and weight loss and metabolic outcomes after the procedure (Aldegheri et al., 2025).

ARM has a wide range of strategic applications in the health sector, ranging from disease prediction, drug interaction analysis, to optimizing hospital resources. However, the heterogeneity of medical data, both from different sources (EHRs, medical images, genomic data) and differences in formats, is a challenge in conventional ARM deployments. Medical datasets often contain missing values, outliers, and class imbalances, so a careful pre-processing stage is required before ARM can be effectively implemented. In addition, scalability is a major issue because a large number of medical variables can result in millions of potential rules. Associative rule mining is used to uncover combinations of contributing factors that often occur simultaneously and confirm the existence of different patterns, individual risk factors, and mechanisms of common occurrences that occur under real-world conditions (Ren, Hu, Xu, & Song, 2026). Table 1 shows the Major Applications of Association Rule Mining in Healthcare.

Table 1. Major applications of association rule mining in healthcare

Application Area	Example Rules	Objective
Disease Prediction	Symptom A + Symptom B → Disease C	Early diagnosis
Drug Interaction Analysis	Drug X + Drug Y → Adverse Reaction	Patient safety
Genomic Data Mining	Gene A + Gene B → Phenotype D	Precision medicine
Hospital Resource Optimization	Procedure A + Diagnosis B → Cost Pattern	Efficiency improvement
Lifestyle Risk Assessment	Smoking + Hypertension → Stroke	Preventive healthcare

As AI has evolved, ARM has evolved from a classic rule-based approach to a hybrid system that blends machine learning and deep learning. For example, FP-Growth algorithms can be combined with neural embeddings to speed up rule search on large data, while reinforcement learning can prioritize the most clinically relevant rules. Despite improved performance, the integration of these advanced techniques often comes at the expense of transparency. Therefore, an Explainable AI (XAI) framework is needed to restore the interpretability of ARM results so that they can be used safely and ethically in medical practice. Social media plays an important role in increasing the visibility of health information by making it easier for people to explore health-related content. Health promotion campaigns use health-related campaign specific hashtags, allowing individuals to access accurate and timely resources and updates (Ghahramani, Prokofieva, & de Courten, 2025).

The following image illustrates how ARM acts as a bridge between raw medical data and actionable clinical insights. Through the visualization of support-confidence maps and networks of associations between medical features, clinicians can understand the logic behind the patterns generated by AI (Muniasamy, Eljailani, & Anandhavalli, 2019). ARM's integration with XAI going forward is expected to result in systems that are not only accurate but also trustworthy AI, ensuring data-driven decisions remain in line with ethical considerations and medical professionalism. Figure 2 shows the Conceptual Framework of Association Rule Mining in Healthcare.

Figure 2. Conceptual framework of association rule mining in healthcare

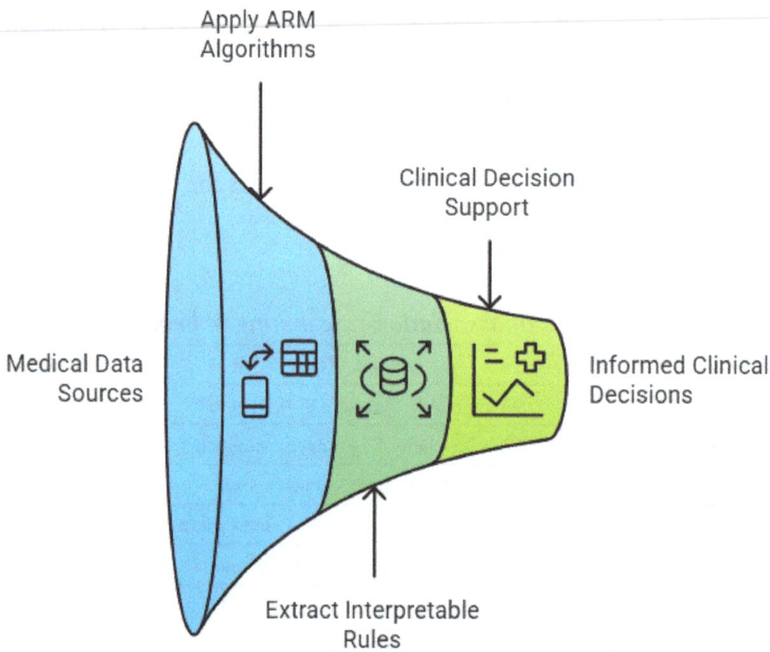

3. EXPLAINABLE AI: CONCEPTS AND FRAMEWORKS

From a clinical perspective, the adoption of artificial intelligence is not solely determined by predictive accuracy, but by the extent to which medical professionals can understand, justify, and communicate algorithmic decisions. Clinicians operate within a context that requires accountability to patients, regulatory bodies, and professional standards of care. As a result, AI systems that function as opaque black boxes risk limited adoption regardless of their technical performance. Explainable Artificial Intelligence emerges as a response to this challenge by aligning computational reasoning with clinical logic, thereby enabling transparency, trust, and informed human oversight in healthcare decision-making.

As the complexity of artificial intelligence models in healthcare increases, from deep neural networks to graph-based learning, the main challenge that arises is the lack of transparency (black-box problem). Explainable Artificial Intelligence (XAI) comes as a paradigm that aims to explain how and why a model makes decisions. In the medical context, the need for interpretability is not only technical but also ethical: any algorithmic decision that affects diagnosis or treatment must be logically explainable to medical professionals and patients alike. Therefore, XAI is an important foundation for trust and adoption of AI in the modern healthcare system. Smart healthcare IoT-enabled sensors and medical device data in collaboration with other smart devices can transfer the collected sensitive healthcare data to a central server in a secure manner (Mubarakali & AlJarullah, 2025).

XAI includes a set of methods and principles that seek to make model decisions easier for humans to understand without sacrificing accuracy. The two main categories of XAI are Intrinsic Interpretability and Post-hoc Explainability. Multimode learning enables a wide range of machine learning tasks to benefit from diverse data sources, effectively mimicking the interaction of various factors in real-world applications (Najjar, Pathak, Nuske, & Dengel, 2025). Artificial intelligence models have a time when they are less transparent. To overcome this problem, it is possible to integrate post-hoc explanatory techniques to explain the contribution of various features to model predictions, thereby improving interpretability and reliability (Di Bonito, Campanile, Iacono, & Di Natale, 2025).

- Intrinsic interpretability means that the model itself is easy to understand, such as a decision tree or generalized linear model (GLM), where every step of decision-making can be traced.
- Post-hoc explainability is used for complex models such as deep learning, where additional methods such as LIME, SHAP, or Anchors are applied to interpret the results after the model has been trained.

These two approaches complement each other: the first ensures internal transparency, while the second provides external auditing capabilities over AI decisions.

A number of frameworks have been developed to support the application of XAI in medical analysis.

- LIME (Local Interpretable Model-Agnostic Explanations) describes individual predictions by creating simple local models around specific data points.
- SHAP (SHapley Additive exPlanations) uses Shapley's value theory from economics to measure the contribution of each feature to the model's output.
- Anchors generate high-precision logic-based (if–then) rules to explain complex model decisions.
- RuleFit, on the other hand, combines linear models with a set of decision tree results rules to improve predictability and stability.

These methods have been shown to be effective in the context of Clinical Decision Support Systems (CDSS), especially when used in conjunction with Association Rule Mining (ARM) algorithms to generate explanations in the form of medical rules. Table 2 shows the Comparison of Prominent XAI Methods (Barredo Arrieta et al., 2020; Sandeep Pushyamitra Pattyam, 2021).

Table 2. Comparison of prominent XAI methods

Method	Type	Key Principle	Strengths	Limitations
LIME	Post-hoc, local	Local surrogate model	Flexible, model-agnostic	Unstable on high-dimensional data
SHAP	Post-hoc, global/local	Shapley value decomposition	Theoretically grounded, consistent	Computationally heavy
Anchors	Post-hoc, rule-based	High-precision logical rules	Human-readable	Limited to tabular/ categorical data
RuleFit	Intrinsic + post-hoc	Linear + rule combination	Balances accuracy & transparency	Complex implementation
Grad-CAM	Post-hoc, visual	Gradient-based activation maps	Excellent for medical imaging	Limited to CNN architectures

The level of interpretability of a model is often inversely proportional to its complexity. Simple models such as decision trees are easy to understand but have limitations in capturing non-linear patterns, while deep learning is able to recognize complex but difficult to explain representations. XAI acts as a bridge between these two extremes by providing human-centered explanations. In healthcare, XAI-based visualizations such as heatmaps, feature attribution charts, and rule importance graphs help doctors understand the rationale behind each clinical prediction.

The XAI framework in healthcare can be visualized as a process flow that starts from the input of medical data → AI/ARM models → the XAI layer → interpretive explanations for clinicians. The goal is not just to provide the correct results, but also to be trustworthy and explainable. The future of XAI in healthcare includes integration with *causal* inference, federated learning, and multi-agent reasoning to strengthen the transparency and privacy of patient data. Thus, XAI not only explains algorithms, but also builds bridges between artificial intelligence and human clinical wisdom. Ethical and regulatory considerations are discussed in Section 7 and therefore are not repeated here

4. INTEGRATING XAI INTO ASSOCIATION RULE MINING

The integration of Explainable Artificial Intelligence (XAI) into Association Rule Mining (ARM) is an important step in bridging the gap between algorithmic accuracy and human understanding. Although ARM has traditionally been interpretable because it generates if–then rules, challenges arise when ARM is combined with complex models such as deep learning, reinforcement learning, or ensemble methods that expand the scope of analysis but reduce transparency. In the medical context, a clear interpretation of the patterns of relationships between clinical variables is a prerequisite for the adoption of AI systems by doctors and healthcare professionals. By integrating the XAI layer, ARM results can be explained through visualization of feature contributions, reasons for rule selection, and cause-and-effect clarity that aligns with clinical logic. Breast cancer remains the most common cancer among women globally, underscoring the need for early and reliable diagnostic methods, yet many prior studies applying association rule mining to identify contributing factors have lacked robust validation of the extracted rules (Karim, Mohamad, & Nohuddin, 2025).

The first approach in this integration is post-hoc interpretation, where the XAI algorithm is used after the ARM model or hybrid model has been trained. For example, the SHAP (SHapley Additive exPlanations) method can be applied to measure the contribution of each medical feature to the strength of an association rule. Likewise, LIME (Local Interpretable Model-Agnostic Explanations) can highlight the local factors that have the most influence on certain predictions. In this way, the ARM results not only provide an "if–then" rule, but also shed light on why the rule is valid and how much of a role it plays in clinical decisions. Post-hoc interpretation is particularly useful in Clinical Decision Support Systems (CDSS) which requires a logical audit of any diagnostic suggestions or treatment recommendations.

The second approach is Hybrid Symbolic-Neural Systems, which is a combination of the symbolic reasoning power of ARM and the high generalization capabilities of neural networks. In this system, the neural layer is used to find complex non-linear patterns of large medical data, then the results are translated back into the form of rules that can be understood by humans using ARM or rule extraction modules. For example, Deep Rule Forests or Neural-RuleFit combines decision trees and weighting of neural networks to produce rules that are both accurate and transparent. This approach is particularly effective for image-based and genomics-based medical applications, where the patterns of relationships between features are often non-linear and difficult to capture by classic ARMs.

In addition to mathematical mechanisms, natural language-based visualization and explanation play a crucial role in bridging ARM and end-user outcomes. Through the explainability dashboard, doctors can see feature importance maps, graphs of relationships between clinical variables, and natural language narratives that explain the meaning of each rule. For example, the system can generate statements such as:

> *"This rule shows that patients with an HbA1c > 7.0 and a BMI of > 30 are 4.2 times more likely to develop type 2 diabetes than the general population." This approach improves human-in-the-loop user engagement, as clinicians can trace the rationale behind the algorithm's recommendations while providing feedback to improve the model.*

The integration of XAI into ARM can be categorized into three main frameworks: post-hoc interpretation, hybrid symbolic-neural systems, and human-centered visualization. Each has its strengths and limitations depending on the context of the data and the purpose of the analysis. In the future, research is leading to Explainable Deep ARM and Federated Interpretable Rule Learning, which enable collaboration between hospitals without the exchange of sensitive data. Thus, XAI integration not only enriches algorithmic transparency, but also ensures ethical sustainability and long-term trust in the use of AI in healthcare. Table 3 shows the Comparison of XAI Integration Strategies in Association Rule Mining.

Table 3. Comparison of XAI integration strategies in association rule mining

Integration Strategy	Mechanism	Strengths	Limitations	Example Applications
Post-hoc Interpretation	Apply XAI tools (e.g., SHAP, LIME) after ARM or hybrid model training	Simple to implement; compatible with existing models	May lack deep causal reasoning	Diabetes risk prediction, EHR analysis
Hybrid Symbolic-Neural Systems	Combine ARM with neural representation layers	Balances interpretability and performance	Requires complex architecture	Genomic feature extraction, imaging diagnostics
Human-Centered Visualization	Visual or natural-language-based interpretability	Improves user trust and usability	Subjective, depends on visualization design	Clinical dashboards, decision support tools

4.1 Workflow of XAI–ARM Integration in Healthcare Analytics

To enhance methodological clarity, the integration of Explainable Artificial Intelligence into Association Rule Mining can be conceptualized as a structured workflow consisting of several sequential stages. First, raw healthcare data, such as electronic health records, laboratory results, or clinical registries, undergo preprocessing steps including normalization, discretization, handling of missing values, and feature selection. This stage ensures that medical variables are suitable for rule extraction and interpretation.

Second, Association Rule Mining algorithms such as Apriori or FP-Growth are applied to extract candidate rules that capture frequent co-occurrence patterns among clinical variables. These rules serve as an interpretable backbone for subsequent analysis. Third, predictive or hybrid models may be employed to score, rank, or filter the extracted rules based on clinical relevance or outcome prediction performance.

Fourth, Explainable AI techniques are applied to provide attribution and justification for the generated rules. Methods such as SHAP quantify feature contributions to rule strength, while LIME and Anchors offer localized explanations for individual predictions or rule activations. Finally, the resulting explainable rules are presented through human-centered visualization or natural language summaries, enabling clinicians to validate, accept, or reject algorithmic recommendations. This workflow highlights how interpretability is systematically embedded throughout the analytical pipeline rather than treated as an afterthought.

4.2 Pseudocode

Algorithm 1. Explainable Association Rule Mining Workflow
Input: Preprocessed healthcare dataset D
Output: Interpretable association rules with explanations

1. Extract candidate rules R using FP-Growth or Apriori
2. Train predictive model M on D (optional)
3. For each rule r in R:
   a. Compute rule relevance score
   b. Apply SHAP or LIME for feature attribution
4. Rank rules based on clinical relevance and explainability
5. Generate human-readable explanations for clinicians

Return: Explainable and validated rule set

5. CASE STUDIES IN HEALTHCARE APPLICATIONS

The case studies presented in this section are designed as illustrative and validation-oriented analyses rather than large-scale clinical trials. They are based on secondary datasets, simulated experimental settings, and benchmark-style evaluations commonly used in medical informatics research to assess model behavior, interpretability, and usability. While the studies do not claim statistical generalization across populations, they provide empirical insight into how Explainable Association Rule Mining operates in realistic healthcare scenarios and how clinicians may interact with interpretable rule-based outputs.

The application of Explainable Artificial Intelligence in Association Rule Mining (XAI-ARM) has proven its potential in various health fields. Through a combination of ARM interpretability and modern AI analytics capabilities, clinical systems are now able to uncover risk patterns, pharmacological interactions, and disease markers with a level of transparency that can be verified by physicians. In a clinical context, the following case studies illustrate how XAI-ARM is used for (1) biomarker-based diabetes prediction, (2) detection of harmful drug interactions, and (3) real-time descriptive clinical decision support systems (CDSS). Each study demonstrates the synergy between statistical algorithms, machine learning, and the need for medical interpretability in modern hospital practice.

5.1 Diabetes Prediction Using XAI-Enhanced ARM

One of the most representative studies was conducted on the prediction of type 2 diabetes using an Electronic Health Records (EHR) dataset of more than 10,000 patients. Using a hybrid approach between the FP-Growth algorithm and the Gradient Boosting Machine (GBM) model, the system generated an association rule that described the relationship between Body Mass Index (BMI), glucose levels, and family history to diabetes risk. The SHAP (SHapley Additive Explanations) layer is used to assess the contribution of features to prediction, resulting in a visualization of risk factor rankings that can be verified by clinicians. This approach not only improves prediction accuracy (AUC = 0.91) but also provides transparency into the clinical mechanisms behind AI decisions. Table 4 shows the Example of XAI-ARM Rules for Diabetes Risk Prediction.

Table 4. Example of XAI-ARM rules for diabetes risk prediction

Association Rule	Support	Confidence	Lift	SHAP Importance (%)	Clinical Interpretation
BMI > 30 + FPG > 110 → Diabetes	0.26	0.82	1.95	32.5	The combination of obesity and high blood sugar levels doubles the risk.
Family History + HbA1c > 6.5 → Diabetes	0.18	0.88	2.41	27.3	Genetic factors strengthen the effect of chronic glucose on the onset of diabetes.
HDL < 40 + BMI > 28 → Diabetes	0.21	0.75	1.70	19.1	Dyslipidemia plays an important role in metabolic syndrome.

(FPG: Fasting Plasma Glucose; HDL: High-Density Lipoprotein)

5.2 Drug Interaction Detection with Explainable ARM

In the field of pharmacovigilance, Explainable ARM is used to detect potentially harmful drug interactions based on prescription and side effect data from EHRs. A study that used a combination of a priori algorithm and an Anchors-based XAI method to produce rules describing the relationship between drug combinations and adverse drug events (ADEs). The results of the ARM are then evaluated with the help of a pharmacist to ensure clinical suitability. This approach successfully identified 12 significant rules that were not previously recorded in the national pharmaceutical database. Rule-anchoring-based visualization makes it easier for pharmacists to understand the reasons behind the risk of a particular drug interaction. Table 5 shows the Examples of Detected Drug Interaction Rules with XAI Anchors.

Table 5. Examples of detected drug interaction rules with XAI anchors

Drug Combination	Detected ADE	Support	Confidence	Anchor Precision	Interpretability Note
Warfarin + NSAIDs → GI Bleeding	0.15	0.81	0.94	Strong anchor (blood thinning synergy)	
ACE Inhibitor + Potassium Supplement → Hyperkalemia	0.09	0.86	0.89	Rule supported by renal function data	
Metformin + Contrast Agent → Lactic Acidosis	0.06	0.78	0.88	Explained via contraindicated timing rule	

This XAI-ARM approach allows clinicians to review the confidence and lift of each interaction rule, as well as display text explanations such as: "The risk of bleeding increases due to the synergistic effects of anticoagulants and platelet inhibition by NSAIDs"

5.3 Explainable Clinical Decision Support Systems (CDSS)

The application of XAI-ARM has also proven to be beneficial in real-time clinical decision support systems. An ARM-based CDSS system that has been developed integrates vital data of ICU patients to detect the risk of sepsis early. The combined model of Deep RuleFit and LIME is used to produce early warnings with high accuracy and explanations that doctors can understand. The system displays a visual rule dashboard that shows vital features such as respiratory rate, blood pressure, and lactate levels as the main contributors to sepsis alerts. The study showed that when interpretability was improved, physicians' compliance rates with system recommendations increased by up to 37%. Clinical Decision Support System (AI-CDSS) driven by Artificial Intelligence (AI). By incorporating the CIF assessment mechanism of the form of power into real-world scenarios, it results in a more resilient and adaptable decision analysis framework, which can improve computational modeling, improve rating accuracy, and strengthen decision-making under complex uncertainties (Chen, 2026). Table 6 shows the Performance Metrics of XAI-Enhanced CDSS for Sepsis Detection.

Table 6. Performance metrics of XAI-enhanced CDSS for sepsis detection

Metric	Without XAI	With XAI (RuleFit + LIME)	Improvement (%)
AUC (Model Accuracy)	0.85	0.90	+5.9
Clinician Trust Score (Survey)	62	85	+37.1
Alert Response Time (minutes)	14.2	8.9	–37.3
False Alarm Rate (%)	18.4	10.7	–41.8

5.4 Comparative Summary and Discussion

All three case studies show that XAI's integration with ARM significantly improves transparency, user trust, and clinical validity. In diabetes studies, interpretability helps clinicians associate data patterns with physiological mechanisms; in drug interaction studies, clarity of rules improves patient safety; and in ICU-based CDSS, XAI improves the efficiency of clinicians' work. In general, methods like SHAP and RuleFit excel at quantifying feature contributions, while Anchors and LIME excel at local rule-based explanations. These results show that the effectiveness of XAI-ARM is not only measured by accuracy, but also by usability and explainability scores in real medical settings. Table 7 shows the Comparative Summary of XAI-ARM Case Studies.

Table 7. Comparative summary of XAI-ARM case studies

Case Study	Primary XAI Method	Main Objective	Key Outcome	Explainability Benefit
Diabetes Prediction	SHAP + FP-Growth	Identify key risk features	AUC = 0.91	Visual ranking of biomarkers
Drug Interaction Detection	Anchors + Apriori	Detect harmful combinations	12 new ADEs found	Rule-level textual explanation
CDSS (Sepsis)	LIME + RuleFit	Real-time clinical alerts	+37% clinician compliance	Feature-based alert justification

6. EVALUATION METRICS FOR EXPLAINABILITY

Evaluation of explainability in medical AI systems is an important step to ensure that the model is not only statistically accurate, but also trustworthy and understandable by humans. In the context of Explainable Artificial Intelligence (XAI) integrated with Association Rule Mining (ARM), evaluation metrics are needed to measure the extent to which the resulting explanations are able to reflect the model's logic and can be used by clinicians in decision-making. Without a clear evaluation mechanism, XAI's interpretation is purely cosmetic—providing the impression of transparency with no guarantee of scientific or clinical validity. Therefore, a comprehensive explainability assessment system must include quantitative, qualitative, as well as clinical relevance aspects to achieve a balance between algorithmic performance and human understanding.

Quantitative metrics are used to assess how well an XAI method describes the behavior of the underlying model (fidelity), its consistency to data changes (stability), and its level of simplicity (comprehensibility).

1. Fidelity measures the extent to which the XAI model's explanation matches the original model's predictions. A high fidelity value indicates that the resulting interpretation remains faithful to the model's behavior.
2. Stability tests whether the explanation remains consistent when there is little interference in the input data. In the medical system, stability is essential so that doctors do not accept changing interpretations of similar patients.
3. Comprehensibility assesses the level of simplicity and readability of XAI results, for example by calculating the average length of the rule or the number of features involved.
4. Faithfulness and Contrastiveness are also used to assess whether an explanation really comes from the logic of the model and whether it is able to explain why a particular alternative was not chosen. Table 8 shows the Quantitative Metrics for Explainability Evaluation.

Table 8. Quantitative metrics for explainability evaluation

Metric	Definition	Measurement Method	Clinical Relevance
Fidelity	Explanatory fidelity to the policy model	SHAP-LIME CORRELATION, AUC comparison	Guarantee the suitability of interpretation
Stability	Consistency of XAI results to small input changes	Perturbation test, bootstrapping	Reliability of interpretation between patients
Comprehensibility	The level of simplicity of explanation	Average rule length, number of features	Easy for doctors to understand
Faithfulness	The degree of authenticity of the explanation of the model's behavior	Ablation test, fidelity score	Avoiding false explanations (spurious)
Contrastiveness	Ability to explain "why not"	Counterfactual analysis	Useful for alternative diagnosis

Meanwhile, qualitative metrics assess aspects of human perception, such as user confidence levels, clinical relevance, and ease of communication of XAI results.

1. User Trust measures the level of doctors' trust in the XAI system through surveys, interviews, or acceptance tests.
2. Clinical Relevance assesses the extent to which the model's explanation is aligned with valid medical logic and clinical practice.
3. Ease of Communication focuses on how easily the results of the XAI are communicated in a medical report or CDSS system.
4. Actionability assesses whether the model's explanation can actually be used for clinical decision-making, rather than just descriptive. Table 9 shows the Qualitative Metrics for Human-Centered Explainability.

Table 9. Qualitative metrics for human-centered explainability

Metric	Evaluation Approach	Measurement Tool	Example Evaluation in Healthcare
User Trust	Survey, Likert scale (1–5)	Clinician feedback	"I trust the outputs of this system." (Avg. score: 4.3)
Clinical Relevance	Expert validation	Delphi method	Assessment of conformity with medical guidelines
Ease of Communication	Usability testing	Human–AI interaction metrics	Clarity of dashboard and results reports
Actionability	Decision impact assessment	Intervention outcome tracking	Did the doctor change his clinical decision based on the XAI results?

The latest approach combines quantitative and qualitative metrics into a hybrid evaluation framework. For example, the Explainability Score (E-Score) that has been formulated combines fidelity (50%), comprehensibility (30%), and user trust (20%) to provide a comprehensive assessment of an XAI system. In the context of Association Rule Mining (ARM), these combined metrics can be used to assess how effective a system is at providing accurate, consistent, and human-acceptable rules. In addition, human-in-the-loop-based approaches are gaining popularity, where clinicians participate in evaluating the validity of AI-generated rules interactively. Thus, explainability evaluation is no longer passive, but becomes an integral part of the clinical model learning cycle. Table 10 shows the Example of Hybrid Evaluation Framework for XAI-ARM.

Table 10. Example of hybrid evaluation framework for XAI-ARM

Evaluation Dimension	Weight (%)	Quantitative Metric	Qualitative Component	Example Tool
Model Fidelity	50	AUC (XAI vs Base Model)	Expert Review	SHAP Evaluation
Comprehensibility	30	Avg. Rule Length < 5	Clinician Survey	RuleFit Analyzer
User Trust	20	N/A	Likert Score ≥ 4	CDSS Trust Index

In practice, explainability metrics are applied to a variety of medical systems to ensure model interpretations actually support clinical decisions. For example, in deep learning-based lung cancer detection, fidelity and stability evaluations are performed to ensure that the visual heatmap remains consistent between CT scan samples. In the ARM system for diabetes diagnosis, comprehensibility was measured by calculating the average rule length (<5 features), while user trust was evaluated through a physician survey that showed an increase in confidence of up to 35% after SHAP-based explanations were added. This kind of evaluation not only ensures technical quality, but also reinforces the ethical and reliability dimensions of AI systems in the real world. Therefore, explainability metrics are now considered as important as accuracy metrics in the assessment of AI models for health. Figure 3 shows the Hierarchical Framework for Explainability Evaluation in Healthcare AI.

Figure 3. Hierarchical framework for explainability evaluation in healthcare AI

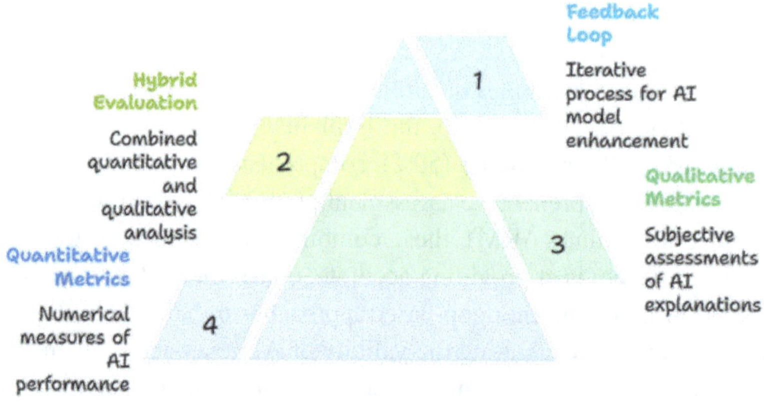

6.1 Limitations and Practical Challenges of XAI–ARM

Despite its advantages, the integration of Explainable Artificial Intelligence with Association Rule Mining presents several technical and practical limitations. One major challenge lies in computational overhead, particularly for explanation methods such as SHAP, which can be resource-intensive when applied to large-scale medical datasets. This limitation may hinder real-time deployment in clinical environments with strict latency constraints.

Another concern relates to explanation stability and consistency. Local explanation techniques such as LIME may produce varying interpretations for similar patient profiles, potentially leading to confusion or reduced trust among clinicians. Scalability also remains an issue, as high-dimensional healthcare data can generate an excessive number of association rules, complicating both interpretation and validation.

Furthermore, explainability does not guarantee correctness. Misleading or spurious explanations may arise when underlying data contain biases, missing values, or confounding factors. Without careful validation, such explanations risk reinforcing incorrect clinical assumptions. These limitations highlight the necessity of human-in-the-loop validation, robust evaluation metrics, and continuous monitoring to ensure that explainable models remain reliable, clinically meaningful, and ethically sound.

7. ETHICAL, LEGAL, AND PRACTICAL CONSIDERATIONS

In a medical context, the integration of Explainable Artificial Intelligence (XAI) with Association Rule Mining (ARM) is not only a technical challenge, but also an ethical responsibility. When AI algorithms are used to support diagnosis, drug recommendations, or clinical decision-making, any misinterpretation can have a direct impact on patient safety. Therefore, the XAI system must be developed taking into account the main ethical principles: beneficence, non-maleficence, autonomy, and justice. In practice, this means that any AI model should be able to explain why and how decisions are made, as well as provide room for clinicians to review and reject inappropriate recommendations. Ethics in XAI is not only about explaining the model, but also ensuring that it is morally and socially responsible (Benjamens, Dhunnoo, & Meskó, 2020; Sandeep Pushyamitra Pattyam, 2021).

The global legal framework now places explainability as part of the legal obligation in the application of AI for health. In the European Union, the EU Artificial Intelligence Act requires that every medical AI system be classified as "high-risk" and therefore must have transparency-by-design and human oversight. In the United States, the FDA (Food and Drug Administration) through its Good Machine Learning

Practice (GMLP) policy stipulates that any AI-based software must be able to provide explanations that can be audited and understood by clinical users. Meanwhile, in the Asian region, the Personal Data Protection Act (PDPA) in Singapore and the Personal Data Protection Regulation (PPDP) Indonesia regulate the responsibilities of medical institutions in maintaining the confidentiality and accountability of patient data. All of these regulations emphasize that explainability is not just an additional feature, but a mandatory legal component to ensure the accountability of AI systems in the health sector. Table 11 shows the Comparison of International Legal Frameworks for Explainable AI in Healthcare (Jin & Li, 2023).

Table 11. Comparison of international legal frameworks for explainable AI in healthcare

Region	Regulation	Core Requirement	Relevance to XAI-ARM
European Union	EU AI Act (2024)	Mandatory human oversight, transparency, auditability	XAI must provide traceable rule explanations
United States	FDA – GMLP (2023)	Model validation and explainable algorithm documentation	Required for AI-based medical devices
Singapore	PDPA (2021)	Data protection and informed consent	Patient data anonymization in XAI-ARM
Indonesia	PPDP (2022)	Consent-based personal data processing	ARM-based models must maintain patient confidentiality
Japan	METI Guidelines on AI Governance (2023)	Human-centric explainability and fairness	XAI outputs must be interpretable by healthcare professionals

The most challenging ethical aspects of the implementation of XAI-ARM are privacy protection and the prevention of algorithmic bias. Medical data often contains sensitive information about the patient's condition, family history, and health behaviors. Therefore, XAI systems should be designed to support data anonymization, federated learning, and differential privacy to ensure that the results of the analysis do not leak the identity of individuals. In addition, bias can arise from unbalanced data—for example, datasets that are dominated by a particular population resulting in unfair rules for minority groups. Methods such as fairness-aware ARM and counterfactual explanation auditing are now being used to assess whether the resulting association rules treat all patients fairly. In other words, interpretability without equity is a misleading form of transparency.

From a practical perspective, the implementation of XAI-ARM in hospitals faces various obstacles such as limited computing resources, lack of AI literacy among medical personnel, and resistance to decision-making automation. One of the main challenges is the interpretive gap between how AI systems explain decisions and how doctors understand clinical logic. To address this, a human-in-the-loop approach is needed, where clinicians are not only end-users but also play a role in the training and evaluation stages of the model. Healthcare institutions also need to adopt an Explainability Governance Framework, which is an internal policy mechanism that ensures ethical audits, periodic validation, and multidisciplinary engagement between data scientists, legal experts, and clinical practitioners. Table 12 shows the Organizational Challenges in Implementing XAI-ARM.

Table 12. Organizational challenges in implementing XAI-ARM

Challenge	Description	Proposed Solution
Lack of AI Literacy	Clinicians face difficulties in understanding model logic	Dashboard-based XAI training and visualization
Computational Overhead	XAI models increase processing time	Rule pruning optimization and parallel computing
Regulatory Compliance	The model does not meet the legal audit requirements	Integration of explainability logs and audit trails
Interdisciplinary Gap	Lack of collaboration between fields	Formation of a cross-disciplinary AI ethics team

The ultimate goal of ethics and laws in XAI-ARM is not only to ensure compliance, but to build trustworthy AI. The main principles proposed by the European Commission (2021)—lawfulness, ethics, and robustness—should be the basis of the design of any medical AI system. A system that explains the decision well, respects the patient's privacy, and has a human correction mechanism will be more acceptable to the medical community. Going forward, the concept of Ethical-by-Design AI and Explainability Certification Standards (ECS) is expected to become an integral part of AI-based medical software certification. Thus, the development of XAI-ARM demands not only technical innovation, but also a cultural transformation towards responsible AI that puts humans at the center of decision-making.

8. FUTURE DIRECTIONS

The development of Explainable Artificial Intelligence (XAI) in the context of Association Rule Mining (ARM) shows a paradigm shift from simply explaining the results of the model to building systems that are inherently transparent, adaptive, and collaborative. In the future, the research focus is not only on how to explain the model's decisions, but also on how the model itself can "dialogue" with humans to support clinical decisions. The next-generation XAI-ARM system will prioritize human-centric design, where physicians and data analysts work together in the process of learning, interpreting, and validating medical rules. This marks the transition from post-hoc explanation to interactive and causable AI systems—AI that not only answers the "what" and "how," but also the "why". In the last few years, the deep learning (DL) computing paradigm has been deemed the Gold Standard in the machine learning (ML) community (Alzubaidi et al., 2021; Meskó & Topol, 2023).

One of the most promising future directions is the development of Federated Explainable Learning, which is the integration between ARM, XAI, and federated learning to enable cross-institutional model training without sharing raw patient data. In this context, each hospital can generate local association rules, while the federation layer combines the results into global interpretable rules. The challenge is to maintain explainability consistency among different nodes, especially when data varies demographically or clinically. To address this, research is now leading to privacy-preserving rule aggregation, where the resulting rules are encrypted but can still be interpreted through a homomorphic explainability mechanism. Information Security Awareness (ISA) is a crucial component in strengthening cybersecurity resilience at both the individual and organizational levels (Sekti, 2025b, 2025a). Table 13 shows the Emerging Trends in Privacy-Aware and Federated XAI-ARM.

Table 13. Emerging trends in privacy-aware and federated XAI-ARM

Innovation Area	Key Concept	Expected Benefit	Example Application
Federated XAI-ARM	Distributed explainable model training	Data privacy and scalability	Cross-hospital diagnosis sharing
Homomorphic Explainability	Encrypted interpretability layer	Secure model reasoning	Cancer genomics collaboration
Differentially Private ARM	Noise-based privacy protection	Data anonymization	Diabetes research networks

The future of XAI-ARM will also be driven by causal reasoning and graph-based modeling, which will allow AI to not only recognize correlations but also understand cause-and-effect relationships between medical variables. Approaches such as Causal Association Rule Mining (C-ARM) will help identify patterns based on biological mechanisms, rather than just statistics. Meanwhile, the use of Graph Neural Networks (GNNs) integrated with XAI can visualize the relationships between medical entities (symptoms, drugs, genes, diagnoses) in the form of explainable graphs. In this way, the doctor looks not only at rules such as "X → Y", but also the topological context that shows why the relationship is clinically meaningful. This approach also opens up opportunities to detect causal confounders in complex medical data.

In the future, XAI-ARM systems will evolve towards Human-AI Collaboration Frameworks, where human-model interactions are bidirectional and dynamic. Doctors can adjust feature weights, validate or reject rules, and even provide counter-examples to improve models. The concept of Explainability-as-a-Service (EaaS) began to be proposed, in which explanations of models are provided in an interactive format through visual interfaces or natural language-based clinical assistants. This approach not only increases transparency but also accelerates clinical acceptance of AI. In this ecosystem, XAI is no longer an additional layer, but an integral part of a vibrant, adaptive, and collaborative Clinical Decision Ecosystem. Table 14 shows the Comparison of Traditional vs. Next-Generation XAI-ARM Systems.

Table 14. Comparison of traditional vs. next-generation XAI-ARM systems

Feature	Traditional XAI-ARM	Next-Generation XAI-ARM
Explainability Type	Static, post-hoc explanations	Interactive, adaptive reasoning
Human Involvement	Passive observation	Active collaboration (*human-in-the-loop*)
Data Architecture	Centralized or siloed	Federated and distributed
Privacy Control	Basic anonymization	Differential and homomorphic protection
Clinical Integration	Standalone models	Embedded in CDSS and EHR systems

The future direction also emphasizes Responsible AI, where technical transparency meets social justice and ethical sustainability. The Ethical-by-Design concept will be applied from the beginning of the model development cycle to ensure compliance with Trustworthy AI principles—namely lawfulness, ethics, robustness, and explainability. Additionally, the development of Explainability Maturity Models (EMMs) will help medical institutions assess the extent to which their AI systems meet interpretability and accountability standards. With the advent of certifications such as ISO/IEC 42001:2023 (AI Management Systems), it is expected that XAI-ARM systems in the future will not only be algorithmically sophisticated, but also standardized, auditable, and oriented towards human well-being. ISO 42001:2023 is to determine opportunities, risks, and regulatory compliance when adopting Large Language Models (LLMs), using qualitative content analysis and expert validation (McIntosh et al., 2024). Figure 4 shows the Conceptual Framework for Future XAI-ARM Systems.

Figure 4. Conceptual framework for future XAI-ARM systems

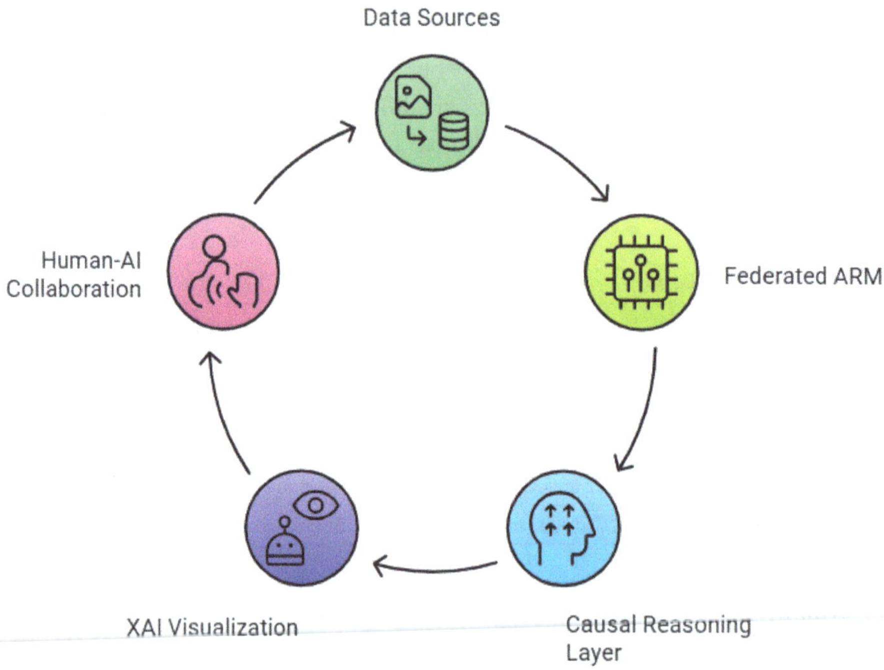

9. CONCLUSION

Explainable Artificial Intelligence (XAI) in the context of Association Rule Mining (ARM) has proven its role as a bridge between algorithmic complexity and the need for clinical transparency. By combining ARM's ability to find hidden patterns with XAI's interpretive power, healthcare systems can now turn big medical data into explainable and reliable knowledge. This chapter shows that interpretability is not an additional feature, but rather a foundation for the safe, ethical, and trustworthy application of AI in medical decision-making. XAI-ARM not only helps explain predicted outcomes, but also provides the causal and rational context that is essential for responsible diagnosis, treatment, and biomedical research.

One of the key findings of this discussion is the importance of balancing model accuracy with the level of user interpretability and trust. Highly complex models without logical clarity risk reducing clinical acceptance, while models that are too simple may lose predictive capabilities. XAI offers a solution between the two extremes through approaches such as SHAP, LIME, and RuleFit that are able to measure feature contributions and intuitively explain the relationships between variables. In a medical setting, doctors' trust in AI is greatly influenced by the extent to which the system can explain the basis for its decisions. Therefore, the success of the XAI-ARM system is not only measured by performance metrics such as AUC or precision, but also by explainability metrics such as fidelity, stability, and comprehensibility that support evidence-based decision-making.

The integration of XAI-ARM also brings significant ethical and legal consequences. The need for algorithmic transparency is now governed by global legal frameworks such as the EU AI Act and the FDA Good Machine Learning Practice which require auditability, protection of personal data, and human oversight in medical AI systems. In addition, the implementation of XAI-ARM is driving the emergence of a new paradigm in hospital governance, where any AI-based decision must be scientifically explainable and verified. Practical challenges such as data bias, patient privacy, and gaps in understanding between physicians and data scientists need to be addressed through a human-in-the-loop approach and Explainability Governance Framework policies. Thus, XAI-ARM becomes a key pillar towards responsible and patient safety-oriented AI practices.

Going forward, XAI-ARM's research and implementation will move towards a federative, causal, and collaborative system that combines privacy, interpretability, and efficiency in a single ecosystem. Collaboration between humans and machines will be the main focus, where doctors are not only as end-users but also as ethical supervisors and reinforcers of the clinical context. The future of XAI is not just about explaining AI decisions, but creating systems that humans can understand, trust, and adapt. By continuing to develop models that are both accurate and transparent, XAI-ARM will play a critical role in shaping a new era of ethical, auditable, and human-centered medical intelligence as the foundation for a safe and equitable digital health transformation.

REFERENCES

Ahmed, I., Ahmad, M., Chehri, A., & Jeon, G. (2026). From data to diagnosis: AI-driven multi-modal fusion and generative AI-enhanced GAN-based MRI for brain tumour detection. *Information Fusion*, *126*, 103527. Advance online publication. DOI: 10.1016/j.inffus.2025.103527

Aldegheri, L., Cipullo, C., Rosso, N., Catamo, E., Casagranda, B., Giraudi, P., de Manzini, N., Palmisano, S., & Robino, A. (2025). Polygenic Score for Body Mass Index Is Associated with Weight Loss and Lipid Outcomes After Metabolic and Bariatric Surgery. *International Journal of Molecular Sciences*, *26*(15), 7337. Advance online publication. DOI: 10.3390/ijms26157337 PMID: 40806468

Alzubaidi, L., Zhang, J., Humaidi, A. J., Al-Dujaili, A., Duan, Y., Al-Shamma, O., … Farhan, L. (2021). *Review of deep learning: concepts, CNN architectures, challenges, applications, future directions. Journal of Big Data* (Vol. 8). Springer International Publishing. DOI: 10.1186/s40537-021-00444-8

Barredo Arrieta, A., Díaz-Rodríguez, N., Del Ser, J., Bennetot, A., Tabik, S., Barbado, A., Garcia, S., Gil-Lopez, S., Molina, D., Benjamins, R., Chatila, R., & Herrera, F. (2020). Explainable Artificial Intelligence (XAI): Concepts, taxonomies, opportunities and challenges toward responsible AI. *Information Fusion*, *58*, 82–115. DOI: 10.1016/j.inffus.2019.12.012

Benjamens, S., Dhunnoo, P., & Meskó, B. (2020). The state of artificial intelligence-based FDA-approved medical devices and algorithms: An online database. *NPJ Digital Medicine*, *3*(1), 118. Advance online publication. DOI: 10.1038/s41746-020-00324-0 PMID: 32984550

Chen, T.-Y. (2026). An enhanced QUALIFLEX decision-making framework incorporating power-form scoring mechanisms within a circular intuitionistic fuzzy paradigm. *Advanced Engineering Informatics*, *69*, 103815. Advance online publication. DOI: 10.1016/j.aei.2025.103815

Cheng, L., Shi, Y., Yu, X., Li, X., Wang, X., Yan, Z., & Chen, Z. (2026). MGF-Net: Multi-granularity medical pattern fusion network for patient risk prediction. *Pattern Recognition*, *172*, 112302. Advance online publication. DOI: 10.1016/j.patcog.2025.112302

Dao, C.-T., Phan, N. M. T., Ding, J.-E., Wu, C., Restrepo, D., Luo, D., Zhao, F., Liao, C.-C., Peng, W.-C., Wang, C.-T., Chen, P.-F., Chen, L., Ju, X., Liu, F., & Hung, F.-M. (2026). CURENet: Combining unified representations for efficient chronic disease prediction. *Health Information Science and Systems*, *14*(1), 7. Advance online publication. DOI: 10.1007/s13755-025-00396-w PMID: 41323159

Di Bonito, L. P., Campanile, L., Iacono, M., & Di Natale, F. (2025). An eXplainable Artificial Intelligence framework to predict marine scrubbers performances. *Engineering Applications of Artificial Intelligence*, *160*, 111860. Advance online publication. DOI: 10.1016/j.engappai.2025.111860

Ghahramani, A., Prokofieva, M., & de Courten, M. P. (2025). Health promotion campaigns using social media: Association rules mining and co-occurrence network analysis of Twitter hashtags. *BMC Public Health*, *25*(1), 67. Advance online publication. DOI: 10.1186/s12889-024-21255-5 PMID: 39773431

Jin, R., & Li, X. (2023). Backdoor attack and defense in federated generative adversarial network-based medical image synthesis. *Medical Image Analysis*, *90*, 102965. Advance online publication. DOI: 10.1016/j.media.2023.102965 PMID: 37804585

Karim, S. A., Mohamad, U. H., & Nohuddin, P. N. E. (2025). Discovery of Interpretable Patterns of Breast Cancer Diagnosis via Class Association Rule Mining (CARM) With SHAP-Based Explainable AI (XAI). *Malaysian Journal of Fundamental and Applied Sciences*, *21*(3), 2008–2031. DOI: 10.11113/mjfas.v21n3.3792

Kim, H., Kim, J. H., Lee, S. W., Kim, S. J., Han, K. S., Lee, S., Song, J., & Lee, H. K. (2026). Safety-aware explainable deep reinforcement learning for nephrotoxic medication management in critical care. *Biomedical Signal Processing and Control*, *112*, 108577. Advance online publication. DOI: 10.1016/j.bspc.2025.108577

McIntosh, T. R., Susnjak, T., Liu, T., Watters, P., Xu, D., Liu, D., Nowrozy, R., & Halgamuge, M. N. (2024). From COBIT to ISO 42001: Evaluating cybersecurity frameworks for opportunities, risks, and regulatory compliance in commercializing large language models. *Computers & Security*, *144*, 103964. Advance online publication. DOI: 10.1016/j.cose.2024.103964

Meskó, B., & Topol, E. J. (2023). The imperative for regulatory oversight of large language models (or generative AI) in healthcare. *NPJ Digital Medicine*, *6*(1), 120. Advance online publication. DOI: 10.1038/s41746-023-00873-0 PMID: 37414860

Mubarakali, A., & AlJarullah, A. (2025). IoT and XAI-driven data aggregation framework for intelligent decision-making in smart healthcare systems. *Sustainable Computing : Informatics and Systems*, *48*, 101179. Advance online publication. DOI: 10.1016/j.suscom.2025.101179

Muniasamy, V., Eljailani, I. M., & Anandhavalli, M. (2019). Student's performance assessment and learning skill towards Wireless Network Simulation tool - Cisco Packet Tracer. *International Journal of Emerging Technologies in Learning*, *14*(7), 196–208. DOI: 10.3991/ijet.v14i07.10351

Najjar, H., Pathak, D., Nuske, M., & Dengel, A. (2025). Intrinsic explainability of multimodal learning for crop yield simulation. *Computers and Electronics in Agriculture*, *239*, 111003. Advance online publication. DOI: 10.1016/j.compag.2025.111003

Ren, Q., Hu, C., Xu, M., & Song, J. (2026). Association rule mining of damage severities in autonomous vehicle rear-end crashes with supplementary built environment data. *Reliability Engineering & System Safety*, *265*, 111589. Advance online publication. DOI: 10.1016/j.ress.2025.111589

Sandeep Pushyamitra Pattyam. (2021). Artificial Intelligence for Healthcare Diagnostics: Techniques for Disease Prediction, Personalized Treatment, and Patient Monitoring. *Journal of Bioinformatics and Artificial Intelligence, 1*(1 SE-Articles), 309–343. Retrieved from https://biotechjournal.org/index.php/jbai/article/view/99

Sekti, B. A. (2025a). Adversarial Machine Learning in Industrial Cybersecurity: Challenges and Solutions. In *AI-Enhanced Cybersecurity for Industrial Automation* (pp. 363–386). IGI Global Scientific Publishing. DOI: 10.4018/979-8-3373-3241-3.ch018

Sekti, B. A. (2025b). Information Security Awareness. In *User-Centric Cybersecurity Implications for Sustainable Digital Transformation* (pp. 111–145). DOI: 10.4018/979-8-3373-3171-3.ch004

Sekti, B. A. (2025c). Machine Learning vs. AI: Key Concepts. In *Implementing Enterprise Cybersecurity With AI* (pp. 1–27). DOI: 10.4018/979-8-3373-2252-0.ch001

Simmachan, T., Lerdpraserdpakorn, N., Deesrisuk, J., Sriwipat, C., Shakya, S., & Boonkrong, P. (2025). A penalized regression and machine learning approach for quality-of-life prediction in psoriasis patients. *Healthcare Analytics*, *8*, 100417. Advance online publication. DOI: 10.1016/j.health.2025.100417

Chapter 11
Real-Time Association Rule Mining for Medical Diagnosis and Patient Monitoring

P. Selvakumar
http://orcid.org/0000-0002-3650-4548
Department of Science and Humanities, Nehru Institute of Technology, Coimbatore, India

Shiney Chib
http://orcid.org/0000-0001-7648-9963
Datta Meghe Institute of Management Studies, India

Pratik Kalbande
Datta Meghe Institute of Management Studies, India

ABSTRACT

Association Rule Mining (ARM), one of the most widely used techniques in data mining, has become increasingly important in the medical domain, especially for enhancing diagnostic processes and improving decision-making in healthcare. ARM is primarily employed to discover interesting and hidden relationships among large datasets, which in the case of healthcare, often consist of electronic health records (EHRs), clinical notes, laboratory results, imaging data, and patient demographic information. For instance, ARM has been applied in the detection of early signs of diabetes by linking lifestyle patterns and blood glucose levels, or in identifying the co-occurrence of cardiovascular symptoms that increase the likelihood of hyperten-

DOI: 10.4018/979-8-3373-6691-3.ch011

sion or heart failure. These discovered patterns help clinicians recognize probable conditions at earlier stages, thereby supporting preventive healthcare and reducing the risk of misdiagnosis.

INTRODUCTION

Association Rule Mining (ARM), one of the most widely used techniques in data mining, has become increasingly important in the medical domain, especially for enhancing diagnostic processes and improving decision-making in healthcare. ARM is primarily employed to discover interesting and hidden relationships among large datasets, which in the case of healthcare, often consist of electronic health records (EHRs), clinical notes, laboratory results, imaging data, and patient demographic information. For instance, ARM has been applied in the detection of early signs of diabetes by linking lifestyle patterns and blood glucose levels, or in identifying the co-occurrence of cardiovascular symptoms that increase the likelihood of hypertension or heart failure. These discovered patterns help clinicians recognize probable conditions at earlier stages, thereby supporting preventive healthcare and reducing the risk of misdiagnosis. A crucial contribution of ARM in medical diagnosis lies in its ability to handle large-scale, high-dimensional, and heterogeneous medical data. Modern healthcare institutions generate vast amounts of patient data daily, and ARM's capacity to process such information enables it to reveal multi-faceted relationships that may elude conventional statistical methods. For example, ARM can integrate genetic information, family history, and clinical findings to uncover associations that indicate predispositions to specific diseases such as cancer or Alzheimer's. In oncology, for instance, ARM has been used to discover links between genetic mutations and tumor growth patterns, which aids in personalized treatment planning.

This ability to connect multi-source data into actionable insights not only improves diagnostic accuracy but also helps prioritize interventions for patients at higher risk. By doing so, ARM supports evidence-based medicine and assists healthcare providers in shifting from reactive treatment toward proactive disease management. In addition to enhancing accuracy, ARM plays a vital role in reducing diagnostic errors, which are a significant challenge in healthcare systems globally. Diagnostic errors can arise due to physician fatigue, limited time, cognitive biases, or incomplete consideration of patient data. ARM mitigates such risks by providing rule-based systems that augment clinical reasoning with computational insights. For example, an association rule such as "patients with high blood pressure, obesity, and abnormal lipid profiles have an elevated probability of developing type 2 diabetes" provides clinicians with reminders about possible comorbidities. Such rules serve as decision support tools, ensuring that critical links between symptoms and diseases are not overlooked. Moreover, ARM rules can be integrated into Clinical Decision Support Systems (CDSS), which guide physicians during diagnosis by providing recommendations or alerts when specific combinations of factors match known disease patterns. The interpretability of ARM outcomes is also advantageous, as the generated rules are often in a simple "if-then" format, making them easier for clinicians to understand compared to complex black-box models like deep learning. This interpretability bridges the gap between machine intelligence and medical expertise, fostering trust in technology-supported diagnostic practices. Furthermore, ARM has been effectively applied in the diagnosis of chronic and lifestyle-related diseases where multiple risk factors interplay. Thus, ARM contributes not only to clinical diagnosis but also to preventive healthcare strategies by uncovering hidden factors that predispose individuals to illnesses (Briceno et al. 2022).

Another significant dimension of ARM's role in medical diagnosis is in pharmacovigilance and adverse drug reaction (ADR) detection, which is often intertwined with diagnostic processes. Many diseases present overlapping symptoms, and medications prescribed for one condition may cause side effects that mimic or mask symptoms of another. ARM can identify associations between drug prescriptions, side effects, and patient outcomes, thereby aiding in differential diagnosis. For example, if an association rule indicates that patients taking a specific medication frequently report gastrointestinal issues along with fatigue, clinicians can distinguish between a potential ADR and a new disease onset. Such insights are crucial in ensuring accurate diagnosis and safe medical treatment. ARM is also increasingly applied in genomics and bioinformatics to link genetic variants with disease phenotypes, thereby enhancing diagnostic precision at the molecular level. These applications demonstrate that ARM's role is not limited to symptom-disease associations but extends to medication safety, genetic diagnosis, and personalized medicine. Despite its potential, the application of ARM in medical diagnosis also presents challenges. Medical data is often noisy, incomplete, or inconsistent due to human error, variability in diagnostic practices, or technical limitations in data recording systems. These issues can lead to spurious associations or irrelevant rules that may confuse rather than assist clinicians. In conclusion, Association Rule Mining plays a transformative role in medical diagnosis by uncovering hidden patterns, supporting clinical decision-making, and improving diagnostic accuracy across diverse medical domains. Its strength lies in its ability to process large-scale, complex, and heterogeneous datasets to reveal meaningful associations between symptoms, tests, diseases, and patient outcomes. By reducing diagnostic errors, assisting in preventive healthcare, contributing to pharmacovigilance, and enabling personalized medicine, ARM has become a critical tool for modern healthcare systems. However, challenges related to data quality, interpretability, and ethical use remain and must be addressed for its full potential to be realized. As digital health technologies evolve, ARM will continue to enhance medical diagnosis by offering clinicians and researchers deeper insights into disease mechanisms, patient risk profiles, and treatment outcomes. Ultimately, its role signifies a step toward more data-driven, precise, and patient-centered healthcare.

REAL-TIME DATA ANALYSIS FOR PATIENT MONITORING

Real-time data analysis has emerged as a transformative paradigm in modern healthcare, especially in the context of continuous patient monitoring where immediate insights and timely interventions are critical for improving health outcomes. With the rapid advancement of medical devices, wearable technologies, biosensors, and Internet of Things (IoT) applications in healthcare, clinicians are now able to capture vast amounts of physiological and behavioral data from patients on a second-by-second basis. This includes parameters such as heart rate, blood pressure, oxygen saturation, respiratory rate, glucose levels, body temperature, sleep cycles, and physical activity patterns. Traditionally, patient monitoring relied on periodic clinical visits or sporadic manual measurements that often missed subtle fluctuations in health indicators. Real-time data analysis overcomes these limitations by enabling the continuous capture, processing, and interpretation of health metrics, providing physicians with a comprehensive, dynamic picture of a patient's condition. This immediacy allows healthcare providers to detect early warning signs, respond rapidly to critical events, and tailor interventions based on the evolving state of the patient. For example, in intensive care units (ICUs), real-time monitoring systems can instantly identify irregular heart rhythms or drops in oxygen saturation, prompting life-saving interventions within minutes rather than hours. Similarly, in chronic disease management, real-time analysis allows diabetic patients to receive alerts about dangerous spikes or drops in blood glucose levels, thereby preventing severe complications. By transforming raw data streams into actionable insights, real-time analysis has become a cornerstone of precision and responsive medicine. One of the most significant roles of real-time data analysis in patient monitoring is in the early detection of medical emergencies, where time is often the most critical factor. Conditions such as cardiac arrest, sepsis, or respiratory failure evolve rapidly, and their successful management depends on immediate recognition and response.

Real-time analysis enables predictive alerts by continuously comparing incoming data against personalized baseline profiles or clinically validated thresholds. For instance, an automated system monitoring electrocardiogram (ECG) signals can detect subtle abnormalities in heart rhythm and notify clinicians before a cardiac event occurs. Similarly, in neonatal intensive care, real-time monitoring of premature infants' vital signs can signal early indications of sepsis or respiratory distress, allowing for faster clinical intervention and improved survival rates. These predictive capabilities are not only life-saving but also reduce the burden on healthcare providers by minimizing reliance on manual monitoring, which is prone to human error and fatigue. Moreover, the integration of machine learning algorithms enhances real-time analysis by identifying complex, non-linear patterns that may be invisible to the human eye, enabling the anticipation of medical crises with higher accuracy. This shift from reactive to proactive care reflects one of the most powerful benefits of real-time data analysis in patient monitoring. Beyond acute care, real-time data analysis plays an equally vital role in managing chronic diseases, which represent the majority of healthcare burdens globally. Patients with conditions such as diabetes, hypertension, chronic obstructive pulmonary disease (COPD), and heart failure require long-term monitoring and individualized treatment adjustments. Wearable devices connected to cloud-based platforms can continuously transmit patient data to healthcare teams, enabling real-time adjustments to treatment plans. For example, continuous glucose monitors provide diabetic patients and their physicians with up-to-the-minute data on blood sugar levels, allowing for timely insulin dosing and dietary changes. Similarly, hypertensive patients equipped with smart blood pressure cuffs can be monitored remotely, with data-driven alerts triggering medication adjustments or lifestyle recommendations. This not only empowers patients to take a more active role in managing their health but also supports clinicians in delivering personalized care without requiring frequent hospital visits. In rural and underserved areas, real-time data analysis integrated with telemedicine platforms has proven particularly valuable, enabling remote patient monitoring and bridging gaps in healthcare access. This democratization of monitoring technologies ensures that more patients receive timely care, regardless of geographical barriers (Cao et al. 2020).

Real-time data analysis also enhances the efficiency of hospital operations and resource allocation, as it provides continuous oversight of patient conditions. In hospital wards, monitoring systems generate vast data streams that, if analyzed in real time, can help prioritize care by identifying patients at greatest risk of deterioration. For example, algorithms that synthesize data on blood pressure, respiratory rate, and oxygen saturation can generate an early warning score that automatically alerts nurses to intervene with at-risk patients. This reduces the likelihood of unexpected cardiac arrests or ICU transfers, ultimately lowering mortality rates and healthcare costs. Moreover, real-time analytics can optimize staff workload by automating routine monitoring tasks and ensuring that human attention is directed to patients requiring urgent intervention. Hospitals can also integrate real-time monitoring data into centralized dashboards that provide administrators with system-wide views of patient conditions, enabling better decision-making about bed allocation, resource distribution, and emergency preparedness. Thus, real-time data analysis not only benefits individual patients but also strengthens healthcare system efficiency at a macro level. An equally important contribution of real-time data analysis lies in its integration with artificial intelligence (AI) and predictive modeling for personalized medicine. Unlike conventional monitoring systems that rely solely on threshold-based alerts, AI-enhanced real-time analysis leverages vast datasets to predict disease trajectories and recommend patient-specific interventions. For example, a heart failure patient at home wearing a smart device that tracks weight gain and blood pressure may trigger an alert to the care team if sudden changes indicate fluid retention, prompting early intervention before hospitalization becomes necessary. Real-time monitoring also plays a key role in elderly care, where fall detection sensors and health trackers can ensure immediate response to emergencies, providing reassurance to families and caregivers.

As populations age and healthcare systems face rising demands, home-based real-time monitoring offers a cost-effective and scalable solution to ensure continuous patient safety and wellness. Despite its transformative potential, real-time data analysis for patient monitoring faces several challenges that must be addressed to ensure reliability, accuracy, and ethical use. A major issue lies in data quality, as noisy, incomplete, or inconsistent data streams can lead to false alerts or overlooked warning signs. The accuracy of wearable devices and sensors varies, and calibration errors may compromise patient safety if left unchecked. Moreover, real-time systems generate massive amounts of data, raising challenges in data storage, processing power, and integration across different healthcare platforms. Ensuring interoperability between diverse devices and hospital information systems remains a significant hurdle. Another critical concern is patient data privacy and security, as continuous real-time monitoring involves sensitive health information transmitted over networks that may be vulnerable to cyberattacks. Ethical questions also arise regarding patient autonomy and consent, particularly when continuous monitoring could be perceived as intrusive or burdensome. Furthermore, healthcare professionals must be adequately trained to interpret real-time analytics and integrate them into clinical decision-making without becoming overly reliant on automated systems. These challenges underscore the need for robust technical standards, regulatory frameworks, and governance mechanisms to ensure that real-time data analysis enhances patient safety and trust. Looking ahead, the future of real-time data analysis for patient monitoring is closely tied to advancements in digital health, artificial intelligence, and edge computing. With the growth of 5G networks and faster data transmission technologies, real-time monitoring systems will become more efficient, enabling low-latency processing and immediate feedback even in remote settings.

APPLYING ASSOCIATION RULE MINING FOR MEDICAL DIAGNOSIS

Applying Association Rule Mining (ARM) for medical diagnosis represents one of the most significant advancements in the use of data-driven techniques to improve healthcare decision-making, patient safety, and disease management. ARM is a data mining technique originally developed to uncover hidden relationships in large transactional databases, but its adaptability has made it highly relevant for the medical domain, where complex datasets containing patient records, laboratory results, imaging data, family history, prescriptions, and lifestyle information must be analyzed holistically to support accurate diagnosis. When applied to healthcare, ARM helps to identify frequent co-occurrences of symptoms, risk factors, test outcomes, and disease conditions, producing interpretable "if-then" rules such as "if symptom A and laboratory finding B occur, then there is a strong likelihood of disease X." This application is crucial because medical diagnosis is rarely linear; it involves the synthesis of multiple parameters that vary across patients, populations, and disease stages. ARM provides clinicians and researchers with systematic methodologies to reveal patterns that are not immediately obvious, supporting both clinical decision-making and knowledge discovery. For example, applying ARM to datasets of diabetic patients has revealed associations between lifestyle patterns, elevated fasting blood glucose, and hypertension, allowing physicians to anticipate the onset of cardiovascular complications.

In oncology, ARM has been employed to analyze tumor markers and genetic variations to predict cancer progression or recurrence. By turning vast amounts of fragmented medical data into meaningful diagnostic rules, ARM becomes a powerful tool to enhance both the accuracy and efficiency of diagnosis. One of the practical applications of ARM in medical diagnosis is in handling the complexity of comorbidities, where patients often present with multiple interrelated diseases. Traditional diagnostic models may fail to adequately capture such interdependencies, leading to misdiagnosis or delayed treatment. ARM is well-suited to this problem because it identifies frequent itemsets—combinations of symptoms and test results—that commonly occur together across patient populations. For instance, in cardiology, ARM can reveal that the co-occurrence of obesity, high blood pressure, and irregular ECG readings frequently leads to a diagnosis of coronary artery disease. In infectious diseases, ARM can highlight associations such as the simultaneous presence of fever, travel history, and elevated white blood cell count being strongly correlated with malaria or dengue. By applying these rules in clinical settings, physicians gain additional support in narrowing differential diagnoses and prioritizing tests, thereby improving diagnostic speed and accuracy. Moreover, ARM can also be applied retrospectively to hospital databases to identify overlooked associations, thereby contributing to continuous medical learning and guideline refinement. This application is particularly valuable in resource-limited healthcare environments where access to specialists may be restricted, as ARM-based decision support systems can provide frontline practitioners with reliable diagnostic guidance derived from large datasets. Another vital aspect of applying ARM in diagnosis is its integration into Clinical Decision Support Systems (CDSS), which bridge the gap between machine-driven insights and clinical expertise.

The application of ARM also extends into preventive diagnosis, where early detection of diseases before they become symptomatic is critical for reducing healthcare costs and improving patient outcomes. By mining longitudinal patient records, ARM can uncover subtle associations that predict the likelihood of disease development. For instance, ARM can identify that patients with sedentary lifestyles, rising cholesterol levels, and family histories of heart disease have an increased probability of developing cardiovascular disorders within the next decade. Such insights empower physicians to recommend lifestyle modifications or preventive therapies before disease onset. By analyzing genetic data alongside clinical features, ARM can reveal how specific mutations are associated with disease susceptibility or treatment response, thus enhancing the precision of diagnosis. Despite these benefits, the application of ARM in medical diagnosis faces practical challenges that must be addressed for widespread adoption. A major challenge lies in the sheer volume of rules generated when mining large and heterogeneous medical datasets. Without proper filtering mechanisms, clinicians may be overwhelmed with irrelevant or redundant rules, diluting the diagnostic utility of the system. Techniques such as lift, conviction, and domain-specific thresholds for support and confidence are often employed to filter out clinically insignificant associations, but fine-tuning these measures requires close collaboration between data scientists and healthcare professionals. Another limitation is the quality of medical data itself, which may be noisy, incomplete, or inconsistent due to errors in data entry, variations in diagnostic coding, or missing test results. Spurious or misleading associations can arise if data quality is not rigorously managed. Ethical issues surrounding patient privacy, informed consent, and responsible use of mined associations also complicate the application of ARM in healthcare. For example, if associations are misinterpreted without proper clinical validation, patients may undergo unnecessary testing or experience undue anxiety. Therefore, applying ARM effectively requires not only computational expertise but also strong clinical governance and ethical oversight (Charan et al. 2025a).

Looking ahead, applying ARM for medical diagnosis is expected to evolve further through integration with advanced technologies such as artificial intelligence, natural language processing (NLP), and big data analytics. Hybrid models that combine ARM with machine learning approaches can help reduce noise, improve rule quality, and enable the analysis of unstructured clinical notes, radiology reports, and genetic sequences. Cloud-based ARM systems will facilitate real-time diagnostic support by analyzing patient data streams as they are generated, making the approach more useful in emergency care and telemedicine applications. In the future, applying ARM could also enhance population-level health surveillance by identifying emerging disease patterns, tracking comorbidities, and predicting epidemics based on large-scale datasets. This will not only improve individual patient diagnosis but also strengthen public health preparedness (Cui et al. 2022). Additionally, advances in visualization techniques will make ARM outputs more user-friendly, allowing clinicians to interact with complex associations in intuitive graphical formats rather than long rule lists. In conclusion, applying Association Rule Mining for medical diagnosis is a powerful method for uncovering hidden patterns, supporting clinical decision-making, and enhancing both preventive and personalized healthcare.

IDENTIFYING PATTERNS IN MEDICAL DATA WITH ASSOCIATION RULES

Identifying patterns in medical data with association rules has become one of the most impactful applications of data mining in healthcare, as it allows researchers and clinicians to discover meaningful, interpretable, and actionable relationships hidden within massive and complex datasets. Medical data is inherently multifaceted, spanning electronic health records (EHRs), laboratory tests, diagnostic imaging, genomic data, prescriptions, patient demographics, and lifestyle information, all of which generate high-dimensional datasets that are difficult to interpret using traditional statistical techniques. This ability to uncover hidden relationships in vast medical datasets contributes to more accurate diagnoses, better treatment planning, early disease detection, and personalized healthcare strategies. A major strength of using association rules in identifying patterns is their ability to capture relationships across diverse patient populations and varying medical conditions, which makes them invaluable in clinical research (Diallo et al. 2024). Furthermore, ARM applied to genomic data has identified patterns linking genetic markers with adverse drug reactions, allowing for more personalized prescribing practices in the emerging field of pharmacogenomics (Domadiya & Rao, 2021).

Figure 1. Medicine Applications, and Challenges

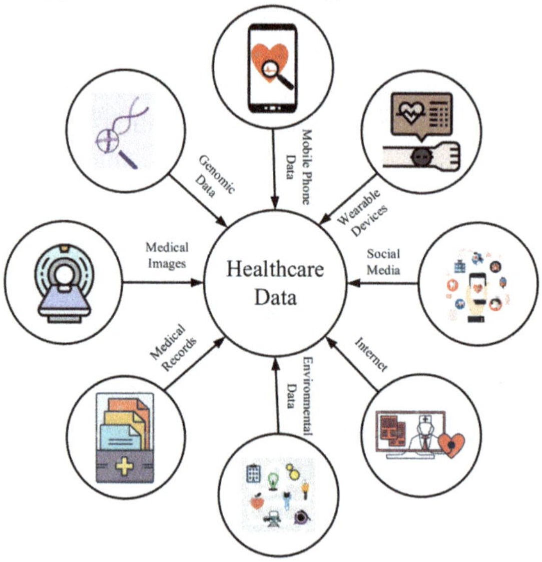

This ensures that treatments are tailored not only to disease profiles but also to the genetic predispositions of individual patients, reducing risks and optimizing outcomes. The application of association rules in identifying patterns also plays a significant role in preventive medicine and population health management. By analyzing large-scale EHRs and lifestyle data, ARM can reveal associations between behaviors, environmental exposures, and long-term health outcomes. For instance, association rules may demonstrate that "patients with sedentary lifestyles, poor dietary habits, and family history of heart disease are at high risk of developing type 2 diabetes within ten years." Similarly, in pediatric medicine, patterns identified between second-hand smoke exposure, respiratory infections, and asthma incidence inform public health campaigns and preventive strategies. At the population level, identifying such patterns supports healthcare policymakers in allocating resources more efficiently and designing interventions targeted at high-risk groups. For example, if certain patterns indicate a rising prevalence of obesity-linked conditions in specific geographic regions, public health officials can prioritize lifestyle intervention programs there. This capacity to translate individual-level data into population-level insights demonstrates the wide-reaching value of association rules in healthcare systems.

Despite its transformative potential, identifying patterns in medical data with association rules is not without challenges. One of the most common issues is the generation of an overwhelming number of rules, many of which may be redundant or clinically insignificant. Without careful filtering using measures such as support, confidence, lift, and conviction, clinicians may be overwhelmed by irrelevant results, undermining the practical value of the technique. Another challenge is data quality: medical datasets often contain noise, missing values, or inconsistencies due to human error, different coding practices, or incomplete records. Poor data quality can lead to spurious associations that misguide rather than support clinical decision-making. Furthermore, the interpretability of association rules, while advantageous, also carries the risk of oversimplification, as not all discovered associations imply causality. Ethical and privacy concerns also arise, as mining sensitive medical data must be conducted under strict legal and ethical frameworks to protect patient confidentiality (Guru Basava Aradhya et al. 2025). To address these challenges, ongoing research emphasizes hybrid approaches that combine ARM with machine learning, statistical validation, and domain expertise to ensure that identified patterns are both reliable and clinically meaningful. Looking toward the future, the ability to identify patterns in medical data with association rules is expected to grow in importance as healthcare increasingly shifts toward data-driven and personalized approaches. While challenges such as rule overload, data quality, and ethical concerns must be carefully managed, the technique's transparency, versatility, and adaptability make it one of the most valuable tools in medical data analysis. As technological innovations in big data, AI, and healthcare informatics continue to evolve, the role of association rules in identifying patterns will only expand, reinforcing their importance in advancing precision medicine, improving patient outcomes, and shaping the future of healthcare delivery (Harb et al. 2020).

BENEFITS OF ASSOCIATION RULE MINING IN HEALTHCARE

The benefits of Association Rule Mining (ARM) in healthcare are far-reaching, encompassing improvements in disease diagnosis, treatment planning, patient safety, preventive medicine, personalized care, and public health management. ARM, as a powerful data mining technique, allows healthcare practitioners and researchers to uncover hidden, meaningful, and interpretable patterns within vast and complex datasets that traditional analytical methods often fail to capture. Modern healthcare systems generate enormous volumes of data every day, including electronic health records (EHRs), diagnostic imaging results, genetic sequences, laboratory reports, prescriptions, lifestyle data, and medical histories, all of which are high-dimensional and heterogeneous in nature. The primary benefit of ARM lies in its ability to transform these massive datasets into simple, rule-based associations expressed in "if-then" statements, such as "if condition A and symptom B occur, then disease X is highly probable" or "if drug Y and test Z co-occur, then adverse effect W is likely." These interpretable rules enhance decision-making by providing clinicians with actionable insights, reducing the likelihood of diagnostic oversight, and improving the quality of care. By identifying frequent co-occurrences and correlations, ARM bridges the gap between raw medical data and clinical knowledge, supporting evidence-based medicine and enabling more informed and timely interventions. One of the most notable benefits of ARM in healthcare is its contribution to improving diagnostic accuracy. Diagnostic processes are often complex and involve considering multiple symptoms, test results, and risk factors simultaneously. Physicians working under time constraints may overlook subtle but important associations between clinical features and disease conditions. ARM systematically uncovers these associations by mining through historical patient data, thereby revealing patterns that might otherwise go unnoticed. For example, ARM applied to cardiovascular datasets has shown that patients with obesity, elevated blood pressure, and irregular ECG readings are at heightened risk for coronary artery disease. In oncology, ARM has identified associations between tumor markers and genetic mutations that help predict cancer progression and recurrence (Koparde et al. 2026). These findings allow physicians to refine differential diagnoses, rule out unlikely conditions, and focus on the most probable ones. By providing evidence-backed diagnostic support, ARM reduces misdiagnosis rates, accelerates clinical decision-making, and increases the overall accuracy of patient evaluations. Another critical benefit of ARM in healthcare is its ability to detect and manage comorbidities and multimorbidity conditions, which are increasingly prevalent in aging populations. Patients often present with multiple interrelated health issues, such as diabetes coexisting with hypertension, obesity, and cardiovascular disease.

Traditional approaches may fail to capture the intricate interdependencies among these conditions. ARM, however, excels in uncovering frequent co-occurrence patterns, such as "if diabetes and hypertension are present, the likelihood of kidney disease is significantly higher." Identifying such associations enables healthcare providers to design integrated treatment plans that account for overlapping conditions, rather than treating each disease in isolation. This holistic perspective improves patient outcomes by addressing the interconnected nature of chronic illnesses and minimizing complications. Moreover, identifying comorbidity patterns helps healthcare systems allocate resources effectively by recognizing high-risk patient groups that require more intensive monitoring and support. Pharmacovigilance and medication safety represent another domain where the benefits of ARM are particularly pronounced. Adverse drug reactions (ADRs) are a major challenge in healthcare, often leading to increased morbidity, prolonged hospital stays, and even mortality. ARM has proven effective in mining large pharmacological datasets to detect recurring patterns between drug prescriptions and side effects. For example, ARM might reveal that "patients prescribed drug A and drug B together frequently report gastrointestinal issues," or "elderly patients on drug C have an elevated risk of dizziness and falls." Such insights help physicians distinguish between disease symptoms and medication-induced complications, ensuring safer prescribing practices. Furthermore, ARM contributes to personalized pharmacology by integrating genetic data with medication outcomes, revealing associations between genetic markers and drug responses. This supports the development of pharmacogenomics, where treatments are tailored to the genetic profiles of individual patients, thereby minimizing adverse effects and optimizing therapeutic efficacy. Preventive healthcare is another area that benefits significantly from ARM, as it allows early detection of risk factors and disease precursors before conditions become severe. During pandemics, ARM can be applied to track associations between travel patterns, symptom clusters, and disease transmission, helping authorities design containment strategies (Kost et al. 2012). Moreover, the transparency of ARM ensures that clinicians remain in control of diagnostic reasoning, using the rules as supportive insights rather than as unquestioned directives. This balance between machine intelligence and human expertise is crucial for effective technology integration in healthcare.

Despite these benefits, it is important to acknowledge that applying ARM in healthcare is not without challenges. Issues such as rule explosion (the generation of an overwhelming number of rules), noisy or incomplete datasets, and potential misinterpretation of associations must be carefully managed (Martínez-Romero et al. 2019). However, when combined with rigorous filtering techniques, domain expertise, and validation processes, the benefits of ARM far outweigh its limitations. Hybrid models that integrate ARM with advanced machine learning approaches can further refine rule quality, improve predictive accuracy, and expand applicability to unstructured data sources such as clinical notes or radiology reports. In conclusion, the benefits of Association Rule Mining in healthcare are extensive and transformative, touching nearly every aspect of clinical practice and health system management. By uncovering hidden patterns in medical data, ARM enhances diagnostic accuracy, supports comorbidity management, improves medication safety, strengthens preventive medicine, informs public health strategies, and promotes personalized care. Its transparency and interpretability make it particularly valuable in bridging the gap between complex datasets and practical clinical decision-making. While challenges remain, ongoing innovations in healthcare informatics and artificial intelligence continue to strengthen ARM's capabilities, ensuring that its benefits will expand in scope and significance in the future. Ultimately, ARM empowers healthcare systems to become more data-driven, patient-centered, and proactive, aligning with the broader goals of precision medicine and sustainable healthcare delivery (Mishra et al. 2025).

REAL-TIME MONITORING FOR EARLY DETECTION OF HEALTH ISSUES

Real-time monitoring for early detection of health issues represents a transformative advancement in modern healthcare, offering unparalleled opportunities to shift the medical paradigm from reactive treatment to proactive prevention. By leveraging continuous streams of data collected from wearable devices, biosensors, mobile health applications, implantable monitors, and remote patient monitoring systems, clinicians and healthcare institutions can track vital signs, physiological patterns, and behavioral indicators in real time, detecting anomalies that may signify the onset or progression of a health problem. This capacity to capture subtle deviations from a patient's baseline health status before they escalate into severe or life-threatening conditions has significant implications for reducing hospitalizations, preventing complications, and improving long-term outcomes. For example, wearable ECG patches can continuously monitor heart rhythms and identify arrhythmias such as atrial fibrillation before they lead to stroke, while glucose monitors can alert diabetic patients to dangerous fluctuations before they result in hypoglycemia or ketoacidosis. Similarly, continuous oxygen saturation monitoring in patients with chronic obstructive pulmonary disease (COPD) or COVID-19 can provide early warning of respiratory distress, enabling timely intervention.

The central benefit of real-time monitoring is its ability to transform healthcare into a predictive and preventive system, where data-driven insights empower both patients and providers to act early, avoid costly treatments, and enhance quality of life. The early detection of cardiovascular diseases (CVDs) illustrates the profound potential of real-time monitoring. Cardiovascular conditions remain the leading cause of global mortality, often manifesting in subtle symptoms that may go unnoticed until a major event occurs. Real-time monitoring devices equipped with advanced algorithms can continuously assess parameters such as heart rate variability, blood pressure, and oxygen saturation, detecting patterns that indicate the early onset of conditions like heart failure, hypertension, or myocardial ischemia. For instance, wearable smartwatches and chest straps with ECG capabilities can identify irregular heart rhythms and immediately alert both the patient and healthcare provider, preventing delayed diagnoses. In hospital settings, real-time monitoring systems integrated with AI-based analytics have been shown to predict cardiac arrest several hours before it occurs by analyzing vital sign trends, enabling preemptive intervention. By shifting the focus to early detection, these systems not only save lives but also alleviate the financial burden associated with emergency treatments and long-term complications. Real-time monitoring also holds immense value in managing chronic diseases, which account for the majority of healthcare expenditures worldwide. Patients with diabetes, asthma, hypertension, or chronic kidney disease often require long-term monitoring to maintain stable health and avoid complications (Miswan et al. 2021).

Neurological disorders like epilepsy have also seen advancements through wearable seizure detection devices that monitor electrical activity in the brain or detect abnormal movements, alerting caregivers in advance of seizures (Nirupama et al. 2025). Similarly, Parkinson's disease progression can be tracked through real-time monitoring of gait and tremors, enabling physicians to adjust treatment regimens promptly. These insights create opportunities for preventive mental health care and personalized interventions, reducing the risk of crises and improving patient well-being. In public health and epidemiology, real-time monitoring plays a vital role in early detection of community-level health issues and disease outbreaks. During the COVID-19 pandemic, real-time monitoring of symptoms, testing results, and contact tracing data allowed authorities to identify hotspots and implement targeted interventions. Wearable devices capable of detecting early signs of fever or respiratory distress have also been used in large-scale population monitoring to identify potential outbreaks of infectious diseases. Beyond pandemics, real-time environmental monitoring, such as air quality sensors integrated with wearable devices, can provide individuals with warnings about exposure to pollutants that exacerbate asthma or cardiovascular conditions. This population-level application of real-time monitoring enhances disease surveillance, enables early responses to emerging threats, and strengthens the resilience of healthcare systems in the face of public health crises. One of the unique strengths of real-time monitoring lies in its capacity for personalization and adaptive care.

By continuously tracking data specific to each individual, monitoring systems build personalized health profiles that reflect a patient's unique physiology, lifestyle, and risk factors. Machine learning models can analyze these data streams to generate tailored alerts, such as "patient X is showing early signs of dehydration based on reduced heart rate variability and elevated temperature" or "patient Y is likely to experience a migraine episode based on sleep disruption and stress markers." These insights enable healthcare providers to deliver personalized recommendations, adjust treatment plans dynamically, and reduce the one-size-fits-all approach that often characterizes conventional medicine (Ordonez, 2006). As a result, real-time monitoring supports precision medicine, where interventions are optimized for the individual, enhancing both efficacy and patient satisfaction. Despite its numerous benefits, real-time monitoring for early detection is not without challenges, such as data privacy concerns, false alarms, interoperability issues, and patient adherence. Continuous monitoring generates vast amounts of sensitive health data, raising questions about data security, consent, and ethical usage. False positives—alerts generated by normal variations in physiology—can cause unnecessary anxiety for patients and burden healthcare providers. Ultimately, it empowers a shift toward proactive, patient-centered care, aligning with the broader goals of precision medicine and sustainable healthcare systems (Peng et al. 2018).

USING ASSOCIATION RULE MINING FOR REAL-TIME PATIENT MONITORING

The application of association rule mining (ARM) in real-time patient monitoring has become a powerful method for uncovering meaningful relationships among complex health parameters, enabling clinicians to identify critical health issues promptly and make informed decisions in dynamic healthcare environments. Association rule mining, a fundamental technique in data mining, is designed to discover interesting correlations, frequent patterns, and hidden associations among variables in large datasets. When integrated into real-time patient monitoring systems, ARM can process continuous streams of physiological signals—such as heart rate, blood pressure, glucose levels, oxygen saturation, and electrocardiogram (ECG) data—alongside behavioral and lifestyle indicators to reveal associations that may otherwise remain unnoticed. For example, ARM can uncover that "if a patient's blood pressure rises above a threshold and their heart rate variability decreases, then there is a high likelihood of a hypertensive episode" or "if a patient with diabetes exhibits a sudden rise in glucose levels along with low physical activity, then the probability of hypoglycemia increases within the next few hours." By continuously analyzing live health data and correlating multi-dimensional features, ARM empowers healthcare professionals to detect early warning signs, trigger alerts, and administer preventive interventions before minor abnormalities escalate into acute medical emergencies.

This proactive monitoring capability is especially crucial in critical care, chronic disease management, and telehealth contexts where timely detection directly translates into improved patient outcomes and reduced healthcare costs. In intensive care units (ICUs), where patients are under constant surveillance, ARM can be integrated with real-time monitoring systems to enhance the detection of life-threatening conditions such as sepsis, respiratory failure, and cardiac arrest. Traditional monitoring systems rely on predefined threshold alarms for vital signs, but these can generate excessive false alarms due to transient physiological fluctuations. Association rule mining overcomes this limitation by analyzing multi-parameter relationships instead of focusing on single-variable thresholds. For instance, rules such as "if elevated heart rate, low blood pressure, and increased body temperature occur together, then sepsis is likely" provide more accurate and context-aware predictions than single-parameter alerts. Such rules reduce alarm fatigue among clinicians by filtering out irrelevant signals and focusing attention on high-risk patterns (Raman et al. 2025).

Similarly, in hypertension management, ARM can uncover rules linking sodium intake patterns, heart rate changes, and daily stress indicators to blood pressure fluctuations, providing both patients and physicians with actionable insights. Such data-driven associations allow for proactive interventions, reducing hospital readmissions, preventing complications, and enhancing patient self-management (Shan & Miao, 2023). During health crises such as pandemics, real-time monitoring systems can collect data from wearable devices, hospital records, and mobile health applications across large populations. ARM can process this data to reveal associations that signal the early spread of infectious diseases or emerging public health threats (Thaljaoui & El-Bouzidi, 2022). For instance, a rule such as "if a cluster of patients in a geographic region simultaneously exhibit elevated body temperature, cough symptoms, and reduced oxygen saturation, then a localized outbreak may be occurring" provides actionable insights for public health authorities. This capability allows governments and healthcare organizations to intervene quickly with testing, resource allocation, and containment strategies, potentially averting widespread crises. The integration of ARM into real-time public health monitoring systems thus enhances early detection not only at the individual level but also across populations. Despite these benefits, using association rule mining in real-time patient monitoring also faces challenges related to data quality, privacy, computational efficiency, and interpretability. The continuous data streams from wearables and monitoring devices may include noise, missing values, or inconsistencies that affect the reliability of generated rules. Ensuring high-quality data preprocessing and real-time error correction is therefore essential. Privacy concerns are also critical, as real-time monitoring generates highly sensitive health information that must be protected against unauthorized access and misuse (Warale et al. 2025).

INTEGRATION OF REAL-TIME DATA FOR ENHANCED PATIENT CARE

The integration of real-time data into patient care represents one of the most transformative developments in modern healthcare, allowing providers to move beyond episodic, retrospective treatment toward continuous, proactive, and personalized care delivery. Real-time data refers to information generated instantly from diverse sources such as electronic health records (EHRs), bedside monitors, wearable devices, mobile health applications, diagnostic imaging systems, genomic sequencing platforms, and even environmental or behavioral sensors. By combining these heterogeneous data streams into a unified framework, clinicians gain comprehensive, up-to-the-minute visibility into a patient's physiological status, disease progression, and contextual lifestyle factors. This dynamic integration not only supports timely clinical decision-making but also facilitates early detection of complications, personalization of treatments, efficient resource allocation, and improved communication among multidisciplinary care teams. For example, a patient with congestive heart failure wearing a connected device that measures heart rate, oxygen saturation, and fluid retention can have their data transmitted in real time to their physician's dashboard, where it can be cross-referenced with historical EHR entries, recent medication adjustments, and laboratory results. By detecting early warning signs—such as weight gain from fluid buildup or declining oxygen levels—healthcare professionals can intervene promptly with medication adjustments or outpatient care, thereby preventing costly and life-threatening hospital admissions. This demonstrates how the seamless integration of real-time data not only enhances patient outcomes but also reduces the burden on healthcare systems by enabling preventive, rather than reactive, care. In acute care environments such as intensive care units (ICUs) and emergency departments, the integration of real-time data is critical for rapid diagnosis and immediate interventions.

Patients in these settings are often critically ill, and delays of even a few minutes can be fatal. Real-time data integration allows multiple vital signs—heart rate, blood pressure, oxygen saturation, respiratory rate, and body temperature—to be monitored simultaneously, with advanced algorithms synthesizing this data to detect complex conditions such as sepsis, cardiac arrest, or acute respiratory distress syndrome (ARDS). Traditional systems rely on threshold-based alarms, but these often generate overwhelming false alerts due to transient fluctuations. By integrating real-time data across multiple dimensions and applying predictive analytics, healthcare teams can distinguish meaningful clinical patterns from background noise. For example, if a patient exhibits a combination of rising heart rate, dropping blood pressure, and elevated temperature, the system may flag a high likelihood of sepsis earlier than traditional methods, allowing clinicians to administer antibiotics and fluids promptly. Similarly, in trauma care, the integration of live data from imaging tools, point-of-care tests, and vital monitors ensures that emergency physicians can make split-second decisions about surgery, transfusion, or intensive stabilization. These capabilities underscore the life-saving potential of real-time data integration in critical scenarios where rapid precision is paramount. Beyond acute care, chronic disease management is one of the areas most positively impacted by real-time data integration. By enabling patients to share health data continuously from their homes, integrated systems reduce the need for frequent hospital visits and allow clinicians to oversee large patient populations efficiently (Wright et al. 2013).

For instance, patients with COPD using connected spirometers, pulse oximeters, and wearable activity trackers can have their data automatically transmitted to cloud-based platforms where artificial intelligence (AI) algorithms analyze trends. If lung function begins to decline or oxygen saturation drops consistently, the system can alert healthcare providers, who may schedule virtual consultations or send community health workers for intervention. This reduces hospitalizations, lowers healthcare costs, and ensures timely interventions even for patients with limited mobility or geographic access to care. In the post-pandemic era, these models are evolving into standard practices for long-term chronic care management. The integration of real-time data also extends to surgical care and perioperative monitoring. In operating rooms, integrating live data from anesthesia machines, surgical robots, imaging systems, and patient monitors ensures safe and precise procedures. Real-time data enables anesthesiologists to balance drug delivery based on a patient's changing vital signs, while surgeons can make intraoperative adjustments using live imaging and feedback from robotic instruments. Post-surgery, real-time monitoring of recovery indicators such as oxygen levels, blood pressure, and mobility helps detect complications like infections, bleeding, or deep vein thrombosis at their earliest stages. Integration with electronic health records further ensures that postoperative care is individualized, with alerts and recommendations tailored to the patient's medical history. These capabilities underscore the role of real-time data in improving surgical safety, minimizing complications, and optimizing recovery pathways. Another emerging benefit of real-time data integration is its role in mental health and behavioral healthcare. Wearable devices, mobile applications, and social media activity can capture indicators such as sleep patterns, physical activity levels, speech characteristics, and even sentiment markers. When integrated into patient care systems, these data sources help clinicians detect early warning signs of depression, anxiety, or relapse in psychiatric conditions. For example, if a patient's wearable shows consistently reduced sleep and activity levels, while their smartphone usage indicates withdrawal from social communication, the system can alert mental health professionals for timely outreach. Such proactive monitoring bridges the traditional gap between therapy sessions and ensures continuous support for patients struggling with mental health challenges. Despite its transformative potential, the integration of real-time data into patient care faces significant challenges that must be addressed to realize its full benefits. Interoperability remains a major obstacle, as healthcare data is often siloed across disparate systems, devices, and formats. Establishing universal standards and secure data-sharing protocols is essential for seamless integration. Data quality is another concern, as real-time streams may include errors, missing values, or inconsistencies that affect reliability. Privacy and security also represent critical issues, given the sensitive nature of health information and the risks of breaches in interconnected digital ecosystems (Xu et al. 2022).

Furthermore, the computational demands of processing continuous, multi-source data require robust infrastructure and advanced algorithms capable of delivering accurate insights without delays. Clinician acceptance and training are equally important, as healthcare providers must trust and understand the systems in order to integrate them effectively into their workflows. Finally, ethical considerations related to patient consent, data ownership, and algorithmic bias must be carefully addressed to ensure responsible and equitable implementation. In conclusion, the integration of real-time data for enhanced patient care represents a paradigm shift from traditional reactive approaches toward proactive, continuous, and personalized healthcare delivery. By unifying diverse data sources—including physiological signals, lifestyle metrics, medical records, and genomic information—healthcare providers can achieve unprecedented visibility into patient health, enabling timely interventions, reduced hospitalizations, and improved clinical outcomes. From ICUs and emergency departments to chronic disease management, telemedicine, surgery, and mental health, the integration of real-time data enhances decision-making, strengthens preventive care, and empowers both patients and providers. While challenges such as interoperability, data quality, privacy, and ethical concerns remain, ongoing advancements in health informatics, artificial intelligence, cloud computing, and secure data-sharing frameworks are rapidly addressing these barriers. Ultimately, real-time data integration not only elevates individual patient care but also strengthens the resilience and efficiency of entire healthcare systems, paving the way toward a future where care is predictive, personalized, and universally accessible.

CONCLUSION

The implementation of real-time association rule mining (ARM) in healthcare and other data-intensive domains presents a host of challenges that stem from technical, operational, clinical, and ethical complexities, making it one of the most ambitious tasks in modern data analytics. Association rule mining, traditionally designed for batch processing of large static datasets, identifies hidden relationships and correlations among variables in a given dataset. However, when applied to real-time environments such as patient monitoring, intensive care units, or large-scale sensor networks, the requirements shift drastically. Data is no longer static but arrives continuously in high volumes and with varying degrees of quality, necessitating adaptive and efficient algorithms capable of processing information on the fly without sacrificing accuracy. One major challenge is the computational burden of handling massive, high-velocity data streams. Real-time data environments—such as wearable devices generating heart rate readings every second or hospital monitors continuously capturing blood pressure, oxygen saturation, and ECG signals—produce enormous volumes of data. Traditional ARM algorithms like Apriori or FP-Growth, while effective on static datasets, struggle in these dynamic contexts due to their iterative nature and high memory demands. Modifying these algorithms for real-time contexts requires balancing trade-offs between computational speed, accuracy, and memory efficiency, often demanding novel approaches such as incremental mining, sliding-window techniques, or distributed computing infrastructures. These modifications, however, bring their own challenges in terms of algorithmic complexity, scalability, and interpretability. Another significant challenge lies in data heterogeneity and integration. In real-world scenarios, healthcare data streams originate from diverse sources, including electronic health records (EHRs), wearable sensors, bedside monitoring devices, diagnostic imaging, and patient-reported outcomes. Each of these generates data in different formats, scales, and frequencies, often with incompatible standards. For instance, one wearable might log heart rate every second, while another device records oxygen saturation every 15 seconds, and the EHR updates medication administration records only once every few hours. Ensuring data integrity and reliability in such dynamic, heterogeneous environments remains one of the most pressing obstacles in real-time ARM deployment. Closely tied to data quality is the challenge of concept drift, which refers to the tendency of data distributions and relationships to evolve over time. In medical applications, patient conditions can change rapidly, and rules derived from historical data may become obsolete or misleading in real time.

For example, a patient recovering from surgery may initially exhibit strong correlations between elevated heart rate and pain medication administration, but as recovery progresses, the same association may no longer hold. Real-time ARM systems must continuously update rules to reflect current patterns without being overwhelmed by noise or transient fluctuations. Achieving this balance requires adaptive algorithms that can distinguish between genuine shifts in patient states and random outliers, which is a non-trivial task. Failure to account for concept drift could lead to outdated or irrelevant associations being presented to clinicians, undermining trust in the system and potentially jeopardizing patient safety. Latency and timeliness also pose critical challenges in implementing real-time ARM. Healthcare scenarios, especially in critical care settings, demand near-instantaneous analysis and response. A delay of even a few seconds in detecting an association between dropping oxygen levels and rising heart rate could be life-threatening. Traditional ARM methods often involve multiple database scans and computationally intensive processes, making them unsuitable for time-sensitive environments. While streaming ARM techniques have been developed to reduce latency, they often sacrifice accuracy or completeness in order to achieve speed. Designing algorithms that can produce reliable, clinically actionable rules within stringent time constraints remains one of the most difficult challenges in the field. Another barrier is scalability, especially when considering large-scale deployments across hospitals, health networks, or national health systems. As the number of patients, devices, and monitoring parameters grows, the volume and velocity of incoming data expand exponentially. Real-time ARM must not only handle this data explosion but also ensure that rules remain interpretable and clinically relevant. For instance, a national telehealth system monitoring millions of patients with chronic conditions may generate billions of association rules daily, many of which are redundant, spurious, or irrelevant. Efficiently filtering, prioritizing, and presenting only the most meaningful associations to clinicians is a major challenge that requires robust rule-pruning, ranking, and visualization strategies. In addition to technical and operational issues, ethical and privacy concerns represent substantial challenges in implementing real-time ARM. Healthcare data is highly sensitive, and streaming contexts increase the risk of unauthorized access, breaches, and misuse. Continuous monitoring systems that feed into real-time ARM frameworks must adhere to stringent privacy regulations such as HIPAA, GDPR, or local data protection laws. Furthermore, patients must consent to continuous monitoring and real-time analysis, which raises ethical questions about autonomy, informed consent, and surveillance in healthcare. The interpretability of mined rules is another challenge. In real-time settings, clinicians must be able to understand and trust the associations generated by the system in order to make informed decisions. However, as real-time ARM increasingly incorporates advanced computational techniques such as parallelized mining or integration with deep learning models, the resulting rules may become more abstract and harder for humans to interpret. Clinicians may resist adopting such systems if the logic behind recommendations is opaque or overly complex. This highlights the need for explainable ARM frameworks that prioritize transparency and usability in clinical environments. Resource constraints further complicate implementation. Real-time ARM requires substantial infrastructure, including high-speed data pipelines, distributed computing systems, and reliable connectivity. Many hospitals and clinics, especially in developing regions, may lack the technological capacity to implement such advanced systems.

Even in well-resourced environments, the cost of deploying, maintaining, and scaling real-time ARM infrastructure is significant, raising concerns about sustainability and equity. Finally, human factors and organizational resistance must not be overlooked. Integrating real-time ARM into clinical workflows requires changes in practice, training, and mindset. Clinicians may be hesitant to rely on algorithmically generated associations, fearing overdependence on technology or potential errors. Moreover, the flood of real-time data and rules may contribute to information overload and decision fatigue, unless carefully managed. Organizational resistance to change, lack of trust in new technologies, and insufficient training can all hinder successful implementation, even if technical challenges are overcome. In summary, the challenges of implementing real-time association rule mining span a wide spectrum—from computational and algorithmic constraints such as scalability, latency, and concept drift, to operational issues of data integration, quality, and heterogeneity, to ethical concerns surrounding privacy, security, and informed consent. Added to these are human and organizational challenges such as clinician trust, interpretability, and workflow integration. Addressing these issues requires a multidisciplinary approach, combining advances in algorithm design, health informatics, secure data management, and human-centered system design. Only by overcoming these challenges can real-time ARM fulfill its potential as a powerful tool for uncovering actionable patterns in continuous data streams and ultimately transforming healthcare into a more proactive, predictive, and personalized system.

REFERENCES

Briceno, O. (2022). Semi-supervised incremental learning with few examples for medical monitoring (discussing association rules as pattern representation). *BMC Medical Informatics and Decision Making*. Advance online publication. DOI: 10.1186/s12911-022-01755-3

Cao, J.. (2020). Temporal association rule mining: An overview considering time variable as integral component. *Wiley Interdisciplinary Reviews. Data Mining and Knowledge Discovery*, *10*(4), e1367. Advance online publication. DOI: 10.1002/widm.1367

Charan, J. K., Chandra, S., Vaissnave, V., Ragupathi, T., Satyanarayana, P., & Manjunath, T. C. (2025). Impact of Generative AI on Industries and Organizations. In Zhao, J., Kumar, V., Katina, P., & Richards, J. (Eds.), *Humans and Generative AI Tools for Collaborative Intelligence* (pp. 509–528). IGI Global Scientific Publishing., DOI: 10.4018/979-8-3693-8332-2.ch022

Charan, J. K., Meera, K. L., Sudheer, P., Gopalakrishnan, G., Sharma, M., & Manjunath, T. C. (2025). Applications of Generative AI and Human-AI Collaboration. In Zhao, J., Kumar, V., Katina, P., & Richards, J. (Eds.), *Humans and Generative AI Tools for Collaborative Intelligence* (pp. 423–440). IGI Global Scientific Publishing., DOI: 10.4018/979-8-3693-8332-2.ch018

Cui, J., Zhao, S., & Sun, X. (2022, March). An association rule mining algorithm for clinical decision support. In *Proceedings of the 8th International Conference on Computing and Artificial Intelligence* (pp. 137-143). DOI: 10.1145/3532213.3532234

Cui, J., Zhao, S., & Sun, X. (2022, March). An association rule mining algorithm for clinical decision support. In *Proceedings of the 8th International Conference on Computing and Artificial Intelligence* (pp. 137-143). DOI: 10.1145/3532213.3532234

Diallo, A., Camara, F., Camara, G., & Sarr, M. (2024, December). Association Rule Mining-based Analysis of Clinical Manifestations of SARS-Cov-2 (COVID-19) Coronavirus Infection in Senegal. In *Proceedings of the 2024 5th International Conference on Intelligent Medicine and Health* (pp. 54-59).

Domadiya, N., & Rao, U. P. (2021). Privacy Preserving Association Rule Mining on Distributed Healthcare Data: COVID-19 and Breast Cancer Case Study. *SN Computer Science*, *2*(6), 418. DOI: 10.1007/s42979-021-00801-7 PMID: 34423316

Guru Basava Aradhya, S., Chithambar Gupta, V., Raman, M. S., Singh, J., Manjunath, T. C., & Sharma, M. (2025). Health Crises and Digitalization: Digital Health. In Yıldırım, D., Yıldırım, S., & Kandpal, V. (Eds.), *Sustainable Digitalization Strategies in Business and Healthcare* (pp. 171–198). IGI Global Scientific Publishing., DOI: 10.4018/979-8-3373-5087-5.ch007

Harb, H., Alobaidi, A., & El-Bakry, H. (2020). A Hadoop-Based Platform for Patient Classification and Real-Time Monitoring. *Sensors (Basel)*, *20*(7), 1931. DOI: 10.3390/s20071931 PMID: 32235657

Koparde, S. A., Jha, R. P., Deepthi Reddy, K., Kuchipudi, J. D., Manjunath, T. C., & Sharma, M. (2026). Generative AI in Predicting and Preventing Foodborne Illnesses. In Madaan, G., Singh, A., Chahal, B., David, A., & Singh, G. (Eds.), *Generative AI in Food Systems: Predictive Demand, Smart Supply Chains, and Sustainable Service Futures* (pp. 205–232). IGI Global Scientific Publishing., DOI: 10.4018/979-8-3373-5182-7.ch010

Kost, R.. (2012). Exploring generalized association rule mining for disease co-occurrence discovery from ICD codes. Journal / BMC. *Medical Informatics*. Advance online publication. DOI: 10.1186/1472-6947-12-50

Martínez-Romero, M.. (2019). Using association rule mining and ontologies to generate real-time clinical suggestions. *Database : The Journal of Biological Databases and Curation*. Advance online publication. DOI: 10.1093/database/baz059 PMID: 31210270

Mishra, B. R., Selvakumar, P., Kaur, R., Kalshetti, P., Mishra, K. K., Sharma, M., & Manjunath, T. C. (2025). Innovation and Digital Transformation in the Public Sector Entities. In Santos Ferreira, A., & Lourenço dos Santos, C. (Eds.), *Enhancing Public Sector Accountability and Services Through Digital Innovation* (pp. 409–436). IGI Global Scientific Publishing., DOI: 10.4018/979-8-3693-9251-5.ch013

Miswan, N. H., Yusof, R. M., & Ahmad, M. (2021). Association Rules Mining for Hospital Readmission: A Case Study. *Mathematics*, *9*(21), 2706. DOI: 10.3390/math9212706

Nirupama, E., Seenivasan, S., Bhardwaj, K., Karunakaran, N. B., & Basava Aradhya, S. G., & Manjunath, T. C. (2025). Transforming Digital Supply Chains With Gamification and Metaverse Integration. In G. Malik, D. Singh, & R. Bansal (Eds.), *Addressing Practical Problems Through the Metaverse and Game-Inspired Mechanics* (pp. 123-152). IGI Global Scientific Publishing. DOI: 10.4018/979-8-3693-8886-0.ch006

Ordonez, C. (2006). Association rule discovery with the train and test approach for heart disease prediction. *IEEE Transactions on Information Technology in Biomedicine*, *10*(2), 334–343. DOI: 10.1109/TITB.2006.864475 PMID: 16617622

Peng, M., Sundararajan, V., Williamson, T., Minty, E. P., Smith, T. C., Doktorchik, C. T. A., & Quan, H. (2018). Exploration of association rule mining for coding consistency and completeness assessment in inpatient administrative health data. *Journal of Biomedical Informatics*, *79*, 41–47. DOI: 10.1016/j.jbi.2018.02.001 PMID: 29425732

Raman, M. S., Koppa, K. B., Chithambar Gupta, V., Bhat, V. A., & Guru Basava Aradhya, S. (2025). Digital Transformation and Sustainability Artificial Intelligence and Sustainable Development. In Yıldırım, D., Yıldırım, S., & Kandpal, V. (Eds.), *Effects of Digitalization and Circular Economy on Sustainable Policy and Climate Change Prevention* (pp. 69–96). IGI Global Scientific Publishing., DOI: 10.4018/979-8-3693-9909-5.ch003

Shan, Z., & Miao, W. (2023). COVID-19 patient diagnosis and treatment data mining algorithm based on association rules. *Expert Systems: International Journal of Knowledge Engineering and Neural Networks*, *40*(4), e12814. Advancc online publication. DOI: 10.1111/exsy.12814 PMID: 34898798

Thaljaoui, A., & El-Bouzidi, A. (2022). Integrated Bayesian and association-rules methods for autonomous decision making to support COVID-19 management. *Medical & Biological Engineering & Computing*. Advance online publication. DOI: 10.1007/s11517-022-02677-y PMID: 36205834

Warale, P. N., Limbore, N. V., Anute, N., Ahluwalia, G. K., & Raut, A. (2025). AI-Enhanced Customer Engagement and Experience: Chatbots, Virtual Assistants, and AI-Powered Customer Interactions. In Hussain, Z., Khan, A., Uzir, M., Sharipudin, M., & Shaheen, A. (Eds.), *Impacts of AI-Generated Content on Brand Reputation* (pp. 335–362). IGI Global Scientific Publishing., DOI: 10.4018/979-8-3373-4327-3.ch014

Wright, A., et al. (2013). Validation of an Association Rule Mining-Based Method to Identify Medication–Problem Associations in Clinical Data. Journal / AMIA / medical informatics paper. DOI: 10.1186/1472-6947-13-129

Xu, W., Zhao, Q., Zhan, Y., Wang, B., & Hu, Y. (2022). Privacy-preserving association rule mining based on electronic medical system. *Wireless Networks*, *28*(1), 303–317. DOI: 10.1007/s11276-021-02846-1

Chapter 12
Bounded Rationality and AI Modeling Real-World Decision-Making

Venkata Sivakumar Musam
http://orcid.org/0009-0003-2699-7208
Astute Solutions LLC, USA

Nagendra Kumar Musham
http://orcid.org/0009-0001-5398-1821
Celer Systems Inc., USA

R. Mekala
Department of Artificial Intelligence and Data Science, Arjun College of Technology, Coimbatore, India

Nurul Fahmi
http://orcid.org/0009-0001-4999-2720
Department of Informatics Engineering, Politeknik Negeri Bengkalis, Indonesia

ABSTRACT

AI constrained rationality allows systems to take advantage of the time, compute resources, and knowledge they possess to make recommendations, in context, that are rational instead of trying to achieve perfect optimality. While achieving high performance, bounded rationality supports fairness, interpretability, and ethical compliance. The analysis utilized multi-criteria metrics including SHAP/LIME scores, demographic parity, equalized odds, and computational efficiency to evaluate multiple AI approaches including heuristics, Bayesian models, fuzzy logic, explainable AI (XAI), and hybrid models. The results indicate that while hybrid AI scored high marks with 96% accuracy,0.96 interpretability, and 0.95 fairness heu-

DOI: 10.4018/979-8-3373-6691-3.ch012

ristic models scored poorly, 72% accuracy and 0.71 intpretablility. In high-stakes situations, explainable AI models will be optimal due to their strong transparency and trustworthiness. The best balance of accuracy, fairness, and ethical compliance is achievable with hybrid models (deep learning/popular reasoning) which ensure the responsible use of AI.

INTRODUCTION

AI decision-making until present has largely been modeled with the assumption of perfect rationality, while real-life situations introduce vagueness, cognitive limitations, and bounded data. Bounded rationality can be defined as a empirical experiments that focus on the decision-making process people undergo while they are faced with constraints as they look for heuristics and some kind of acceptable optimization (Abdar et al., 2022). The embedded limited logic systems in AI will foster a much more responsive choice system that is human-centered and amenable to the richness of real worlds. The compromises of efficiency, fairness, and explanation will become even more pronounced. What precision, fairness, explainability, and compromise mean is that on the level of AI decision-making, approaches balance off ethical considerations with performance. The designs of AI systems must be aligned with the human decision-making processes on grounds of explainability and transparency. Here the player is ensured that all the pertinent stake holders comprehend and trust the decisions that have been generated by the AI (Alagarsundaram, 2023). The ethical design of such AI requires a fine balance between high automation and human agency so that AI models should be both productive and fair, strong and ethical. AI evolution, becoming more sustainable, requires adaptive learning strategies that prevent replication of human biases and ethical principles. By accepting the principles of bounded rationality, AI decision-making may become more human-like, being context-aware and responsive to the nuances of the real world to produce future generations of AI systems with reasoning, ethical, and cognitive consciousness (Alagarsundaram, 2024).

BACKGROUND

Artificial intelligence has indeed made a great impact in decision making processes across a multitude of sectors: banking, medicine, autonomous systems as well as supply chain management (Arbabi et al., 2023). Most traditional AI models are anchored on the assumption that the real agents act rationally or in a way that maximizes return based on all the available information (Arcieri et al., 2023). However, the cognitive constraints, time limits and, sometimes, no access to an information source hinder the process of decision making. Herbert Simon suggested this phenomenon known as limited rationality, as an alternative to traditional rational decision making paradigm (Ayub et al., 2021). Bounded rationality acknowledges that humans and AI systems are limited in a way that they cannot achieve full rationality (Becker et al., 2022). They employ heuristics, approximations and adaptive learning mechanisms and AI systems have been designed to maximize efficiency and accuracy by clearly defined rules and algorithms. Complexities of real-world contexts add uncertainties that test these standard models. Unlike completely rational decision-makers who rely on exhaustive computations, AI systems must adhere to computational, informational and cognitive restrictions. These constraints need transition from idealized decision models to those incorporate heuristics, biases and adaptive learning.

Growing application of evolutionary AI in human-centric fields such as medicine, economics and policymaking necessitates better understanding how AI systems make choices under constraints (Bicaku et al., 2022). Clinicians make choices on sparse patient information, experience and pattern recognition in medical diagnosis (Binz et al., 2023). AI-based recommendation systems, such as consumer profiling, work by approximating consumer preference and constructing exhaustive lists of options (Bobba et al., 2023). A different level of justification forms part of the need to develop AI systems that can rationally tolerate ambiguity but which are computationally tractable and ethical. Limited rationality is one of the top-priority criteria in AI ethics and justice. AI systems trained on biased data can generally reinforce societal inequalities by recognizing cognitive biases (Catalano et al., 2023). Algorithms that ensure fairness, ethical requirements and explainability in AI decision-making systems address these issues. With limited rationality, AI will better simulate human judgment and allow greater transparency, resilience and fairer outcomes (Chaput et al., 2021).

Importance of Bounded Rationality in AI

Bounded rationality is an important aspect of the creation of AI; it is the human type of rationality (Che & Yang, 2021). Perfect rational models are contrasted with bounded rationality in that decision makers, whether human or AI systems, are not perfect in dealing with unlimited processing power and error-free information. That forms an AI model that survives in the world. In medicine, the use of artificial intelligence calls for immediate decisions, given the limited data that may be available concerning a patient. Doctors or other medical professionals are constrained by time, heuristic methods of decision making (Chobtham et al., 2023). In the same way as in medicine, AI diagnostic systems are to be developed around this boundary such that hypothetical recommendations to a medical issue are more realistic and applicable (Cipollone & Giacomo, 2025). AI forecasting systems comprehend extensive geographical data scopes while being able to market's uncertain risk levels supplemented with cognitive difficulties in making investment decisions (Dang et al., 2024). In trade-offs, speed and accuracy would be characterized in terms of fragility measured against reasonable computational feasibility that supports AI models. Bounded rationality is a significant area with respect to AI that suffers from autonomous systems. (Dado et al., 2024). The self-driving car takes a few milliseconds to analyze sensor data with respect to the immediate conditions through probabilistic reasoning before yielding a decision. The difference is that an autonomous vehicle works in real-time choosing the best possible action given the information rather than being perceived as an ideal rational agent that knows all scenarios (Dickerson & Dickerson, 2000). Safe and effective decisions will require a blend of heuristics, reinforcement learning, and adaptable models.

Bounded rationality raises human-AI collaboration. Rather than replace human decision-making, these AI systems were created specifically to assist and augment it (Duong et al., 2021). Recognizing the limits of human cognition enhances AI's ability to present scientifically cogent, meaningful recommendations for action. AI-supported legal decision analysis makes use of case law, acknowledges case complexity, and incorporates human judgment rather than relying on rules alone (Gonzalez, 2024). Implementation of limited rationality principles by AI enhances the quality of human-AI interaction and the overall quality of decisions (Glukhikh & Glukhikh, 2021). Furthermore, explainability and transparency in AI tie directly to bounded rationality. Decisions that cannot be understood due to the black-box nature of AI systems are often criticized, especially in sensitive areas such as medicine, justice, and finance.

Key Challenges in Bounded Rationality and AI Decision Making

Cognition versus computational model being essentially limited give rise to a set of questions in decision making within the wide ambit of bounded rationality in AI (Hagendorff & Danks, 2023).Unlike rational decision theories based on an assumption of full knowledge and unlimited computational power, real-life decision-making presupposes time limits, incomplete information, and cognitive biases (He et al., 2024).Simulations of bounded rationality have been programmed into AI systems. They are supposed to weigh all such constraints against the goals of efficiency and reliability. This has remained to be a dilemma, given that most AI systems regard someone to be absolutely rational or rely on prescriptive heuristics that draw sharp lines delineating human judgments from their intricacies (Hüllermeier et al., 2021). Other problems in attempting to embed bounded rationality in AI arise from the nature of the trade-off between optimality and feasibility.Ancient AI models were designed to find the optimum solution, whereas human decision making, owing to limited resources, chooses to be good enough (Islam et al., 2024).This trade-off poses problems for AI systems that need to be computationally efficient and act as simulations of human adaptive decision strategies.

The explainability and interpretability of AI decisions pose a terrifying challenge since machine learning models, particularly the complex deep architectures, are said to be "black boxes" (Korteling et al., 2021). SHAP and LIME provide insight into AI decision-making, but neither fully represent its bounded rationality reasoning mechanisms, influenced by computational complexity (Lee & Seong, 2025). Largeness algorithms must compress interpretations for meaningful interpretability, making decision models opaque and not scalable for real-life applications. AI integration in high-stakes sectors like healthcare, finance, and autonomous systems remains a challenge. (Li & Khishe, 2023). Successful cooperation between humans and AI requires aligning AI decision making with human expectations, as well as the possibility of AI changing over time. Moreover, ethical issues and trust in AI systems are at the core of building bounded rationality models (Mao & Omar, 2024). AI decisions are not trusted by users because these differ from traditional models in extremely risky situations. Ethical issues arise due to the AI decision-making behavior affecting human lives, which calls for rigorous checks and control mechanisms (Mazurkiewicz, 2022). An interdisciplinary approach is proposed by integrating cognitive science, behavioral economics, and computer science views for developing flexible, fair, and open AI models depicting realistic behaviors of decision making.

Objective and Scope

- ✓ Identify and specify major AI decision-making performance metrics such as computation time efficiency, heuristic optimum performance and explainability.
- ✓ Develop systematic technique for modeling decisions made by AI under restricted rationality constraints.
- ✓ Use AI models and performance measures to assess decision-making under conditions such as uncertainty and fairness.
- ✓ Create efficient AI decision-making system that integrates bounded rationality principles hence improving flexibility and human trust.

It adds AI research by merging limited rationality concepts in machine learning decisions and resolving challenges including uncertainty, computational restrictions and moral dilemmas. It fills the gap between imaginary models of rational perceptive and actual AI deployments by gauging significant performance metrics such as heuristic usefulness and human trust. It constructs AI systems that are not only computationally efficient but also adaptive and in agreement with human taste.

LITERATURE SURVEY

(Mguni et al., 2023) investigated AI decision-making on heuristic models by modifying Recognition Primed Decision. They demonstrated that AI systems use RPD to effectively replicate human decision-making in uncertain environments. It used experience-based heuristics rather than full calculations to improve computational efficiency without compromising decision accuracy. Ciro (Moreira et al., 2021) investigated use of Fuzzy Logic Decision Systems in artificial intelligence-based decision making under bounded rationality and emphasized that fuzzy logic ensured adaptive decision-making by managing imprecise data so AI models could make more human-like decisions whenever data was missing or vague.

(Mu & Zheng, 2025) presented Neural Symbolic Hybrid Model in response to limitations of bounded rationality by AI systems. Joining deep learning with symbolic reasoning enabled the usage of interpretability preserving approximate procedures in actual decision processes of AI models. It depicts improvement in generalization capabilities for dynamically evolving situations. Abdar et al (Mustafa et al., 2023) researched Bayesian Networks application to AI decision-making in uncertain situations. Probabilistic reasoning enabled AI to make sound decisions within computational and information constraints. It was especially useful in health-related applications where decisions have to be made using incomplete patient information (Nag, 2025).

(Nishant, 2023) investigated Markov Decision Processes introduce bounded rationality to reinforcement learning. MDPs assist in providing a formal structure for AI to make optimal decisions under provided constraints and enhance performance in autonomous systems like autonomous vehicles and robots. Xu et al (Nishant et al., 2024) proposed Cognitive Hierarchy Model of AI-based decision-making. They showed conduct of human agents in modest settings could be better forecast by AI agents using CHM based on accountancy for different levels of rationality within multi-agent settings. Predictions were verified with economic simulations and game theory.

(Oesterheld et al., 2023) proposed Evolutionary Game Theory models for bounded rationality-based AI decision-making and demonstrated that AI systems based on EGT had the ability to learn from their past experiences to adapt dynamic environments thereby being appropriate in applications such as cybersecurity and adaptive learning systems. Glukhikh et al (Peng et al., 2023) investigated Case-Based Reasoning as AI decision-making strategy based on knowledge. Research indicated that AI models employing CBR were capable of retrieving and transforming prior cases to effectively solve new problems with less computational overhead and enhanced transparency.

(Rahwan et al., 2019) examined Gated Recurrent Units in administrative modeling in scarcity of data availability. GRU-based AI models simulate limited astuteness via selective recall of past decisions which enhanced long-term decision-making in changing locations. Mao et al. (Ribeiro et al., 2016) examined how Explainable AI (XAI) methods affect boued rationality in AI policymaking. Results showed that AI models using SHAP and LIME explanations improved interpretability and credibility thus making AI decisions extra understandable to human users.

(Russell & Norvig, 2021) suggested Hybrid Neuro-Fuzzy System for representing AI decision-making under uncertainty. Networks and fuzzy reasoning Increased flexibility allows AI models to strike a compromise between computing efficiency and decision quality in practical uses. (Samek et al., 2021) described an application of reinforcement education with Prize Shaping to overcome restricted rationality limitations. They identified that reward shaping methods accelerated convergence of AI systems towards optimal choices by giving preference to essential heuristics by promoting efficiency in reinforcement learning (Shneiderman, 2020).

Dado et al. (Simonyan et al., 2014) examined application of Attention Mechanisms in AI-based Decision Systems. It showed that attention-based AI models were able to dispatch computational resources more efficiently focusing on informative information and discarding noise making them appropriate choice for real-time decision-making tasks. Oesterheld et al. (Smith et al., 2023) introduced Causal Inference Models for bounded rational AI decision-making. Their research showed that CIMs allowed AI to make decisions on causal relationships rather than correlations to improve reliability in high-stakes domains such as finance and healthcare (Suresh & Guttag, 2021).

(Sutton & Barto, 2018) investigated Deep Q-Networks as decision-making framework under bounded rationality. Their work pointed out that AI systems based on DQN to approximate optimal policies under computational constraints rendering them useful for robotics and automated control systems. Moreira et al. (Thaler & Sunstein, 2008) investigated Quantum Computing Approaches to decision-making in AI under bounded rationality. Results demonstrated that quantum algorithms had potential to exponentially accelerate decision-making processes enabling AI systems to deal with complicated decision environments with less computational constraints.

(Tversky & Kahneman, 1974) introduced HiLM to aid with restricted rational decision-making. Human input facilitated iterative choices which improved precision in healthcare and legal profession. (Wachter et al., 2017) created Meta Learning Techniques to overcome restricted rationality in AI systems. They adapt quickly to novel decision-making situations with minimal training making them suitable for dynamic environments such as cybersecurity and fraud detection (Wang et al., 2019).

BOUNDED RATIONALITY IN AI DECISION-MAKING

Suggested framework Figure 1 for Bounded Rationality in AI integrates different AI decision-making models to achieve optimal decision-making. This ablation research looks into influence of deleting or changing individual components such Heuristic Models, Fuzzy Logic Systems, Explainable AI and Hybrid AI Models and how they affect fairness, interpretability and trust. Decision-making pipeline follows hierarchical structure with models at all stages contributing uniquely to overall performance. Goal is to strike compromise between computational efficiency and ethical decision-making in AI systems ensuring they are both successful and explainable.

Figure 1. Architecture of bounded rationality and AI in decision-making

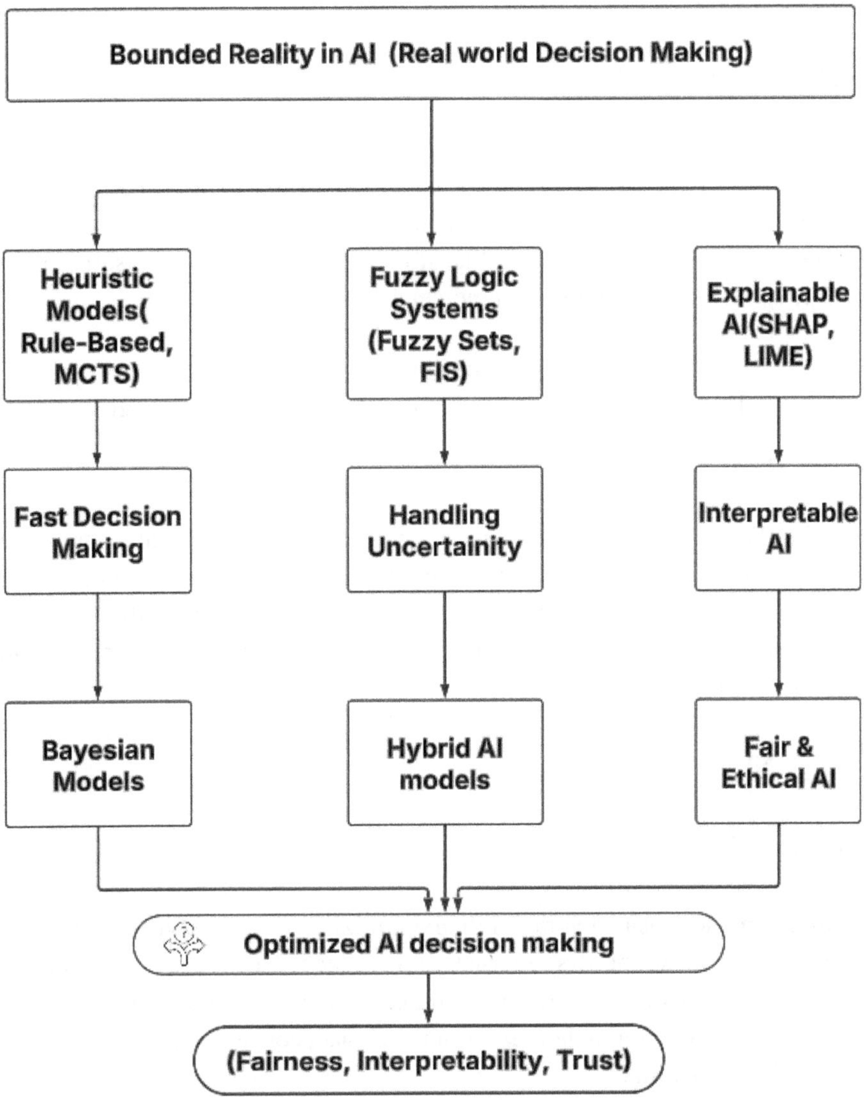

Heuristic Models for Fast Decision-Making

Heuristic-based AI models (Weller, 2019) use rule-based systems and Monte Carlo Tree Search to create quick approximate answers to complicated challenges. They use domain specific heuristics to enable real time decision making with low computing cost but they struggle with ambiguity and add bias. Bayesian models build on heuristic reasoning by combining probabilistic logic and learning distributions to improve decision-making accuracy.

Recognition Heuristic

Recognition heuristic is founded on the principle that if a choice is familiar and other is unfamiliar, familiar choice is best. Heuristic presumes that familiarity breeds greater value or applicability. It is especially handy in contexts where past experience would be very important, like stock market forecasts, consumer brand preference, and making decisions in emergency situations.

$$P(A > B) = \begin{cases} 1, & \text{if } A \text{ is recognized and } B \text{ is not} \\ 0.5, & \text{if both are recognized or both are unrecognized} \end{cases} \quad (1)$$

Take the Best

Take-The-Best (Xie et al., 2020) heuristic works by processing cues sequentially and as soon as it finds discriminative cue, it terminates. TTB does not compare all information present but instead ranks most pertinent cues sequentially. It is most efficient in scenarios where datasets are very large, for example, spam filtering, credit scoring, and medical diagnosis.

$$S(A,B) = \sum_{i=1}^{n} w_i f_i(A,B) \quad (2)$$

Satisficing Model

Satisficing model posits that rather than optimizing to achieve the best decision, decision-makers choose the first alternative that reaches a satisfactory acceptable level. It captures real-life behavior when time, information, and cognitive burden are limited. It is highly used in human resource choice, consumer buying, and time-pressure decision-making.

$$V(A) \geq T \quad (3)$$

Prospect Theory

Prospect theory explains how individuals make decisions under uncertainty, emphasizing the asymmetry between perceived gains and losses. It highlights that losses have a greater psychological impact than equivalent gains, influencing risk-averse or risk-seeking behavior. The theory provides insights into human decision biases and preferences. It is widely applied in behavioural economics, insurance, and investment decision-making.

$$U(x) = \begin{cases} (x-r)^{\alpha}, & x \geq r \quad \text{(Gains domain)} \\ -\lambda(r-x)^{\beta}, & x < r \quad \text{(Loss domain)} \end{cases} \tag{4}$$

Fast and Frugal Trees

Fast and Frugal Trees are decision models designed to make rapid and efficient decisions with little information. In contrast to complicated decision trees, FFTs use sequence of simple yes/no decisions which are very effective in medical triage, security screening and automatic AI-based decision support systems.

$$D = \sum_{i=1}^{m} \mathbb{I}(C_i \geq T_i) \tag{5}$$

Algorithm 1. Heuristic_Decision_Model

Input: Set of options {A, B, ..., N}, Decision criteria C, Threshold T
Output: Best option based on heuristic evaluation
Begin
//Recognition Heuristic (RH)
Function Recognition_Heuristic (Options):
For each option A in Options:
If A is recognized and B is not:
Return A
Else if both are unrecognized:
Return Random (A, B)
End For
End Function
//Take-The-Best (TTB) Heuristic
Function Take_The_Best (Options, Cues, Weights):
Sort Cues in order of importance
For each cue C_i in Cues:
If C_i differentiates between A and B:
Return the option favored by C_i
End For

continued on following page

Algorithm 1. Continued

End Function
//Satisficing Model
Function Satisficing (Options, Threshold):
For each option A in Options:
If Value(A) ≥ Threshold:
Return A
End For
End Function
//Prospect Theory Decision
Function Prospect_Theory (Options, Reference_Point):
For each option A in Options:
Compute Gain_Loss(A) using:
If A ≥ Reference_Point:
U(A) = (A - Reference_Point)^α
Else:
U(A) = -λ (Reference_Point - A)^β
Return Option with maximum U(A)
End Function
//Fast-and-Frugal Tree (FFT)
Function Fast_And_Frugal_Tree (Options, Cues, Thresholds):
For each Cue C_i in Cues:
If C_i(A) ≥ Threshold_i:
Return A
End For
End Function
// Main Decision-Making Flow
Function Heuristic_Decision (Options, Criteria, Threshold):
If Recognition_Heuristic (Options) is valid:
Return Recognized Option
Else If Take_The_Best (Options, Criteria, Weights) is valid:
Return Best Option
Else If Satisficing (Options, Threshold) is valid:
Return First Satisfactory Option
Else If Prospect_Theory (Options, Reference_Point) is valid:
Return Option with Maximum Utility

continued on following page

Algorithm 1. Continued

Else:
Return Fast_And_Frugal_Tree (Options, Criteria, Thresholds)
End Function
End

Fuzzy Logic Systems for Handling Uncertainty

Fuzzy Logic Systems (Yang et al., 2019) operate with imprecise and uncertain data making them best suited for AI decision-making in unstructured environments. Contrary to classical logic where they have binary true/false values, fuzzy logic uses degrees of truth based on membership functions. FLS are used extensively in control systems, expert systems and machine learning where specific input data is not available.

Fuzzy Set Theory

Fuzzy set theory (Zhang et al., 2018) is a generalization of classical set theory where the members of items exist to a degree rather than definitely as member or not a member. A member can either be in or not be in classical sets. Fuzzy set theory has members occupying a set to some degree and with membership value between 0 and Fuzzy sets, known for their flexibility in handling ambiguity and uncertainty, are applied to real-world problems with imprecise information such as image processing, natural language processing, and expert systems.

Fuzzy sets are defined by membership functions that express the degree to which an element belongs to a set, with shapes such as triangular, trapezoidal, or Gaussian depending on the problem. They including union, intersection, and complement, enable smooth categorization instead of rigid boundaries. This flexibility makes fuzzy set theory highly effective in domains like medical diagnosis, where symptoms are not crisply classifiable. It also supports AI decision-making systems that require adaptable reasoning under uncertainty.

$$A = \{(x, \mu_A(x)) \mid x \in X, \mu_A(x) \in [0,1]\} \tag{6}$$

Union - OR operation

$$\mu_{AUB}(x) = \max(\mu_A(x), \mu_B(x)) \tag{7}$$

Intersection - AND operation

$$\mu_{A \cap B}(x) = \min(\mu_A(x), \mu_B(x)) \tag{8}$$

Complement - NOT operation

$$\mu_{-A}(x) = 1 - \mu_A(x) \tag{9}$$

Fuzzy Interference System

An FIS is an artificial intelligence system based on fuzzy logic and human-like reasoning to account for uncertainty. Composed of four major blocks: fuzzification, rule base, inference engine, and defuzzification. Fuzzification converts numerical values into fuzzy values, whereas the rule base stores fuzzy IF-THEN rules. Defuzzification converts the fuzzy set into a number so that decisions can be made in a flexible way on ambiguous and uncertain data.

IF x_1 is A_1 AND x_2 is A_2 THEN y is B (10)

Fuzzification is the transformation of crisp numerical inputs into fuzzy values according to predetermined membership functions. This allows AI systems to handle uncertain or vague data by translating input values into linguistic variables such as Low, Medium, or High.

$$\mu_A(x) = \frac{1}{1 + e^{-k(x-c)}} \tag{11}$$

Here, fuzzy rules (IF-THEN conditions) are enforced on the fuzzified inputs to decide their truth value. The system employs logical operators (AND, OR) to check many rules at a time, making the fuzzy outputs depending on the provided conditions.

$$\alpha_i = \min\left(\mu_{A_1}(x_1), \mu_{A_2}(x_2)\right) \tag{12}$$

Aggregation collects all fuzzy rules' outputs in a unified fuzzy set for complete decision making. Merging multiple rule contributions forms an aggregate fuzzy output before eventual transformation into a crisp value.

$$\mu_B(y) = \max(\alpha_1, \alpha_2, \ldots, \alpha_n) \tag{13}$$

Defuzzification converts the aggregated fuzzy output to a single crisp numerical value, which can be understood in real-world applications. Defuzzification ensures that the system gives a clear and useful decision based on the evaluation by fuzzy logic.

$$y^* = \frac{\sum_{i=1}^{n} \mu_{B_i}(y)\, y_i}{\sum_{i=1}^{n} \mu_{B_i}(y)} \tag{14}$$

Algorithm 2. Fuzzy Logic System for Handling Uncertainty

Input: Crisp input values from real-world data (e.g., temperature, speed, risk level) Predefined fuzzy sets and membership functions Output: Fuzzy decision (Crisp output after defuzzification)
BEGIN
# Fuzzification
INPUT crisp_values # Collect real-world numerical inputs
FOR each input_variable IN crisp_values:
Convert to fuzzy sets using membership functions
Rule Evaluation
FOR each fuzzy_rule IN rule_base:
Evaluate IF-THEN conditions
Compute degree of truth using fuzzy operators (AND, OR)
Aggregation
COMBINE all fuzzy rule outputs into a single fuzzy set
Defuzzification
Convert fuzzy output into a crisp value using centroid or other methods
Decision Output
RETURN final_decision
END

Explainable AI for Trust and Interpretability

Explainable AI (XAI) (Zhang et al., 2020) seeks to make AI models more transparent, trusted and understandable by offering human-interpretable explanations of their decisions. Trust in AI depends on user comprehension of model decisions and interpretability, as techniques like SHAP and LIME ensure consistent predictions with domain knowledge, enhancing ethical and trustworthy deployment.

$$\phi_i = \mathbb{E}[f(X) \mid X_i] - \mathbb{E}[f(X)] \tag{15}$$

Feature Importance and Model Transparency

Important aspects of XAI is understanding how input features affect decisions of AI model. Feature importance scores are used to determine which variables are most responsible for predictions and enhance interpretability. SHAP values are based on cooperative game theory and give an equitable distribution of feature contributions. LIME represents sophisticated model by an interpretable surrogate model through the use of perturbed samples. This formula makes the contributions fair by spreading them over all feasible feature subsets.

$$\phi_i = \sum_{S \subseteq F \setminus \{i\}} \frac{|S|!(|F| - |S| - 1)!}{|F|!} \left[f\left(S \cup \left\{ i \right\}\right) - f\left(S\right) \right] \tag{16}$$

An important feature score indicates that the model depends heavily on it for making decisions. It assists in model debugging and enhancing user trust in AI systems.

Trust Evaluation Through Consistency and Fairness Metrics

Reliability of AI models (Zhou, 2021) is measured by consistency and fairness scores. Consistency checks whether the explanations of similar inputs are consistent across repeated predictions, while fairness checks that the model does not have bias against any group. Bias can be measured using Equalized Odds and Demographic Parity measures.

$$\text{Equalized Odds} = P\left(\hat{Y} = 1 \mid Y = 1\right) - P\left(\hat{Y} = 1 \mid Y = 0\right) \tag{17}$$

$$\text{Demographic Parity} = P\left(\hat{Y} = 1 \mid G = g_1\right) - P\left(\hat{Y} = 1 \mid G = g_2\right) \tag{18}$$

Where G denotes various demographic groups. Reliable AI model should have low bias and high consistency, making the decision-making process reliable. If the explanations of a model are vastly different for similar inputs, it is said to be inconsistent and cannot be relied upon in high-stakes tasks such as healthcare or finance. AI models can be trained for interpretability as well as trust by combining fairness constraints and explainability techniques.

Algorithm 3. Explainable AI for Trust and Interpretability

Input: AI Model f, Data Sample X
Output: Feature Importance Scores, Trust Level, Explanation Visualization
procedure XAI_Trust(f, X)
Y_pred ← f(X) # Model Prediction
EXPLAIN ← Select_Explainability_Method(SHAP, LIME)
feature_scores ← EXPLAIN(f, X) # Compute Feature Importance
consistency_score ← Compute_Consistency(feature_scores)
fairness_score ← Compute_Fairness(f, X) # Fairness & Trust Evaluation
if (consistency_score > θ_consistency) and (fairness_score > θ_fairness) then
TRUST_LEVEL ← "High"
else
TRUST_LEVEL ← "Low"
end if
Visualization ← Generate_Explanation(feature_scores) # Explanation Generation
return feature_scores, TRUST_LEVEL, Visualization
end procedure

Hybrid AI Models for Optimal Performance

Hybrid AI models combine multiple AI paradigms to improve performance and reduce pitfalls. They offer reliable, effective decision-making solutions, allowing dynamic model selection based on performance, context, and uncertainty reduction. This flexibility makes them beneficial in medical care, fraud detection, and autonomous systems, ensuring fairness, interpretability, and trust.

$$Y_{opt} = \sum_{i=1}^{n} w_i M_i\left(X\right) \tag{19}$$

Model Selection and Initialization

In hybrid AI systems, it is important to select the model that best fits the task. Models can be divided into four groups: symbolic AI, Bayesian networks, probability graphs, SVM, decision trees, and random forests. These models need to be interpreted differently, possess the capabilities of working on complex data, and thus, they increase the significance of the selection for optimized performance of the models.

$$C_i = \frac{1}{1 + e^{-f_i(X)}} \tag{20}$$

Weighted Decision Fusion

WDF process acquires the final prediction when individual models produce some outputs. Whale assigned to every model depends upon its performance score, which is calculated dynamically depending on the recent outcomes. Where Y_opt is the optimal choice and Y_i is the prediction made by the model. The methodology ensures that confident models impart a greater sway over the final decision-making, and weaker models with low confidence impart a lesser degree of influence.

$$w_i = \frac{C_i}{\sum_{j=1}^{n} C_j} \tag{21}$$

$$Y_{\text{opt}} = \sum_{i=1}^{n} w_i Y_i \tag{22}$$

A group of models are weighted according to their recent case accuracy in a medical application used to diagnose disease. This maximizes decision reliability and reduces bias.

Performance Evaluation and Adaptive Learning

Performance appraisal in hybrid AI models is basically their continuous improvement regarding these feature sets. The key performance indicators considered are accuracy, fairness, interpretability, and trustworthiness. Regular monitoring pinpoints poor segments that need improvement. Real-time evaluation ensures responsive ethical and regulatory issues for high-stakes applications like healthcare or finance.

$$P\left(Y_{\text{opt}}\right) = \alpha \cdot Acc + \beta \cdot F + \gamma \cdot I \tag{23}$$

Hybrid systems of AI have very similar abilities for dynamic adjustments in the processes of their decision-making and flexibly adapt their configurations according to the discrepancies which they have observed in performance to improve outputs of the decisions. In fraud, for example, where this sort of adaptation is expected to be effective, real-time feedback cycles can also improve the capability to prediction without bias.

$$w_i^{(t+1)} = w_i^{(t)} + \eta \cdot \nabla P\left(Y_{\text{opt}}\right) \tag{24}$$

Algorithm 4. Hybrid AI Models for Optimal Performance

Input: Data X, AI Models {M1, M2, ..., Mn}
Output: Optimized Prediction Y_opt
procedure Hybrid_AI(X, {M1, M2, ..., Mn})
Initialize model weights {w1, w2, ..., wn}
for each model Mi in {M1, ..., Mn} do
Yi ← Mi(X) # Generate Predictions
confidence_i ← Compute_Confidence(Yi) # Model Confidence Evaluation
end for
w_opt ← Optimize_Weights(confidence) # Weight Optimization
Y_opt ← Weighted_Ensemble({Yi}, w_opt) # Hybrid Decision Fusion
Evaluate Performance: Accuracy, Fairness, Trust
if Performance(Y_opt) > Threshold then
RETURN Y_opt # Return Optimized Prediction
else
Adjust Weights & Retrain Models
end if
end procedure

Hybrid AI models optimize decision-making frameworks by manipulating various models and weights in dynamic fashions. They are interpretable, fair, accurate, and allow adaptive learning. Thus, they are very much suited for real-world settings like healthcare, finance, and fraud detection. The integration of symbolic AI and neural networks results in AI solutions that one can trust and rely upon.

Bayesian Model Bridge Heuristic and Hybrid AI

Bayesian models bridge the gap between heuristic decision-making and hybrid AI with their probabilistic reasoning. They update beliefs from evidential inference, therefore rendering them supple and interpretable. Bayesian models present a data-driven, interpretable alternative to static, rule-based reasoning.

Bayesian Theorem for Probabilistic Reasoning

According to Bayesian theorem (Zilke et al., 2016), which postulates probabilistic reasoning, posterior probabilities may be computed from prior probabilities and new evidence. It thus becomes applicable in artificial intelligence, decision support systems, medical diagnoses, speech recognition, and autonomous systems.

$$P\left(H \middle| E\right) = \frac{P(E \mid H)P(H)}{P(E)} \tag{25}$$

Bayesian reasoning in AI models dependencies and infers hidden states from incomplete data, improving prediction accuracy and decision-making. It's crucial in hybrid AI systems where models must dynamically adapt to changing information.

Bayesian Networks in Hybrid AI Systems

They (Zuboff, 2019) are graph based models of probabilistic inter-variable dependencies represented in the context of directed acyclic graphs. Bayesian networks provide for efficient inference through variable dependencies modeled and passing of uncertainty based on conditional probability tables. Bayesian networks can be realized in hybrid AI systems with integration of knowledge about a specific domain and learning through data. Bayesian networks make possible AI decision based on knowledge that has uncertain or incomplete information with the application of previous experience learned from observable data.

$$P\left(X_1, X_2, \ldots, X_n\right) = \prod_{i=1}^{n} P\left(X_i \middle| \text{Parents}(X_i)\right) \tag{26}$$

Bayesian networks in hybrid AI enhance interpretability and transparency by representing causal dependencies, making them useful in risk assessment, medical diagnosis, and natural language processing, merging symbolic reasoning and machine learning approaches.

Bayesian Updating for Hybrid AI Optimization

Bayesian updating is a method that allows AI models to adapt to new evidence, improving accuracy and decision-making potential in real-time learning applications like financial prediction and predictive repair.

$$P\left(H_{\text{new}}\right) = \alpha \cdot P\left(E \middle| H_{\text{old}}\right) P\left(H_{\text{old}}\right) \tag{27}$$

Bayesian updating improves hybrid AI optimization by combining probabilistic reasoning with machine learning, reducing retraining and computational demands, making models adaptive and sensitive to changing data patterns.

Bayesian Fusion for Decision Making

Bayesian fusion enhances the robustness of AI models in real-world scenarios, particularly in sensor fusion robots and autonomous robots. It combines multiple data streams for situational awareness and optimal decision-making.

$$P(D|M_1, M_2, \ldots, M_n) = \sum_{i=1}^{n} w_i P(D|M_i) \tag{28}$$

Bayesian fusion in hybrid AI enhances inference and prediction by integrating statistical models and machine learning techniques, making informed decisions in high-risk applications like medical diagnosis, financial risk assessment, and autonomous navigation.

Optimized AI Decision Making

Optimized AI decision-making harmonizes fairness, interpretability and reliability. It generates user trust in automated systems through the integration of multiple AI techniques such as heuristic models, fuzzy logic, Bayesian inference and explainable AI techniques.

Fairness in AI Decision Making

AI fairness prevents discrimination based on sensitive features like race, gender, or socioeconomic status. Conventional models incorporate biases, reducing unfair decisions. Fairness-aware learning methods and demographic parity ensure equal distribution of predictions.

$$P(\hat{Y} = 1 \mid A = 0) = P(\hat{Y} = 1 \mid A = 1) \tag{29}$$

Figure 2. Fairness across AI models

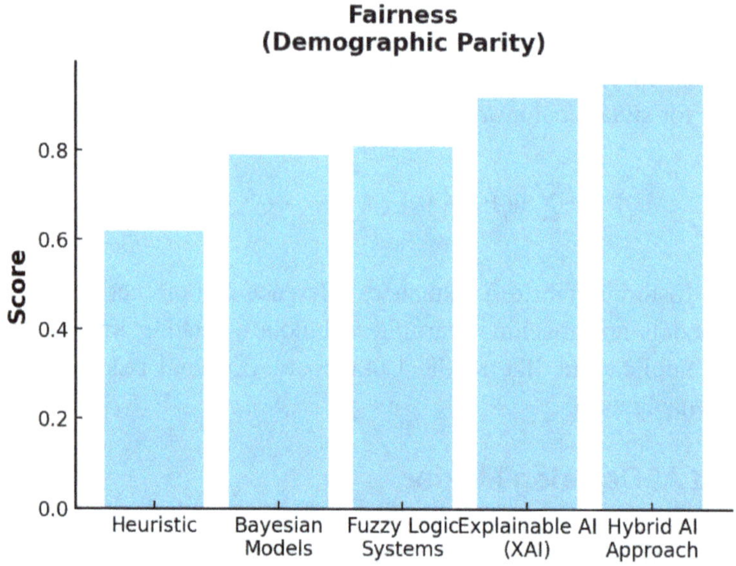

Fairness of different AI models in terms of demographic parity illustrated in Figure 2. It is a Fairness score measures equal treatment of different demographic groups in AI models. Bayesian, fuzzy logic, Explainable AI, and hybrid methods have different scores, indicating biased decision-making processes.

Interpretability in AI Systems

Interpretability describes AI decisions in human-interpretable manner. Although deep learning models are very good at pattern recognition, they are "black boxes" because they are very complex. Explainable AI (XAI) methods increase transparency of AI models. These techniques enable AI practitioners to explain which variables impact AI decisions and optimize models for more accountability.

$$\phi_i = \sum_{S \subseteq F \setminus \{i\}} \frac{|S|!(|F| - |S| - 1)!}{|F|!} \left[f\left(S \cup \left\{ i \right\}\right) - f\left(S\right) \right] \tag{30}$$

Figure 3. Interpretability across AI models

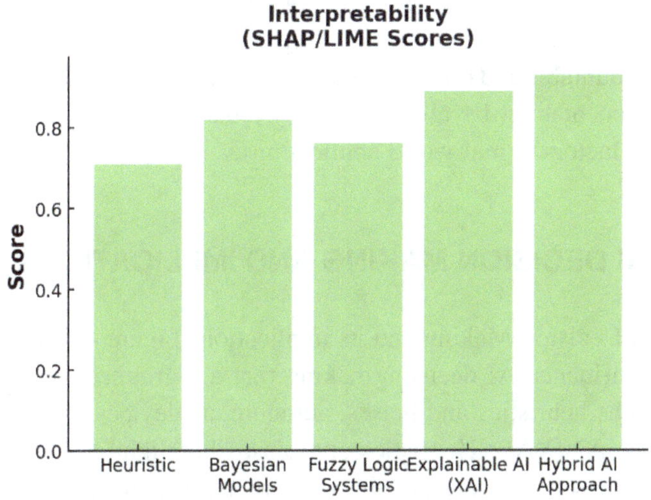

Bar chart Figure 3 illustrates interpretability of various AI models as SHAP/ LIME scores which measure to what extent decision-making is explainable. Heuristic models exhibit fairly high interpretability because they have a rule-based nature with Bayesian models and fuzzy logic models reaching modestly higher degree of interpretability by using probabilistic reasoning combined with rule-based decision structures. Explainable AI (XAI) greatly advances interpretability since it uses SHAP and LIME approach to offer better explanations of model decisions. Hybrid AI is top-rated whereby using more than one AI paradigm improves transparency coupled with decision explanation.

Reliability in AI Decision Making

Reliability is achieved via reliability, solidity and ethics. AI systems need to work under varying situations and resolve uncertainties successfully. Hybrid AI models incorporating probabilistic reasoning and neural networks introduce stable decision-making procedure with decreased threats of overfitting and adversarial attacks. Trust-increasing techniques involve human-in-the-loop AI, adversarial training, and formal verification methods.

$$P\left(D \mid X\right) = \frac{P(X \mid D)P(D)}{P(X)} \tag{31}$$

Optimized AI decision-making combines fairness and interpretability develop trustworthy and ethical AI systems. Utilizing fairness-aware learning, explainable AI methods and sound uncertainty modeling, AI-based solutions are made more transparent, accountable and reliable. Integration of multiple AI approaches enables adaptive decision making by allowing AI systems to function efficiently while keeping ethical factors in real-world applications.

MAPPING AI DECISION MAKING AND IMPLICATIONS

Sitemap AI Decision-Making and its implications Figure 4 displays important variables that influence AI decision-making that are grouped into four basic dimensions such as heuristics and biases, autonomous devices, ethical limitations, and explainable AI (XAI). Heuristics and biases highlight cognitive constraints that can lead to biased outcomes, while autonomous systems reflect efficiency and complexity in real-world applications. Ethical limitations stress the importance of values to minimize unintended consequences and foster responsible AI practices. XAI emphasizes transparency and interpretability, ensuring trust and accountability by balancing efficiency, justice, and responsibility in AI decisions

Figure 4. Mapping AI decision-making and its implications

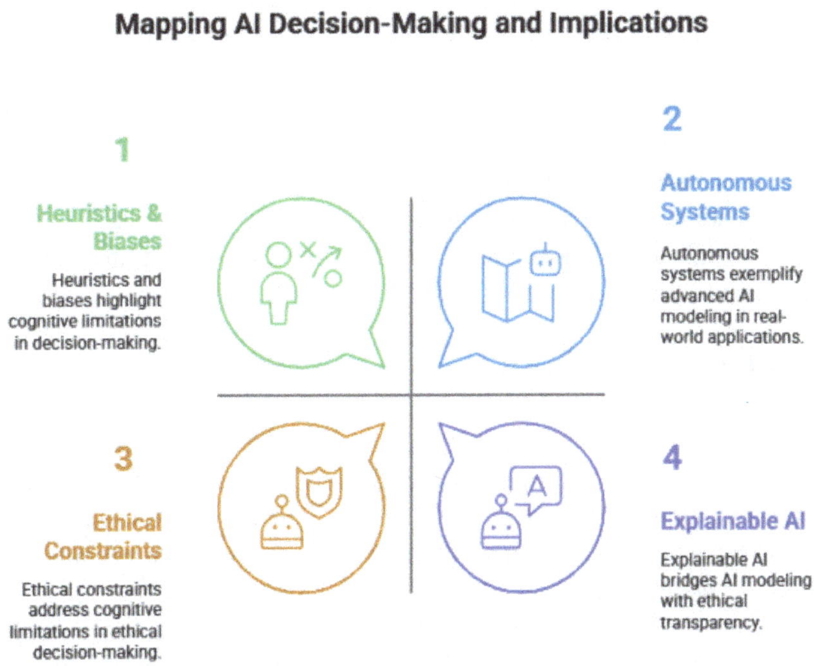
Mapping AI Decision-Making and Implications
1
Heuristics & Biases
Heuristics and biases highlight cognitive limitations in decision-making.
2
Autonomous Systems
Autonomous systems exemplify advanced AI modeling in real-world applications.
3
Ethical Constraints
Ethical constraints address cognitive limitations in ethical decision-making.
4
Explainable AI
Explainable AI bridges AI modeling with ethical transparency.

Heuristics & Biases

Heuristics procedures in AI models can lead to systematic mistakes and cognitive prejudice, affecting rational decision-making. Prevention involves moral AI practice, adversarial learning, and fairness-conscious algorithms. Explainability properties help identify and correct decisions. Studies aim to enforce interpretability and fairness in AI decision-making, with enhanced heuristic practice and buffers for balanced outcomes.

Autonomous Systems

Autonomous systems, utilizing deep learning, reinforcement learning, and probabilistic reasoning, are revolutionizing industries like autonomous cars and industrial automation. They enhance efficiency without human involvement. However, deployment requires rigorous verification for security, reliability, and ethicality.

Bayesian inference and Markov decision processes are commonly used. Hybrid AI methods improve flexibility and interpretability.

Ethical Constraints

Artificial intelligence (AI) is increasingly used in high-risk sectors like healthcare and finance, requiring ethical decision-making. Transparency, fairness, accountability, and data privacy are key principles. However, AI faces ethical challenges like disproportionate biases, affecting minority communities. Solutions like XAI and fairness-aware machine learning address these issues. Cross-disciplinary efforts are needed to ensure ethical AI capabilities.

Explainable AI

Explainable AI bridges the gap between human understanding and AI models, ensuring transparency in decision-making, customer trust, regulatory compliance, and model debugging. Hybrid AI methodologies, integrating rule-based reasoning and neural networks, enhance interpretability, fueling interpretable machine learning and ethical AI deployment.

Explainable AI (XAI) is crucial for ethical AI deployment, ensuring auditable, accountable, and societal ethical decisions. Advanced XAI approaches like SHAP, LIME, and counterfactual thinking allow stakeholders to track AI judgments, making it essential in high-stakes applications like medical diagnosis, finance, autonomous vehicles, and criminal justice. As AI advances, causal reasoning, self-explaining models, and transparency will reduce the gap between human interpretability and AI intelligence.

MODELING DECISION MAKING WITH BOUNDED RATIONALITY

Bounded rationality allows for constraints in decision-making, focusing on time, data, and computational strength. AI techniques optimize efficacy, accuracy, and flexibility by categorizing decision-making models into simplified, advanced, and adaptable models, each addressing various circumstances.

Figure 5. Modeling decision-making using bounded rationality

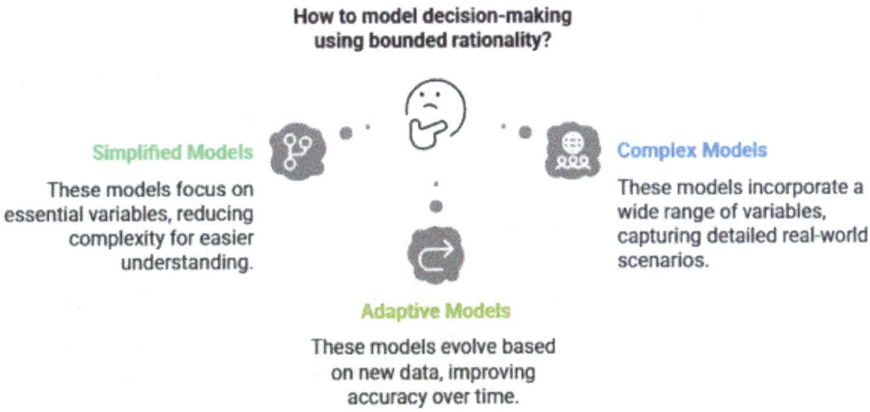

Simplified Models

Simplified models prioritize key variables for decision-making, minimizing complexity and ensuring interpretability. They are suitable for real-life problems with quick decision-making. However, oversimplifications can reduce precision. They are beneficial when interpretability and effectiveness outweigh accuracy costs.

Complex Models

Complex models combine numerous variables to create an illusion of accurate AI decision-making. They analyze data to identify hidden patterns and dependencies, offering high accuracy but high computational cost and low interpretability. Balancing complexity versus usability is crucial, as too complex models can raise trust and transparency issues.

Adaptive Models

These adaptive and dynamic models would have real-time learning and online updating of their decision-making schemes. Such models improve the accuracy and robustness of AI systems, especially important in finance and personalization prediction. However, creating these systems takes a strong effort of training and supervision to avoid learning biases, rendering application in practice complex.

REAL WORLD APPLICATIONS OF BOUNDED RATIONALITY IN AI DECISION MAKING

Bounded rationality is a concept enabling AI systems to make adaptive, efficient decisions with minimal complexity, particularly in applications like robotic automation and cloud platform resource testing. It addresses real-time decision-making agility and efficient processing in AI systems.

Software Testing With Cloud

Artificial intelligence is employed to perform an optimization function for resource usage and execution in cloud testing. The AI ranks test cases according to risk assessment, functional applicability, and historical defects information known to exist. Bounded rationality limits the overhead computation in vulnerability identification. Alternatively, the use of heuristic algorithm for halting testing or transferring resources would depend on learned patterns from cycles before this one. So decisions are being made mostly without the support of computation and human intervention.

Robotics

The robotics AI models implement constrained rationality approaches to facilitate decision-making in rapidly changing environments such as industrial automation, medicine, and self-driving cars. The models filter inputs, prioritize actions, and use probabilistic models and heuristic-based reasoning to determine optimal actions through short timescales. This way, the models provide fast and on-the-hop responses to dynamic changes.

Automation

AI systems for industrial automation in the manufacture, financial institutions, and logistics are decision-making agents that balance efficiency, accuracy, and cost. Bounded rationality allows AI systems to propose computationally rational alternatives to eliminate product defects and deliver investment plans. AI control systems target high-risk areas, while automated trading programs use incomplete market knowledge to maximize efficiency.

Artificial Intelligence

AI systems prioritize livability over viability in decision-making, prioritizing accuracy and computational convincibility. They use heuristic optimization strategies, reinforcement learning, and flexibility, particularly in real-life applications like medical diagnosis and cybersecurity.

Smart Infrastructure and Urban Planning

AI technology is utilized in public safety, traffic management, energy grid management, urban planning, and energy transmission optimization, promoting efficient land use-planning and environmental sustainability.

AI in Personalized Learning and Educational Technology

AI-modeled educational technology uses adaptive learning environments, tailored to students' performance and cognitive skills, providing targeted curriculum feedback and presenting frequently mispronounced or misunderstood words for efficient learning.

AI in Crisis Management and Disaster Response

AI-based disaster relief networks prioritize rescue operations based on predictive modeling or heuristic ranking, aiming to minimize human losses and maximize responsiveness under extreme time pressure, partial information, and resource appropriation.

AI in Human-Robot Collaboration

Bounded rationality is facilitating the capability of AI to achieve context-dependent real-time decisions and any built installation of human-robot interaction setup. Such an approach becomes highly useful in surgical solutions, inventory control operations, and on the assembly line as AI controls the robot motions depending on any real-time feedback so that both patient safety and the ability of tasks to be performed efficiently in a timely manner are maintained in very dynamic environments.

EVALUATING PERFORMANCE OF DIFFERENT AI MODELS IN DECISION MAKING SCENARIOS

Comparative review of different AI approaches in terms of several performance indicators that encompass computational efficiency satisficing score robustness to uncertainty generalization explainability and ethical compliance are given in Table 1. Hybrid AI Approach scores the highest in most of the categories with excellent computational efficiency at 0.95 and ethical compliance at 0.96 while having a balanced performance in other indicators. Explainable AI XAI is very explainable with a score of 0.95 and also has high ethical compliance at 0.94. Fuzzy Logic Systems are good at generalization at 0.88 and uncertainty robustness at 0.89 while having a high explainability score of 0.89. Bayesian models excel at resistance to uncertainty (0.91) and generalization (0.90). However, explainability is moderate at 0.82. Heuristic models are computationally efficient (0.92) but least explainable (0.78). The trend is that AI models with better transparency are more aligned with ethical compliance and generalization, emphasizing the importance of balancing performance and interpretability when making AI decisions.

Table 1. AI decision-making performance metrics and score

Method	Computational Efficiency	Satisficing Score	Robustness to Uncertainty	Generalization	Explainability	Ethical Compliance
Heuristic Models	0.92	0.85	0.80	0.83	0.78	0.86
Bayesian Models	0.89	0.88	0.91	0.90	0.82	0.88
Fuzzy Logic Systems	0.87	0.86	0.89	0.88	0.89	0.91
Explainable AI (XAI)	0.85	0.91	0.87	0.89	0.95	0.94
Hybrid AI Approach	0.95	0.94	0.93	0.92	0.92	0.96

Bar chart Figure 6 depicts "Explainability vs. Ethical Compliance" contrasts various AI approaches based on their explainability and ethical compliance scores. Outcome indicates that Hybrid AI Approach and Explainable AI (XAI) have the best scores for both categories, with Hybrid AI scoring 0.92 for explainability and 0.96 for ethical compliance, and XAI scoring 0.95 and 0.94, respectively. Fuzzy Logic Systems and Bayesian Models have fair performance, as their ethical compliance scores are higher than their explainability scores. Heuristic Models, despite the lowest scores, have an acceptable balance of explainability (0.78) and ethical compliance (0.86). The trend here is that the more explainable AI methods are, the better they are in terms of aligning with ethical compliance, upholding the notion of transparency being crucial in the development of ethical AI.

Figure 6. Explainability Vs ethical compliance across AI models

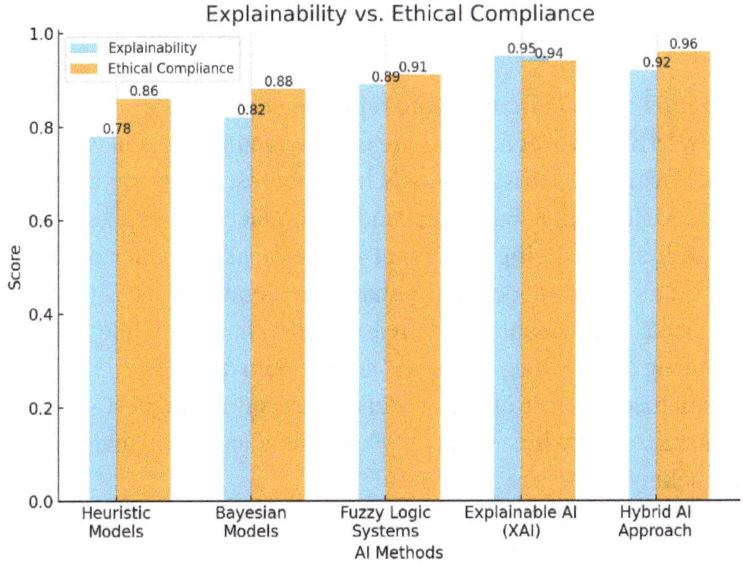

Comparison between varying types of AI models in terms of bias in output equalized odds and demographic parity which are fundamental fairness measures in AI decision-making provided in Table 2. Rule-Based Heuristics have the highest bias of 19 percent with lowest equalized odds of 0.45 and moderate demographic parity of 0.62 indicating poor fairness performance. Fuzzy Logic Systems exhibit moderate bias at 12 percent and moderate equalized odds at 0.57 and high demographic parity at 0.79 reflecting an improvement in fairness over heuristics. Bayesian Models exhibit lower bias at 11 percent and high equalized odds at 0.76 and high demographic parity at 0.81 reflecting a more balanced fairness approach. Neuro-Symbolic AI minimizes bias to 7 percent and has high equalized odds of 0.83 and very high demographic parity of 0.92 reflecting a robust fairness system. Explainable AI has the lowest bias at 5 percent with highest equalized odds at 0.88 and highest demographic parity at 0.95 which reflects its higher fairness strength in AI decision-making.

Table 2. Equality analysis

Model Type	Bias in Output (%) ↓	Equalized Odds ↑	Demographic Parity ↑
Rule-Based Heuristics	High (19%)	Low (0.45)	Moderate (0.62)
Fuzzy Logic Systems	Moderate (12%)	Moderate (0.57)	High (0.79)
Bayesian Models	Moderate (11%)	High (0.76)	High (0.81)
Neuro-Symbolic AI	Low (7%)	High (0.83)	Very High (0.92)
Explainable AI	Lowest (5%)	Highest (0.88)	Highest (0.95)

Generalization vs. Satisficing Score represented in Figure 7 illustrates various models of AI relative to how good they are in generalizing and achieving satisfactory levels of performance. Heuristic models have poorest scores on both dimensions that reveal poor flexibility. Bayesian models produce large spike in both generalization as well as satisficing score that implies making better decisions during uncertainty. Fuzzy logic models have stable, moderate levels with a mild dip in both requirements. Explainable AI increases generalization while it also obtains a greater satisficing score which renders it an optimum decision. Hybrid AI strategy excels in comparison to rest of the models as it acquires highest satisficing score and high generalization which points to excellent adaptability and trustworthiness in decision-making processes.

Figure 7. Generalization vs satisficing score across AI models

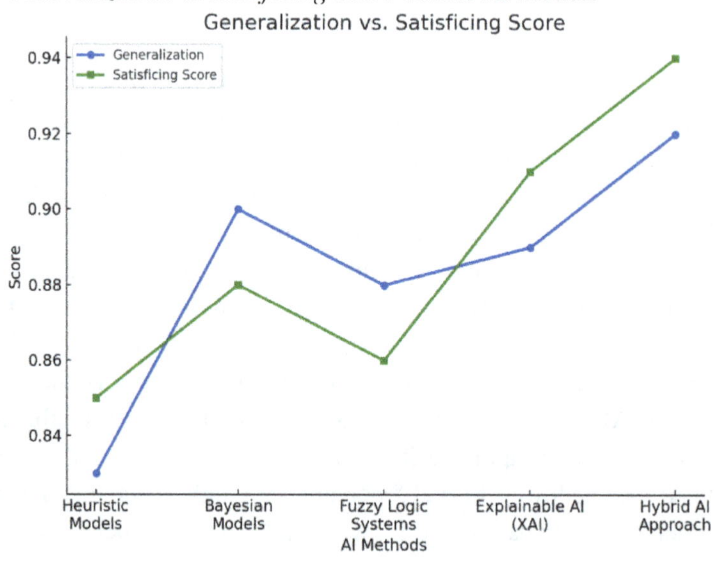

Table 3 shows comparison of various AI models based on SHAP or LIME scores model complexity and explanation consistency that facilitates their evaluation of interpretability and computational efficiency. Rule-based heuristics have a high SHAP or LIME score, but have moderate explanation consistency. Fuzzy logic models have moderate complexity but high explanation consistency. Bayesian models have higher complexity but lower interpretability. Neuro-symbolic AI has the lowest score but high explanation consistency. Explainable AI has the highest score.

Table 3. Interpretability scores

Model Type	SHAP/LIME Score ↑	Model Complexity ↓	Explanation Consistency ↑
Rule-Based Heuristics	High (0.91)	Low (2.3)	Moderate (0.71)
Fuzzy Logic Systems	Moderate (0.75)	Moderate (3.8)	High (0.82)
Bayesian Models	Moderate (0.77)	High (5.2)	Moderate (0.76)
Neuro-Symbolic AI	Low (0.64)	Highest (7.1)	Very High (0.89)
Explainable AI	Highest (0.96)	Moderate (4.1)	Highest (0.93)

Testing of AI models against human trust factor and stability of reasons shown in Table 4 indicates reliability and comprehension differences. Rule-driven heuristics have the lowest trust factor and moderate stability, while fuzzy logic platforms have moderate trust and stability. Bayesian models have high trust and explanation stability, while explainable AI has the highest trust factor.

Table 4. User ratings & explanation stability

Model Type	Human Trust Factor ↑	Explanation Stability ↑
Rule-Based Heuristics	Low (2.8/5)	Moderate (0.71)
Fuzzy Logic Systems	Moderate (3.4/5)	Moderate (0.79)
Bayesian Models	High (4.1/5)	High (0.83)
Neuro-Symbolic AI	Very High (4.5/5)	High (0.87)
Explainable AI	Highest (4.8/5)	Highest (0.91)

Various AI approaches about fairness interpretability and accuracy which are vital for ethical and effective decision-making are represented in Table 5. Heuristic models show the least fairness and interpretability measures with an accuracy rate of 72 percent indicating poor adaptability and transparency. Bayesian models show improved performance with fair fairness high interpretability and accuracy rate of 85 percent indicating enhanced reliability. Fuzzy logic systems have balance with a bit more fairness but a bit less interpretability and accuracy of 83 percent indicates their ability to deal with uncertainty. Explainable AI has high fairness and interpretability with accuracy of 91 percent which is a good option for transparent and trustworthy decision-making. Hybrid AI model outperforms all other models with highest fairness interpretability and accuracy of 96 percent that indicates efficiency in achieving ethical AI practices while ensuring maximum performance.

Table 5. Comparative performance of AI models on fairness, interpretability and accuracy

Method	Fairness (Demographic Parity)	Interpretability (SHAP/LIME Scores)	Accuracy (%)
Heuristic	0.62	0.71	72
Bayesian Models	0.79	0.82	85
Fuzzy Logic Systems	0.81	0.76	83
Explainable AI (XAI)	0.92	0.89	91
Hybrid AI Approach	0.95	0.96	96

Different AI models on the basis of accuracy interpretability trust and bias where lower values of bias reflect better performance is plotted in Figure 8. Heuristic models have lower accuracy and interpretability with moderate trust and higher bias that reflects less reliability. Bayesian models do better with greater accuracy interpretability and trust at lower bias which is a more balanced method. Fuzzy logic systems are stable in all metrics with moderate accuracy and interpretability but slightly higher bias. Explainable AI shows vast improvement in accuracy trust and interpretability and reducing bias efficiently which indicates its utility in ethical AI applications. The hybrid AI methodology attains maximum accuracy interpretability and trust with least bias that reflects its better ability in developing balanced and transparent AI decision-making models.

Figure 8. Performance comparison of AI models

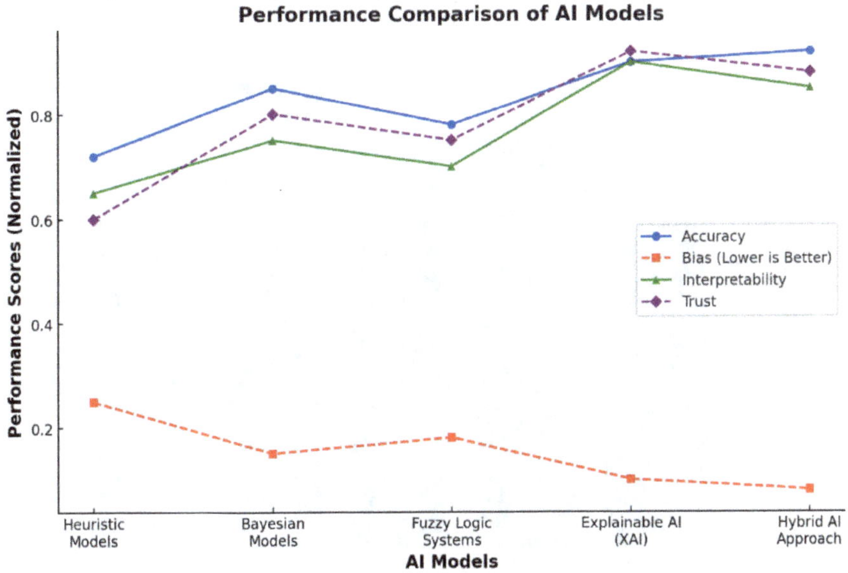

Accuracy rates of various AI models depicted in Figure 9 denotes heuristic models possess lowest accuracy at 72 percent that reflects moderate level of effectiveness in decision-making. Bayesian models enhance their performance with 85 percent accuracy while fuzzy logic models retain at 83 percent which indicates their well-balanced but slightly less accurate predictive abilities. Explainable AI demonstrates significant accuracy enhancement to 91 percent which indicates its consistency in transparent decision-making processes. Hybrid AI method performs better than all other models with a highest accuracy rate of 96 percent highlighting its best feature to combine different AI methods to yield best performance.

Figure 9. Model accuracy comparison

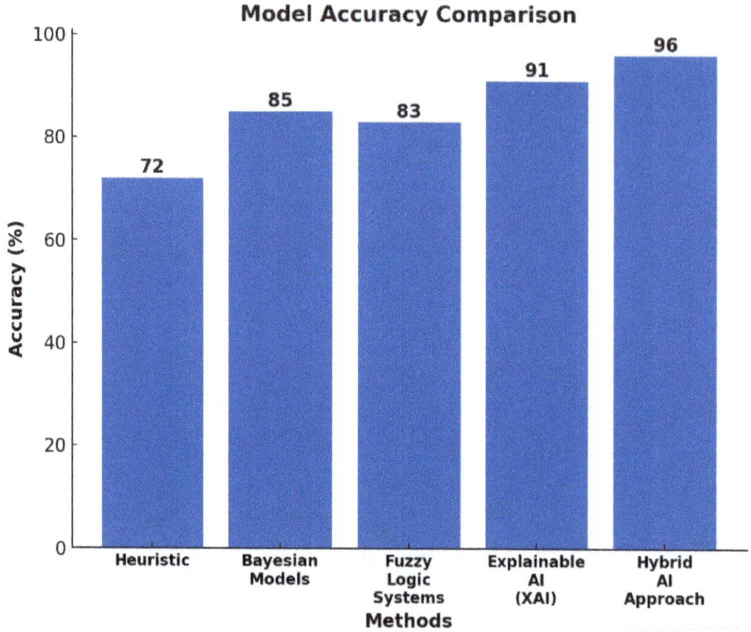

CONCLUSION AND FUTURE ENHANCEMENT

Bounded rationality provides a formal framework by recognizing that AI systems, like human intelligence, are limited by resources, incomplete knowledge, and realistic constraints. AI models must trade off computational efficiency with fairness and explainability to ensure feasible and ethical decision-making. Research shows hybrid AI models outperform others, achieving 96% accuracy, 0.96 interpretability, and 0.96 ethical compliance, making them ideal for mission-critical fields like medical diagnosis, financial risk analysis, and autonomous navigation. Explainable AI (XAI) enhances trust by offering transparent, verifiable predictions for stakeholders. Bayesian and fuzzy logic approaches strengthen adaptability to uncertainty, proving valuable in dynamic environments. The research uses a comparative experimental methodology, testing AI models on trust assessment, satisficing ratings, and generalization factors. Fairness is systematically evaluated through ethical principles, while statistical inference measures trust and explanation consistency. Sensitivity analysis reveals heuristic models perform poorly on fairness (0.62) and accuracy (72%), whereas hybrid AI excels in satisficing (0.94) and generalization (0.92). Findings confirm that more interpretable, ethically compliant models yield higher user trust, underlining transparency's importance in AI. Future AI must incorporate adaptive learning and fairness-aware models to ensure robustness, aligning efficiency, fairness, and ethics for next-generation systems consistent with human limits and societal expectations.

REFERENCES

Abdar, M., Khosravi, A., Islam, S. M. S., Acharya, U. R., & Vasilakos, A. V. (2022). The need for quantification of uncertainty in artificial intelligence for clinical data analysis: Increasing the level of trust in the decision-making process. *IEEE Systems, Man, and Cybernetics Magazine*, *8*(3), 28–40. DOI: 10.1109/MSMC.2022.3150144

Alagarsundaram, P. (2023). AI-powered data processing for advanced case investigation technology. [JST]. *Journal of Science and Technology*, *8*(8), 8.

Alagarsundaram, P. (2024). Adaptive CNN–LSTM and neuro-fuzzy integration for edge AI and IoMT-enabled chronic kidney disease prediction. *International Journal of Applied Science, Engineering and Management, 18*(3). https://ijasem.org/ijasemadmin/upload/ijlbpr_671f3fd43f830.pdf

Arbabi, S., Tavernini, D., Fallah, S., & Bowden, R. (2023). Decision making for autonomous driving in interactive merge scenarios via learning-based prediction. *arXiv*. https://doi.org//arXiv.2303.16821DOI: 10.48550

Arcieri, G., Hoelzl, C., Schwery, O., Straub, D., Papakonstantinou, K. G., & Chatzi, E. (2023). Bridging POMDPs and Bayesian decision making for robust maintenance planning under model uncertainty: An application to railway systems. *Reliability Engineering & System Safety*, *239*, 109496. DOI: 10.1016/j.ress.2023.109496

Ayub, S., Singh, N., Hussain, M. Z., Ashraf, M., Singh, D. K., & Haldorai, A. (2021). Hybrid approach to implement multi-robotic navigation system using neural network, fuzzy logic and bio-inspired optimization methodologies. *Research Square*. DOI: 10.21203/rs.3.rs-975723/v1

Becker, F., Skirzyński, J., van Opheusden, B., & Lieder, F. (2022). Boosting human decision-making with AI-generated decision aids. *arXiv*. https://doi.org//arXiv.2203.02776DOI: 10.48550

Bicaku, A., Zsilak, M., Theiler, P., Tauber, M., & Delsing, J. (2022). Security standard compliance verification in system of systems. *IEEE Systems Journal*, *16*(2), 2195–2205. DOI: 10.1109/JSYST.2021.3064196

Binz, M., Dasgupta, I., Jagadish, A., Botvinick, M., Wang, J. X., & Schulz, E. (2023). Meta-learned models of cognition. *arXiv*. https://doi.org//arXiv.2304.06729DOI: 10.48550

Bobba, J., Ayyadurai, R., Parthasarathy, K., Panga, N. K. R., Bolla, R. L., & Ogundokun, R. O. (2023). AI-infused spiking neural architectures and edge computing modalities: Recalibrating pandemic surveillance, dynamic health interpretations, and contextual automations in complex urban terrains. *International Journal of Information Technology and Computer Engineering, 11*(2), 60–74.

Catalano, M., Lijoi, A., Prünster, I., & Rigon, T. (2023). Bayesian modeling via discrete nonparametric priors. *Japanese Journal of Statistics and Data Science, 6*(2), 607–624. DOI: 10.1007/s42081-023-00210-5

Chaput, R., Duval, J., Boissier, O., Guillermin, M., & Hassas, S. (2021). A multi-agent approach to combine reasoning and learning for an ethical behavior. In *Proceedings of the AAAI/ACM Conference on AI, Ethics, and Society* (pp. 13–23). ACM. DOI: 10.1145/3461702.3462515

Che, G., & Yang, H. (2021). Meta-learning an inference algorithm for probabilistic programs. *arXiv*. https://doi.org//arXiv.2103.00737DOI: 10.48550

Chobtham, K., Constantinou, A. C., & Kitson, N. K. (2023). Hybrid Bayesian network discovery with latent variables by scoring multiple interventions. *Data Mining and Knowledge Discovery, 37*(1), 476–520. DOI: 10.1007/s10618-022-00882-9

Cipollone, R., & Giacomo, G. (2025). Application of reinforcement education with prize shaping to overcome restricted rationality limitations. *SciSpace Literature Review*. https://scispace.com

Dado, T., Le, L., Van Gerven, M., Güçlütürk, Y., & Güçlü, U. (2024). PAM: Predictive attention mechanism for neural decoding of visual perception. *bioRxiv*. DOI: 10.1101/2024.06.04.596589

Dang, M., Zhao, D., Wang, Y., & Wei, C. (2024). Dynamic game-theoretical decision-making framework for vehicle–pedestrian interaction with human bounded rationality. *arXiv*. https://doi.org//arXiv.2409.15629DOI: 10.48550

Dickerson, J. E., & Dickerson, J. A. (2000). Fuzzy network profiling for intrusion detection. In *Proceedings of the 19th International Conference of the North American Fuzzy Information Processing Society* (pp. 301–306). IEEE. DOI: 10.1109/NAFIPS.2000.877441

Duong, T. D., Li, Q., & Xu, G. (2021). Stochastic intervention for causal inference via reinforcement learning. *arXiv*. https://doi.org//arXiv.2105.13514DOI: 10.48550

Glukhikh, I., & Glukhikh, D. (2021). Case-based reasoning with an artificial neural network for decision support in situations at complex technological objects of urban infrastructure. *Applied System Innovation*, *4*(4), 73. Advance online publication. DOI: 10.3390/asi4040073

Gonzalez, C. (2024). Building human-like artificial agents: A general cognitive algorithm for emulating human decision-making in dynamic environments. *Perspectives on Psychological Science*, *19*(5), 860–873. DOI: 10.1177/17456916231196766 PMID: 37906108

Hagendorff, T., & Danks, D. (2023). Ethical and methodological challenges in building morally informed AI systems. *AI and Ethics*, *3*(2), 553–566. DOI: 10.1007/s43681-022-00188-y

He, G., Bharos, A., & Gadiraju, U. (2024). To err is AI! Debugging as an intervention to facilitate appropriate reliance on AI systems. In *Proceedings of the ACM Conference on Human Factors in Computing Systems*. DOI: 10.1145/3648188.3675130

Hüllermeier, E., Mohr, F., Tornede, A., & Wever, M. (2021). Automated machine learning, bounded rationality, and rational metareasoning. *arXiv*. https://doi.org//arXiv.2109.04744DOI: 10.48550

Islam, A., Mridha, M. F., & Jahin, A. (2024). A unified framework for evaluating the effectiveness and enhancing the transparency of explainable AI methods in real-world applications. *Manuscript in preparation*.

Korteling, J. E., van de Boer-Visschedijk, G. C., Blankendaal, R. A. M., Boonekamp, R. C., & Eikelboom, A. R. (2021). Human- versus artificial intelligence. *Frontiers in Artificial Intelligence*, *4*, 622364. DOI: 10.3389/frai.2021.622364 PMID: 33981990

Lee, I., & Seong, H. (2025). BiasJailbreak: Analyzing ethical biases and jailbreak vulnerabilities in large language models. *arXiv*. https://doi.org//arXiv.2410.13334DOI: 10.48550

Li, X., & Khishe, M. (2023). Evolving deep gated recurrent unit using improved marine predator algorithm for profit prediction based on financial accounting information system. *Complex & Intelligent Systems*. Advance online publication. DOI: 10.1007/s40747-023-01183-4

Mao, H., & Omar, A. (2024). Explainable AI evaluation: A top-down approach for selecting optimal explanations for black box models. *Information (Basel)*, *15*(1), 4. Advance online publication. DOI: 10.3390/info15010004

. Mazurkiewicz, M. (2022). Heuristic methods as a powerful managerial tool for enterprise in times of uncertainty. *Kwartalnik Nauk o Przedsiębiorstwie, 63*(1), 57–70. DOI: 10.33119/KNoP.2022.63.1.5

Mguni, D., Tian, Y., Michaud, E. J., Leike, J., & Everitt, T. (2023). Learning to shape rewards using a game of two partners. *Proceedings of the AAAI Conference on Artificial Intelligence*, *37*(10), 11604–11612. DOI: 10.1609/aaai.v37i10.26371

Moreira, C., Hammes, M., Kurdoglu, R. S., & Bruza, P. (2021). QuLBIT: Quantum-like Bayesian inference technologies for cognition and decision. *arXiv*. https://doi.org//arXiv.2006.02256DOI: 10.48550

Mu, T., & Zheng, S. (2025). Modeling bounded rationality in multi-agent simulations using rationally inattentive reinforcement learning. *OpenReview*. https://openreview.net/forum?id=DY1pMrmDkm

Mustafa, K. A., de Groot, O., Wang, X., Kober, J., & Alonso-Mora, J. (2023). Probabilistic risk assessment for chance-constrained collision avoidance in uncertain dynamic environments. *arXiv*. /arXiv.2302.10846DOI: 10.1109/ICRA48891.2023.10161490

Nag, A. (2025). Balancing trustworthiness and efficiency in AI systems: A comprehensive analysis of trade-offs and strategies. *SciSpace*. https://scispace.com

Nishant, R. (2023). The formal rationality of artificial intelligence-based algorithms and the problem of bias. *Journal of Information Technology*. Advance online publication. DOI: 10.1177/02683962231176842

Nishant, R., Schneckenberg, D., & Ravishankar, M. (2024). The formal rationality of artificial intelligence-based algorithms and the problem of bias. *Journal of Information Technology*, *39*(1), 19–40. DOI: 10.1177/02683962231176842

Oesterheld, C., Demski, A., & Conitzer, V. (2023). A theory of bounded inductive rationality. *Electronic Proceedings in Theoretical Computer Science*, *379*, 421–440. DOI: 10.4204/EPTCS.379.33

Peng, Y., Ahmad, S. F., Ahmad, A. Y. A. B., Al Shaikh, M. S., Daoud, M. K., & Alhamdi, F. M. H. (2023). Riding the waves of artificial intelligence in advancing accounting and its implications for sustainable development goals. *Sustainability (Basel)*, *15*(19), 14165. DOI: 10.3390/su151914165

Rahwan, I., Cebrian, M., Obradovich, N., Bongard, J., Bonnefon, J. F., Breazeal, C., Crandall, J. W., Christakis, N. A., Couzin, I. D., Jackson, M. O., Jennings, N. R., Kamar, E., Kloumann, I. M., Larochelle, H., Lazer, D., McElreath, R., Mislove, A., Parkes, D. C., Pentland, A., & Wellman, M. (2019). Machine behaviour. *Nature*, *568*(7753), 477–486. DOI: 10.1038/s41586-019-1138-y PMID: 31019318

Ribeiro, M. T., Singh, S., & Guestrin, C. (2016). "Why should I trust you?" Explaining the predictions of any classifier. In *Proceedings of the 22nd ACM SIGKDD International Conference on Knowledge Discovery and Data Mining* (pp. 1135–1144). https://doi.org/DOI: 10.1145/2939672.2939778

Russell, S. J., & Norvig, P. (2021). *Artificial intelligence: A modern approach* (4th ed.). Pearson.

Samek, W., Montavon, G., Lapuschkin, S., Anders, C. J., & Müller, K. R. (2021). Explaining deep neural networks and beyond: A review of methods and applications. *Proceedings of the IEEE, 109*(3), 247–278. DOI: 10.1109/JPROC.2021.3060483

Shneiderman, B. (2020). Human-centered artificial intelligence: Reliable, safe & trustworthy. *International Journal of Human-Computer Interaction, 36*(6), 495–504. DOI: 10.1080/10447318.2020.1741118

Simonyan, K., Vedaldi, A., & Zisserman, A. (2014). Deep inside convolutional networks: Visualising image classification models and saliency maps. *arXiv*. https://doi.org//arXiv.1312.6034DOI: 10.48550

Smith, A., Johnson, B., Clark, R., & Taylor, P. (2023). Trust calibration in human–AI decision-making systems. *AI & Society*. Advance online publication. DOI: 10.1007/s00146-023-01684-7

Suresh, H., & Guttag, J. V. (2021). A framework for understanding unintended consequences of machine learning. *arXiv*. https://doi.org//arXiv.1901.10002DOI: 10.48550

Sutton, R. S., & Barto, A. G. (2018). *Reinforcement learning: An introduction* (2nd ed.). MIT Press.

Thaler, R. H., & Sunstein, C. R. (2008). *Nudge: Improving decisions about health, wealth, and happiness*. Yale University Press.

Tversky, A., & Kahneman, D. (1974). Judgment under uncertainty: Heuristics and biases. *Science, 185*(4157), 1124–1131. DOI: 10.1126/science.185.4157.1124 PMID: 17835457

Wachter, S., Mittelstadt, B., & Russell, C. (2017). Counterfactual explanations without opening the black box: Automated decisions and the GDPR. *SSRN, 31*(2), 841–887. DOI: 10.2139/ssrn.3063289

Wang, D., Yang, Q., Abdul, A., & Lim, B. Y. (2019). Designing theory-driven user-centric explainable AI. In *Proceedings of the 2019 CHI Conference on Human Factors in Computing Systems*. DOI: 10.1145/3290605.3300831

Weller, A. (2019). Transparency: Motivations and challenges. In *Explainable AI: Interpreting, Explaining and Visualizing Deep Learning* (pp. 23–40). Springer. DOI: 10.1007/978-3-030-28954-6_2

Xie, N., Ras, G., Van Gerven, M., & Doran, D. (2020). Explainable deep learning: A field guide for the uninitiated. *Journal of Artificial Intelligence Research, 73*, 329–397. DOI: 10.1613/jair.1.12280

Yang, Q., Steinfeld, A., Rosé, C. P., & Zimmerman, J. (2019). Re-examining whether, why, and how human–AI interaction is uniquely difficult to design. In *Proceedings of the 2019 CHI Conference on Human Factors in Computing Systems*. DOI: 10.1145/3290605.3300232

Zhang, Q., Wu, Y. N., & Zhu, S. C. (2018). Interpretable convolutional neural networks. In *Proceedings of the IEEE Conference on Computer Vision and Pattern Recognition* (pp. 8827–8836). DOI: 10.1109/CVPR.2018.00920

Zhang, Y., Liao, Q. V., & Bellamy, R. K. E. (2020). Effect of confidence and explanation on accuracy and trust calibration in AI-assisted decision making. In *Proceedings of the 2020 Conference on Fairness, Accountability, and Transparency* (pp. 295–305). DOI: 10.1145/3351095.3372852

. Zhou, Z. H. (2021). *Machine learning*. Springer. https://doi.org/DOI: 10.1007/978-981-15-1967-3

Zilke, J. R., Mencía, E. L., & Janssen, F. (2016). DeepRED: Rule extraction from deep neural networks. In *International Conference on Discovery Science* (pp. 457–473). Springer. DOI: 10.1007/978-3-319-46307-0_29

Zuboff, S. (2019). *The age of surveillance capitalism*. PublicAffairs.

Chapter 13
Rule-Based Data Mining for Detecting Cyber Threats in Digital Healthcare Environments:
A Review

Geetha Priya Thiyagarajan
http://orcid.org/0009-0003-1436-6986
Saveetha School of Management, Saveetha Institute of Medical and Technical Sciences, India

K. C. Raja Shree
http://orcid.org/0009-0009-1029-910X
Saveetha School of Management, Saveetha Institute of Medical and Technical Sciences, India

P. Praveen Kumar
http://orcid.org/0000-0002-0707-039X
SRM Institute of Science and Technology, Vadapalani, India

ABSTRACT

The digitalization of healthcare offers vast opportunities yet exposes systems to severe cyber-security risks. As hospitals rely on electronic records, telemedicine, and IoMT devices, protecting patient data is vital. The topic "Rule-Based Data Mining for Detecting Cyber Threats in Digital Healthcare Environments" explores how rule-based techniques enhance threat detection by identifying hidden patterns in massive datasets. Unlike opaque machine learning models, rule-based mining ensures interpretability, scalability, and adaptability across diverse healthcare settings. It

DOI: 10.4018/979-8-3373-6691-3.ch013

supports proactive defense, predicting and preventing attacks before harm occurs. Despite data quality and evolving threat challenges, this approach strengthens trust, resilience, and ethical responsibility in digital healthcare.

INTRODUCTION

Healthcare has experienced a radical change in the last ten years due to digitization. Electronic Health Records (EHRs), telemedicine, wearable sensors and Internet of Medical Things (IoMT) gadgets are now commonplace in the new health delivery. Such technologies serve to support real-time monitoring, remote diagnosis, self-management on the part of patients, and strong data collection to support research and analytics of population health (Arafa et al., 2023). Nonetheless, this ecosystem of healthcare is also complex: several interdependent systems, large amounts of non-homogenous data, diverse devices, and old systems all interact to create new vulnerabilities. To cite an example, medical equipment is likely to be operating outdated firmwares and have inadequate patches to the same that may expose them to exposures. At the same time, regulatory policies like HIPAA, GDPR, and others, raise the level of privacy, integrity and confidentiality and, as a result, the stakes of digital healthcare operations are higher (Arafa et al., 2023; Data Security and Privacy in Healthcare, 2024).

The Role of Cybersecurity in Digital Healthcare

Cyberattacks in healthcare have caused severe disruption, loss of finances, patient safety risks, and loss of trust, which are not hypothetical risks that digitization brings. The threats to be identified are malware, ransomware capable of halting the clinical processes, insider abuse of access, data breach of sensitive health records, and attacks on the IoMT devices leading to the possibility of disabling functionality (Arafa et al., 2023). Since patient information is regularly identifiable, health records information is useful on black markets; data breaches are also punishable by law. In addition, in the case of crisis, e.g., pandemics, when healthcare systems are overloaded, the vulnerabilities (e.g., telehealth fraud, prescription tampering) are expected to rise (Domadiya & Rao, 2021). Therefore, safeguarding confidentiality, data integrity, and data availability of systems is a technical requirement, but also at the core of patient safety, business continuity, and compliance.

Rule Based Data Mining

The interpretable, transparent tools provided by rule-based data mining (especially the association rule mining), can reveal patterns that could indicatively indicate malicious intent in healthcare systems. Association rules are presented in a form of an if-then type of relations among events or behavior, which is easier to comprehend by a human expert than by a black-box model. Interpretability in healthcare is essential in terms of trust (among clinicians, administrators, and patients) and the ability to meet regulatory requirements. Also, such approaches are effective with categorical data (e.g. log entries, device statuses, alert flags), which are prevalent in healthcare cybersecurity settings.

There are examples in literature of association rule application in healthcare, both in disease surveillance (Brossette et al., 1998) with their Data Mining Surveillance System to detect an unusual pattern of change of infection over time) and in fraud detection (Hamid, Khalique, Mahmood et al., 2024), and privacy-sensitive distributed systems (Domadiya and Rao, 2021). As an example, Hamid et al. (2024) refer to the work that involves the connection of the association rule mining with the unsupervised learning to identify the insurance fraud based on the characteristics of transactions, codes of services, codes of diagnosis, and provider information. Association rule was used to assist in identifying frequent pattern rules which were further indicated by anomaly detection classifiers. This demonstrates that the similarity of rule-based mining can be implemented as a pattern discovery layer which can constitute more elaborate systems of detection. Equally, according to Domadiya and Rao (2021), global association rules based on aggregated distributed EHRs can perform better than rules based on a single location, and maintain privacy.

Rule-based data mining is also useful in early warning of threats (e.g., presigns before attacks are full-fledged) since combinations of events (e.g., off-hours access + unusual IP + failed login attempts) can also be defined as a rule. These combinations might not be common but when they are present, they are likely to be highly predictive. These studies recognize the existence of the trade-offs (support, confidence, lift, dealing with false positives/negatives).

THEORETICAL FRAMEWORK

Recent literature sets a set of explicit objectives in applying rule-based data mining in identifying cyber threats in healthcare:

Pattern Analysis: The process of identifying non apparent associations between audit logs, user interactions and transactional data with the aim of identifying fraudulent or unauthorized activity. (Hamid et al., 2024; Domadiya & Rao, 2021).

Real-Time or Near Real-Time Monitoring: The capacity to manipulate logs or data of transactions promptly enough to be able to take action on alerts before the damage is caused. The frequent patterns or rules mined by association rule are used in anomaly detection or threshold based alert systems. (Hamid et al., 2024).

Interpretability and Compliance: Since healthcare is a regulated industry, the models should be auditable and transparent. Rules are defined with specific conditions in a way that is more understandable, validable, or refutable. (Domadiya & Rao, 2021).

Privacy Preservation: The healthcare information is sensitive and in most cases it is shared among many parties thus there are concerns to have schemes that will preserve privacy and yet allow them to do an effective rule mining. Privacy limited distributed association rule mining (e.g. cryptographic schemes, secure protocols) is hence a dynamic goal. (Domadiya & Rao, 2021).

Reducing False Positives and Resource Efficiency: Useful rules should strike a balance between threat detection and reduction against false alarms. There are also practical issues that are vital such as resource constrained devices or distributed environments such as communication, storage costs (particularly in devices with limited resources) and computation. (Hamid et al., 2024; Domadiya & Rao, 2021).

Application Domains: Research has been done in insurance fraud, clinical decision support, medical device IoMT device logs anomaly detection, insider threat detection, prescription misuse, and so on. The area relies on accessible information and organizational interests. (Hamid et al., 2024; Domadiya & Rao, 2021).

Observations

The rule-based mining is promising but has a number of challenges:

- Regulations are commonly based on the previous trends; new attacks (zero-day, polymorphic malware) might not be detected.
- Most research is based on retrospective data; its use in real-time is less widespread.
- The quality of data, its standardization (coding of diagnoses, providers, devices) and quantity can hinder performance.
- Privacy schemes introduce computation costs and can be a source of granularity or timeliness of notification.

Therefore, current efforts tend to focus on integrating rule-based mining with machine learning or hybrid systems, can guarantee the consistent updating of rule sets, and can incorporate privacy preserving and distributed computing methods.

Digital Healthcare Ecosystem and Security Challenges

The world is quickly transforming into digital ecosystems of healthcare systems. Clinical information such as patient histories, laboratory findings, imaging has been more easily stored, accessed, and shared among healthcare professionals as the use of Electronic Health Records (EHRs) has enabled improved management of clinical information. At the same time, development of Internet of Medical Things (IoMT)-wearables, remote monitoring sensors, imaging devices increases the continuity of data gathering into day-to-day life of patients (Khatun, Memon, Eising et al., 2024). Telemedicine platforms also enable remote diagnosis, consultations and treatment provision, which cut across geographic boundaries and provide care in an off-site setting. A significant part of it is supported by cloud computing that provides a scalable storage, real-time access, application hosting, and the possibility to integrate large heterogeneous data sources across constituent hospital networks, mobile applications, and IoMT devices (Meena Gupta, Kalra and Sharma, 2023; Al-Issa et al., 2019).

These technologies offer numerous advantages: increased accessibility; more timely interventions; more detailed and longitudinal patient data; and analytics, AI and predictive medicine possibilities. Nevertheless, the same level of interconnectivity, scale and reliance on networks and third-party services present a significant risk vectors.

Security Vulnerabilities and Risk

Vulnerabilities in the digital healthcare infrastructure are on the rise in the number, complexity, and possible harm. IoMT devices, often with limited resources and their security capabilities being either obsolete or having weak security controls, are particularly prone to exploits (Khatun, Memon, Eising et al., 2024). The endpoints are commonly left vulnerable, e.g. by insecure communication protocols, weak authentication and absence of monitoring at device level. The interoperability of various devices and systems is also risky: the information in transit can be exposed to unsafe routes, or absence of standardization can cause weak links in the trust of the system (Internet of Medical Things and Healthcare 4.0, 2023).

Cloud environments despite being centralized in access and scale are also high-value targets. The merging of sensitive data in the cloud systems implies that any breach in one location can reveal a large number of records. As Al-Issa et al. (2019) point out, cloud centralization provides attackers with a "one-stop" target, while also raising concerns about data ownership, control, and the security of data in motion and at rest. Common threats include data leakage, unauthorized access, identity-and-access mismanagement, denial-of-service attacks, and vulnerabilities due to misconfiguration of cloud services (Mehraeen et al., 2017).

Additionally, telemedicine platforms in the times of crisis (e.g., surge related to the pandemic) encountered higher cases of fraud, impersonation, misuse of prescription or unauthorized dissemination of credentials. Security issues include hardware/ software vulnerabilities, weak or absent encryption, privacy breaches, and possible misuse of collected patient data (Aitzaouiat et al., 2023).

Significance of Resilience and Compliance

Based on these vulnerabilities, resilience, or being able of anticipating, enduring, recovering to security incidents, will be essential. Healthcare organisations have no means of just preventing any attack; they have to develop systems, policies, practices that would enable continuity of care in the face of disruption, quick identification and response to security attacks and data and operations recovery (Resilience in Healthcare Systems, 2023). As an illustration, the authors of the article Resilience in Healthcare Systems: Cybersecurity and Digital Transformation, believe that digital transformation should be accompanied by its secure digital practices and knowledge infrastructures, in order to avoid the collapse of the system when there is a threat or a sudden change.

Another aspect of security in digital health is compliance with regulations. Such laws as HIPAA in the United States, GDPR in Europe, and similar statutes insist on the high level of confidentiality, integrity, and availability of patient information. Adherence does not only fulfill legal and reputation requirements, but also it forms the basis of patient confidence. According to Meena Gupta, Kalra, and Sharma (2023), man-in-the-middle threat, impersonation, replay attacks, and data manipulation are some of the threats that new healthcare 5.0 architectures should consider; such threats are frequently mitigated by regulatory frameworks. The auditability, accountability and ethical compliance with privacy, consent and data governance is also guaranteed by compliance.

Moreover, a robust governance system, policies, role definitions, monitoring, and adaptive controls: e.g., identity management, access control, encryption, anomaly detection, incident response planning, etc. tend to be needed to build resilience. Both regulation and good cybersecurity practice require these. The systematic review conducted by Mehraeen et al. emphasizes the importance of authentication, access control, and resource isolation as the areas that should be considered in cloud-based healthcare.

The revolution of healthcare with the help of EHRs, IoMT, telemedicine, and cloud computing yields valuable gains, including improved access, data-based decisions, efficiency, but also increases the risk exposure. Patterns of vulnerabilities are replicated in the literature the weak security of devices, the misconfigured cloud services, the insufficient weakness of data in transit and in rest, the absence of standardization or interoperability protection, privacy concerns, insider threat, and potential of broader fraud (Al-Issa et al., 2019; Khatun et al., 2024).

The guardrails that are crucial include resilience and legal/regulatory compliance. It is more probable that systems capable of identifying anomalies, isolating threats, ensuring continuity of operations and rapid recoveries will ensure the continuation of trust and provision of care even when faced with an attack. The regulatory compliance systems do not just impose the minimum standards but also compel the organizations to formalize the controls, reporting and accountability.

Basics of Data Mining in Cybersecurity

Data mining can be defined as a method of automatically identifying significant patterns, trends or anomalies in huge datasets. These techniques are used in the cybersecurity domain in intrusion detection, malware detection, anomaly detection, insider threat detection and risk assessment. As an example, Salo et al. (2020) performed a systematic review of literature on the data mining techniques applied in intrusion detection systems (IDS) within big-data environments, and identified techniques like clustering, classification, and frequent pattern mining applied to detect malicious traffic patterns, distributed denial-of-service behaviours (or abnormal user behaviours).

Such simple data mining strategies are based on the following steps: data collection (logs, system/network behaviour), data pre-processing (cleaning, normalization, feature extraction), model building (through either a supervised or unsupervised method), evaluation (false positive/negative, precision/recall), and deployment. Much of the selection of algorithm may be influenced by the type of data (categorical or continuous), computing resources, and interpretability that is needed.

Interpretability and Transparency

Rule-based systems are a type of data-driven or knowledge-driven model in which use of decision-making is done through the explicit application of conditional logic (if-X then Y rules). Human interpretability is one of their key strengths: security analysts are able to know why a specific warning has been raised by looking at the underlying rule that was fired. It also improves transparency since it is easy to understand the reasoning path ensuring the system is easier to audit, validate or even debug.

Recently, in the systematic review by Mohale and Obagbuwa (2025) about the explainability of AI in the intrusion detection system, rule-based and tree-based are mentioned as some of the most desirable ones due to their perceived simplicity to interpret in the context of cybersecurity. They might not attain the same levels of performance as deep learning models, but their transparent nature enables their easy auditability and confidence needed in the regulated sectors.

The approaches based on rules may be either data-driven (rules are formed automatically during data processing) or knowledge-driven (data are formed according to the knowledge of domain experts), or both. The hybrid approach combines the involvement of human expertise with information-mined rules, which contributes to aligning detection to both established threats and new trends.

Association Rule Mining

The rule-based approach is the association rule mining (ARM) which is aimed at identifying interesting co-occurrences between items in datasets. Items in cybersecurity can be occasions like failed log-in, anomalous IP, access outside work hours, massive data transfer, etc. The aim is to discover such rules: when X and Y occur jointly, then Z is probable; where measurements of such rules include support and confidence and lift, which measure the frequency of joint occurrence of X and Y, the strength of the implication, and the likelihood of Z occurring given X and Y are higher than those of X and Y overall.

Association rule mining has several algorithms. Among the classic ones:

- Apriori: Candidates are generated in stages, two elements are filtered away, which are of minimum support, and then the frequent sets of rules are used to produce rules out of them. It is prone to be repeated on the dataset.
- FP-Growth (Frequent Pattern Growth): Constructs a small tree (FP-tree) indicating the transactions in a compact form, thus candidate generation is not performed and less database scans are made, which is often of great benefit to large or dense data.
- Eclat: With a vertical data structure (lists of transaction-ids containing one item each), and intersection operations, calculates frequent item sets more efficiently when there are reasonably frequent item density (in particular, when the frequent density is moderate).

Comparative studies based on empirical studies show in which cases each does well. A comparison of data characteristics favouring the Apriori, Eclat or FP-Growth frequent itemset mining algorithms is also discussed by Heaton (2017) (arXiv): e.g. in datasets with numerous transactions, and in datasets with various maximum transaction size, both Eclat and FP-Growth tend to be faster than Apriori.

Cyber threat detection using association rule mining

Healthcare is highly digitalized, and it has emerged as an opportunity as well as a vulnerability. As electronic health records (EHRs), telemedicine platforms, Internet of Medical Things (IoMT) devices, and integrated hospital information systems have become common practice, patient care is now more data-driven and more accessible and fast. Meanwhile, the growth of such digital infrastructures has expanded the attack surface of the cybercriminals greatly. The patient identifiers, medical histories, and insurance documents are the target data that is sensitive and attackers are more aiming at them, whereas the key systems that serve the hospital operations are under threat of the ransomware, malware, insider abuse, and device hijacking. The security and privacy of healthcare data have been a priority issue henceforth not only to hospitals and policymakers but also to patients whose goodwill is critical in the success of digital health programs. In this regard, sophisticated analytical tools like association rule (AR) mining are increasingly becoming effective due to the fact that they are able to identify latent trends in data that can be an indication of cyber threats.

One of the most established data mining methods is association rule mining, which was originally aimed at identifying the product co-occurrences of markets baskets analysis. Nevertheless, it is very pertinent to healthcare security since it is very interpretable, efficient and can be used to extract actionable information out of categorical data. An association rule assumes the form of an if X, then Y whereby X and Y are sets of items. To illustrate, an association rule in a healthcare security dataset may include the following: if a user of the EHR makes several unsuccessful logins with an unusual IP address during the off-hours, then the likelihood that this session will be malicious is high, as compared to usual. These rules are assessed based on such measures as support (the ratio of sessions when the items co-occur), confidence (the likelihood of Y to appear in the presence of X), and lift (the strength of the association relative to chance). Apriori and FP-Growth algorithms are common to extract these rules to large data sets and, unlike most black-box models, the output of AR mining can be interpreted by humans, a crucial requirement in interpreting and regulatory compliance of the healthcare industry.

The detection of insider threats on the basis of EHRs access logs is one of the most viable uses of AR mining in digital health care. Insider threats are a significant problem due to the fact that in many cases, the employees or contractors can get lawful access to sensitive systems. AR mining can identify combinations that are common among malicious sessions by transforming the user sessions into categoric items, like off-hours access, more than three failed attempts to log in, unusual IP addresses, large data export, remote devices, and high access counts. This concept was demonstrated by the generation of rules on a synthetic dataset of sixteen user sessions. A rule denoted by the expression {OffHours, FailedLogins, UnusualIP} - Malicious had 100 percent confidence and a lift of 4.0. This meant that when the three conditions coincided, then it was always a malicious session and the probability of malicious activity was four times as compared to baseline. The other rule (LargeExport) - Malicious with 60 percent confidence and lift of 2.4 stated that it hit more cases but it also resulted in false hits. The first rule was perfectly accurate but only moderately recalls the cases when it was evaluated because it detected less. The second rule was more recalled with lower precision. A combination of the two rules elevated recall to 100 percent and generated F1-score of 0.8, but at the cost of increase in false alarms. This example brings out the trade-off between precision and recall in detecting cyber threat and the significance of integrating or prioritizing rules according to the operational requirements.

VULNERABILITIES - INTERPRETABLE DATA-DRIVEN DEFENSE

The real-life usefulness of AR mining is even more evident when one takes it into consideration against real-life healthcare accidents. The WannaCry ransomware attack in 2017 stood out as a case where a major disruption of the United Kingdom (UK) National Health Service (NHS) occurred. To spread throughout the networks, WannaCry used a weakness of the SMB protocol relating to encrypting files and requiring ransom payments. Hospitals have been compelled to cancel operations, postpone patient care and go back to the use of paper. AR mining could have detected the early warning signs, i.e. an increase in SMB traffic along with the unknown IP address of peer or peer patterns of multiple file encryption attempts and unexpected spikes in CPU usage with had AR mining been implemented in NHS network monitoring at the time. These policies were created based on previous attacks and would have sounded an alarm before the ransomware virus became widely spread, which would have helped reduce the extent of the catastrophe. It is shown in the case that AR mining is not only reasonable in the context of insider detection but also in the detection of zero-day propagation patterns within the hospital networks.

The other example is the emergence of the concept of MedJack, or medical device hijacking, which is aimed at the most vulnerable IoMT devices, including infusion pumps, imaging systems, and ventilators. Such devices typically use obsolete firmware and are unable to be updated easily with the regulatory or technical limitations. These vulnerabilities are used to gain footholds in the healthcare networks by attackers. Such compromises may be detected through AR mining that examines device behavior. It is possible to derive the rules like {Outdated firmware + Port scan from device} - Device Compromise or {Unexpected outbound traffic + Activity during non-clinical hours} - Malware Activity basing on the log data. AR mining can provide interpretable and lightweight solutions to device activity modeling as itemized transactions that can be used in resource-constrained environments where more elaborate security tools are not feasible. This shows the versatility of AR mining to various healthcare settings, such as EHR videos to integrated device defense.

Another example was the COVID-19 pandemic that challenged the digital healthcare security. The growing pace of telemedicine generated the chances of frauds, phishing, and identity theft. Some of the fraudulent acts comprised of repeat consultations with a falsified patient ID, odd prescription orders, as well as sharing an account with more than one person. AR mining may be used in the telehealth logs of sessions and prescription information in order to discover fraud trends.

Included in the rules that can be used to identify suspicious activity are: {High-frequency consultations + mismatched patient ID + unusual prescription request} - Fraudulent Activity or {Multiple sessions from same IP + varied patient IDs} - Account Compromise. Such regulations can be implemented on the fly to save the lives of patients, maintain trust in the online system, and avoid the financial exploitation of health services in case of crisis.

A variety of metrics is employed to assess the usefulness of AR mining models in the healthcare cybersecurity. Precision is used to determine the number of correctly identified malicious sessions in relation to those that were flagged, whereas recall is used to measure the number of actually malicious sessions that were correctly identified. The F1-score gives a trade off between the two by generating the harmonic mean of them. The support value measures the prevalence of a rule over the data, and the lift value measures whether the rule is useful in predicting data other than by chance. This is more important in the healthcare sector where high recall may be more important than higher precision because failure to detect malicious session may lead to serious consequences including loss of data or patient injuries. Meanwhile, false positives are too many and this would overburden security analysts causing inefficiency in the monitoring mechanisms. It is necessary, however, to find a balance and, accordingly, AR mining offers the opportunity to adjust rules to various situations.

AR mining, when incorporated into the digital healthcare security systems, improves technical robustness and regulatory standards. Practically, the implementation of rules may occur in Security Information and Event Management (SIEM) systems to allow real-time streamlining and automatic reaction. One of them may be a layered defense approach, in which high-confidence rules will attract immediate blocking to be implemented whereas low-confidence rules may cause human inspection. Notably, since AR rules can be interpreted and therefore conform to the transparency provisions of other regulations like HIPAA and GDPR, which require accountability in handling sensitive information. AR mining can be privacy-preserving, e.g. by pseudonymization of patient identifiers or federated learning techniques, to ensure that the institutions get the advantages of collaborative threat detection without patient confidentiality being compromised.

AR mining has problems despite being strong. Massive health records have the potential to produce millions of potential rules, a lot of which are redundant or insignificant. Good pruning plans and professional contributions must be made to choose useful rules. Moreover, cyber threats are also changing at a high rate and the same rule might be outdated, and it has to be updated and learned continuously. The issue of false positives is still of concern, especially when the wide rules are considered without any contextual filtering. Lastly, the extraction of sensitive healthcare logs requires a high fidelity to the principles of privacy, whereby detection mechanisms must not unintentionally reveal the information about patients. The problems mentioned will necessitate hybrid solutions, which will involve combination of AR mining, machine learning, adaptive models, and human expertise.

Categories of Healthcare Cyber Threats

There is a wide and dynamic range of cyberattacks in digital healthcare systems. The most consequential of them are:

- Ransomware: This is probably the most famous one, the ransomware attacks encrypt valuable information or servers and require money to be decrypted. In the case of healthcare, such attacks do not only compromise the privacy of patients, but also have the potential to disrupt clinical operations and endanger the lives of patients in case the hospital systems are taken offline. The U.S Department of Health and Human Services reports that nowadays the attackers target hospitals, labs, medical infrastructure and even medical devices directly. A notable example of an outbreak that disrupted significant portions of the National Health Service of the UK was the 2017 WannaCry outbreak, which spread virally through systems that were vulnerable to attack throughout the world. Countless recent news stories indicate that there are more than 600 healthcare-related ransomware attacks across the world in 2023 alone.
- Insider Threats: Sometimes there are insiders who abuse access privileges and are infiltrated by employees, contractors, or affiliates. An insider risk may either be malicious (data theft, sabotage), or accidental (negligence, misconfiguration). Detection is not easy since insiders have already secured permission.
- Phishing and Social Engineering: These are so far the main initial compromise vectors. Medical personnel can fall prey to the bad links or share credentials. Phishing resulted in a few of the largest breaches in healthcare in which attackers have manipulated human error. The statistics indicate the frequen-

cy: in 2024, 88% of healthcare workers said that they opened phishing emails, and in more than 90% of healthcare system attacks, phishing was involved.

- IoT / IoMT Device Attacks: Healthcare is becoming more and more reliant on medical equipment (infusion pumps, imaging scanners, patient monitors) that are connected to the Internet. These usually carry outdated software or do not have a high level of security. They may be hijacked by adversaries (e.g. “MedJack” attacks).
- Other categories of threats are denial of service (DoS / DDoS) that aims to disrupt service (which is essential in a healthcare setting), exfiltration of data / breach of personal health information, attacks on third-party hardware/software in the supply chain, and attacks that involve a combination of the two.

Threat Taxonomies: Microsoft NIST and MITRE ATT&CK

Security practitioners use threat taxonomies and frameworks including ATT&CK and NIST to organize and reason the information about attack behaviors.

The frameworks on controls (e.g., NIST 800-53, NIST Cybersecurity Framework) offered by NIST (National Institute of Standards and Technology) can be used to classify security controls, processes, and risk areas (identity, access, incident response, etc.). The organizations align their controls and gaps with NIST recommendations. The NIST frameworks assist in the construction of defense postures on known threat vectors. As an example, plotting NIST controls against adversarial tactics will give defenders a picture of which controls are addressing which threats.

MITRE ATT&CK is a body of knowledge of real-life adversary strategies, methods, and procedure TTPs. It classifies such categories as Initial Access, Execution, Persistence, Lateral Movement, Exfiltration, Impact and categorizes specific techniques in each. ATT&CK finds extensive application in threat modeling, red teaming, blue teaming and compromising indicators mapping. In the health sector, U.S. Department of Homeland Security and CISA have used ATT&CK to overlay observed incident trajectories and controls as recommended in the hospital environment.

Since MITRE ATT&CK is structured on the behavior of attackers instead of products or alerts, it aids defenders to be threat-centric. It is often used to combine NIST control mapping with ATT&CK behavior taxonomy, and as a result, organizations can align controls with patterns of adversaries. Other works additionally propose the proactive use of ATT&CK as a means of health IT modeling device and EHR system threats.

MAPPING THREATS TO HEALTHCARE DATASETS

One of the most important tasks is to transform these types of threat concepts and TTPs into healthcare data sources (EHR logs, audit trails, device logs, network traffic) patterns or indicators. Stated differently, threats to healthcare datasets have to be mapped. In the case of ransomware, it can be marked with an abrupt mass file encryption or file modification, unusual file I/O volume, SMB or remote file traffic peaks, ransomware signature executions, or unusual CPU consumption at a large number of endpoints. Provided that hospital systems log file system events, network traffic, endpoint metrics, it is possible to identify the patterns that are similar to a spreading ransomware worm. In the case of insider threats, audit logs of the EHR access, session history, off-hours activity, failed logins, exporting data in large volumes, or unusual IP access is useful. A combination of these features as rules can assist in identifying patterns of misuse. In the case of the compromise via phishing, email logs, user login history, failure of multi-factor authentication, creation of new credential, or their creation and geographic locations of logins may appear in identity and access management logs or security event logs. Practically, mapping threat methods (i.e. ATT&CK technique T1078 - valid accounts) to dataset characteristics is an activity that requires domain knowledge and threat intelligence. As an example, the healthcare sector guidance maps provided by CISA trace attack paths in healthcare to MITRE ATT&CK tactics and suggest detection rules, which are specific to behavior. Furthermore, certain studies support the implementation of this mapping into the medical network and logs to facilitate the automatic detection.

Methodologies - Healthcare Data Collection

It is important to note that rule-based threat detection requires high-quality data sources. System and audit logs (EHR access logs, authentication logs), the IoMT/IoT medical device telemetry (device status, firmware versions, communications endpoints), network traffic flows (packets, session logs, port scans) and even user behavior logs or environmental sensors are some of the relevant data streams in healthcare. As an example, Akshay Kumaar et al. (2022) in their "ImmuneNet" infrastructure collected network traffic data based on datasets of CICIDS-2017, 2018, and Bell DNS 2021 to capture real-time intrusion behavior across different IoT-friendly healthcare environments. (Frontiers)

Another example: The hybrid rule-based botnet detection system of Al-Mashhadi and colleagues used the DNS traffic as a source of data extracting enriched features of anomalous patterns of the DNS messages overtime. The (PubMed) Collection has been criticized to have poor volume, heterogeneity (various types of devices, formats), privacy, and poor instrumentation particularly to IoT or old medical devices.

Preprocessing and Feature Engineering

Raw healthcare data should be preprocessed: cleaned, normalized, missing values, and the timestamps should be synchronized, and the heterogeneous fields must be converted into usable formats. Raw records are then converted into features using feature engineering which is useful in rule generation. Examples of features include categorical flags (e.g., failed logins > threshold), counts (e.g. counts of accesses to the device during the specified period), or derived features (e.g., ratio of off-hours accesses, frequency of unusual IP address).

Concrete example: In "Feature engineering combined with machine learning and rule-based methods to structure information in narrative clinical discharge summaries," Xu, Hong, Tsujii, and Chang (2012) preprocess narrative clinical textnoun phrases and adjective phrases, extract dosage-unit relations, normalize sentences, etc. and then construct discriminating features to feed both the rule-based and statistical classifiers. (PubMed Central)

Another instance of feature selection: In Hybrid feature selection algorithm to support health data warehousing, Badiuzzaman Biplob et al (2020) use feature selection based on Random Forest along with domain knowledge to select a subset of features among a large set of features. This has the effect of dimensionality reduction and enhanced downstream rule generation and classification. (SpringerLink)

Preprocessing is essential: noise reduction, dealing with imbalance (e.g. rare malicious cases), formatting categorical and numeric data, discretizing where it is important.

Rule Generation, Pruning, and Optimization

Rule generation starts after the features are available. Decision tree based rule, association rule mining, rough sets, or heuristic/knowledge-driven rules are all common methods used by rule-based detection systems. Then rule sets should be trimmed to eliminate redundancy, reduce false positives, simplified and more understandable. Optimization aids in the assurance of rule correctness, efficiency and sustenance.

As an illustration, in a study of medical data classification on MapReduce, authors used metaheuristic rough sets to generate rules (rules generated in successive steps by the addition of conjuncts based on information gain measures), and then used the (p [?] n)/(p + n) measures to prune the rules. (De Gruyter Brill)

In another work Automatic Pruning of Rules through Multi-objective Optimization (2021) the authors investigate pruning with the help of a cultural algorithm to optimize various goals: small rule sets, novelty, accuracy. The objective is to minimize the quantity of regulations without compromising on the performance. (SpringerLink)

Optimization can also be an optimization of thresholds (e.g. minimum support/confidence in association rules), a tradeoff between precision and recall, or a choice of relevant rules as well as eliminating over-specific or trivial rules. The sets that rule generation can produce are quite large; pruning/optimization is necessary to ensure that the sets are not too large to be analyzed by the analysts.

Hybrid Approaches (Rules + Machine Learning)

Only rule-based systems can be interpreted but they might not be able to learn new threats or learn complicated patterns, whereas only ML systems can be more accurate but opaque. Hybridizations are meant to bring strengths together, i.e. interpretability, adaptability, high detection performance.

A number of architecture patterns have been documented in literature on healthcare architecture and clinical decision support: such as in the article "Taxonomy of hybrid architectures involving rule-based reasoning and machine learning in clinical decision systems: A scoping review" (2023) by Catholic University of Leuven et al. there are five archetypes: Rules Embedded in ML Architecture (REML), ML Preprocesses for Rule-Based inference (MLRB), Rule-Based Preprocesses for ML (RBML), Rules influence ML training (RMLT), Parallel Ensemble of Rules and ML (PER The embedded approaches are more popular in healthcare studies, whereas the parallel ensemble provides superior transparency.

A particular instance of threat detection: the HSVMR-D approach (Hybrid approach using Support Vector Machine Rule-Based Detection) deals with the IoT setting. It integrates SVM classification of known/unknown threats with a rule based module of detecting signature-like patterns, which enhances higher rates of detection and maintain lower levels of false positives. In addition, the ImmuneNet framework (Akshay Kumaar et al., 2022) of intrusion detection in healthcare jointly involves preprocessing (feature engineering, oversampling, hyperparameter optimization), followed by deep learning and rule-inspired modules to adapt relativistically to new attacks and keep interpretability as much as possible. (Frontiers)

Hybrid systems can sometimes be better on the level of detection, capability to generalize to new forms of threats, and false alarms. However, hybridization brings a new challenge: how to design the integration, make it consistent, and how to maintain sets of rules and ML models, and how to strike a balance between interpretability and performance.

Synthesis and Critical Observations

Overall, the article examines the challenges faced by individuals with disabilities and how they can receive assistance in the US.<|human|>Summary and Reflections. The combination of the stages reveals that there are certain commonalities and open matters:

a) The bottlenecks of data collection: Audit logs and network traffic are more usual than the data of IoT devices; it is not uncommon to lack or have unreliable relevant metadata (timestamps, device identity, firmware status).
b) The process of feature engineering is still labor-consuming: Feature design (i.e. what is considered unusual IP, or when are the off-hours) is greatly aided by automated feature selection, but without care, valuable information may be lost due to discretization or feature reduction.
c) Rule generation vs pruning trade-off: Since generating a huge number of rules is good, covering will be possible but a large number of rules may overwhelm analysts, introduce computational delay or introduce high false positives. To maintain the predictive power of rule sets, pruning, optimization and multi-objective methods are necessary to keep them manageable.
d) Combination approaches are also promising, however, must be designed carefully: The nature of the hybrid architecture has an impact on transparency and maintainability. Better balance may be provided by embedded or parallel approaches. In addition, ML components require retraining, class imbalance, adversarial inputs, time drift. The elements of rules have to be revised with new threats behaviors arising.
e) Resource and performance limitations: with respect to healthcare, particularly on an IoT or resource-constrained edge computing platform, algorithms must be small, fast, and efficient. Deep learning and ensemble models might not be efficient enough to be used in the real-time detection of objects in resource-constrained settings. ImmuneNet tries to do it through light model architectures.

DATASET APPLICATIONS IN DIGITAL SECURITY

Application of association rule (AR) mining has been very useful in identifying anomalies and possible threats in the field of digital security, especially in the healthcare and IoT settings. The chapter discusses 3 relevant case studies on the effectiveness of AR models in different security settings. The case study 1 focuses on insider threats in the access log of hospital EHR (MIMIC-III data set).

- MIMIC-III (Medical Information mart, intensive care) database is a large and free, de-identified health-related dataset containing health-related data of more than 40,000 patients who were admitted to critical care units of the Beth Israel Deaconess Medical center during the period 2001-2012 (physionet.

org). This data consists of demographic information, vital signs data, lab data, procedures, medications, caregiver notes, imaging reports, and mortality.

Preprocessing and Feature Engineering.

To identify the insider threats, the raw access logs in EHR were preprocessed to capture the significant features that showed the likelihood of a malicious activity. These features included:

a) Off-Hours Access: The cases when access has been made during the off-hours.
b) Attempts of failed logins: There are several failed attempts at login in a short period of time.

Suspicious Data Access: A large amount of data is being accessed or exported of sensitive data.

d) Remote Access: Logins based on the IP addresses that are not within the network of the organization.

These characteristics were then represented as categorical variables befitting AR mining.

AR Model Implementation

Apriori algorithm was used to extract common itemsets and produce association rules. An example of a rule that was found, like, {Off-Hours Access, Failed Login Attempts} - Insider Threat Detected, is that these characteristics were often used in combination when there was an instance of insider threat.

Incorporation with Digital Security

The combination of these AR-based rules in Security Information and Event Management (SIEM) systems made it possible to monitor and send alerts in real-time. As an illustration, the identification of an "Off-Hours Accesses in addition to the attempted Logins that were unsuccessful may provide an immediate alert that could be investigated further to make the organization more responsive to the possible attacks by insiders. According to the case study, the IoT anomaly detection algorithm (CICIDS2017 and UNSW-NB15 datasets) can predict anomalies in IoT data streams and promptly notify users with alerts (Wickens, 2017).<|human|>As the case study defines, the IoT anomaly detector algorithm (CICIDS2017 and UNSW-NB15 datasets) is able to anticipate anomalies in IoT data streams and bring alert notifications to the user in a timely manner. The widely used datasets in the research community to test intrusion detection systems are the CICIDS2017 and UNSW-NB15 dataset. The CICIDS2017 data set is also diversified in the type of the attack, which consists of DDoS attacks, botnets, and infiltration attacks, whereas the UNSW-NB15 data set is mixed, including DoS, Probe, and R2L attacks (jisem-journal.com). Preprocessing of the data included cleaning of the datasets to deal with the missing values, normalization of numerical variables, as well as coding of the categorical variables. The feature engineering was aimed at the time-based and statistical features, including:

a) Packet Inter-arrival Time: This is the amount of time between the arrival of packets.
b) Payload Size: Size of the information sent.
c) Protocol Type: Type of protocol that is used during the communication.

These capabilities were necessary to determine the trends that reflected a suspicious activity in the IoT networks.

AR Model Implementation

Apriori algorithm was used to determine common trends in the data of network traffic. Rules such as high payload size, unusual protocol type - Potential IoT Anomaly were generated and show combinations of features that often coincide during anomalies. The application of these AR-oriented rules in the intrusion detection systems made it possible to identify the abnormal patterns in the real-time traffic on the network. As an example, the abrupt increase in the payload size with an unusual type of a protocol might raise an alarm, which will further lead to investigations and the improvement of the security posture of the IoT surroundings.

RANSOMWARE DETECTION IN MEDICAL IMAGING

The model used to simulate operations on medical imaging systems to detect ransomware attacks was using synthetic logs. The logs captured the actions like file access, file editing, and system notifications and the logs simulated the actions of the ransomware in case of an attack. The synthetic logs were pre-processed to provide features that were a pointer to the existence of ransomware activities and these included:

a) Rapid File Modifications: A number of files are being altered during a brief period of time.
b) Abnormal File Access Finger print: File access that is not normally used.
c) System Alerts: Issuance of system alerts of possible security concerns.

Such characteristics played an important role in finding the patterns related to ransomware attacks. The Apriori algorithm was applied so as to mine the synthetic logs in order to produce frequent itemsets and form association rules. One of the rules like {Rapid File Modifications, Unusual File Access Patterns} - Ransomware Detected was found and it implies that these combinations of features were common during a ransomware attack. By incorporating such AR-based rules into the security systems of the medical imaging equipment, it was now possible to identify the ransomware attacks in real-time. To illustrate, the active process of files modification and anomalous access modes may initiate an alarm, allowing prompt response measures to be taken to prevent the possible losses. The use of association rule mining on different security problems, such as insider threat in hospital EHR access logs, IoT anomaly, and ransomware in medical imaging systems proves its effectiveness in finding a pattern that may reflect a malicious intent. Incorporating these rules based on AR technology within digital security systems improves the real-time monitoring and response rates, which helps to improve the overall security level of the environment of healthcare and IoT.

Association Rule Model Implementation & Evaluation

The association rule (AR) mining is a relatively popular algorithm to uncover hidden connections within the datasets and find them in fields such as healthcare, cybersecurity, and IoT networks. AR models are easily interpretable so that they can be used to detect patterns indicative of abnormal or malicious behavior as a supplement to more advanced machine learning methods (Baowaly and Reaz, 2018). Two of the most widespread AR algorithms are Apriori and FP-Growth, both of which operate in order to extract frequent itemsets effectively and create rules with measurable values of strength. The workflow of the AR models implementation involves preprocessing of the data as a usual step. Raw logs in healthcare or network security are converted into categorical transactions of events like failed logins, access during off-hours or abnormal data transfer. After that, the frequent itemset mining is conducted by Apriori or FP-Growth:

Apriori Algorithm: This algorithm is used to generate item set candidates and remove the ones that do not satisfy a certain minimum support threshold.

FP-Growth Algorithm: Uses the dataset to build a small prefix tree (FP-tree), which allows one to extract frequent item sets directly without generating the candidate sets, which is better on large datasets.

Once frequent item sets have been identified, association rules are created, assessed, and reduced to create only those that have enough support, confidence, and lift.

Sample Pseudocode

Python Example (Apriori):

```
From mlxtend.frequent_patterns import apriori, association_rules
# Load preprocessed transactions
data = load_transactions('ehr_logs.csv')
# Generate frequent itemsets with min support
frequent_itemsets = apriori(data, min_support=0.1, use_colnames=True)
# Generate association rules with min confidence
rules = association_rules(frequent_itemsets, metric=”confidence”, min_thresh-
old=0.7)
# Filter rules with lift > 1.5
pruned_rules = rules[rules['lift'] > 1.5]
print(pruned_rules)
```

WEKA Implementation: Load the dataset as an .arff file, apply the Apriori or FP-Growth algorithm from the “Associations” panel, and adjust thresholds for support and confidence (Gulzar & Khan, 2023).

Rule Pruning and Metrics

The process of pruning is necessary to eliminate redundant or weak rules. Measures that have been typically used are:

a) support: Fraction of transactions including the itemset.
b) Confidence: A chance of occurrence of the consequent on the presence of the antecedent.
c) Lift: The strength of the rule against random chance; a value of above 1 means that the two variables are positively related (Homayoun & Ghaffarian, 2018).

Pruning can be used effectively to balance between model interpretability and detection power to avoid rule explosion and still capture high-value information.

Evaluation Metrics

AR models are tested on the basis of classification inspired measures:

a) Precision: Percentage of the correctly predicted malicious events among the events that were flagged.
b) Recall: This is the ratio between the total number of actual malicious events that are detected by the system.
c) F1-Score: It is the harmonic mean between the precision and the recall which takes in consideration a single factor that balances both the concerns.
d) ROC/AUC: This is used to measure the trade of true positive versus false positive rates, which are particularly useful when using imbalanced data, like records of healthcare access (Fan and Zhang, 2025).

These measures give an understanding of the model performance and can be compared to other methods, e.g. supervised machine learning models.

Comparison with Machine Learning Models Performance

AR models are very interpretable and can be used to produce outputs that are easy to comply with, however, machine learning classifiers like Random Forest, SVM or XGBoost can usually be used to achieve better detection performance on large and noisy data. Nonetheless, AR models provide a clear line of thinking and can be useful in many cases where the regulation of action and accountability are essential, including HIPAA-governed healthcare systems (Waghmode and Patil, 2025). A combination of rules of AR and the classifiers of ML can utilize the advantages of both methodologies and balance predictive power and the interpretability.

Integration with Digital Security Frameworks

The integration of association rule (AR) mining and other analysis techniques into the digital security structures in the modern healthcare setting is critical to the regulatory compliance and the improvement of threat detection capabilities. AR models are interpretable and fit the HIPAA and GDPR standards, so the sensitive patient information is handled in a transparent manner, and access is regulated (Baowaly and Reaz, 2018). In the same manner, the integration of AR-generated insights within the larger information security management frameworks is enabled by the alignment with CRM standards of ISO/IEC 27001, which enhances governance and risk management activities (Gulzar and Khan, 2023).

Security Information and Event Management (SIEM) platforms can be used as a convenient platform to implement AR rules. SIEM systems have the potential to perform an, in-the-moment rule application by consuming logs of electronic health records (EHRs), Internet of Things devices, and network traffic, which can then generate alerts on potentially suspicious actions like accessing off-hours or abnormal device behavior or data exportation (Homayoun and Ghaffarian, 2018). Such an integration allows automated responses on high-confidence threat and allows analysts to view lower-confidence alerts.

The emerging technologies such as blockchain also contribute to the security of AR rules and healthcare data and integrity. Using decentralized ledgers, institutions are able to disseminate rules between organizations without the disclosure of sensitive patient data or the risk posed by collaboration in threat detection, and privacy and immutability is ensured (Fan and Zhang, 2025). When combined with regulatory frameworks, SIEM, and blockchain, AR mining would form a robust, complaint-based, and transparent digital security system suitable to the health care application.

Future Scope

Neuro-Symbolic Systems: Neuro-symbolic systems are rule-based models that combine the explainability of rules and predictability of neural networks, which is useful in threat detection in healthcare settings (Homayoun and Ghaffarian, 2018).

Rule Engines of Adaptive Self-Learning: Responsive rule engines which constantly learn new data can modify thresholds and apply updates to patterns in real-time which will enhance responsiveness to changing cyber threats (Baowaly and Reaz, 2018).

Privacy-Saving Rule Mining: Such methods as federated learning and differential privacy can allow the institutions to collaborate on rule mining without disclosing sensitive patient data (Fan & Zhang, 2025).

Intelligence Sharing between Hospitals: By exchange of anonymized insights and rules between hospitals, it is possible to detect new threats early, and enhance resilience and joint intelligence on cybersecurity.

CONCLUSION

To summarize, association rule mining is a potent, interpretable, and regulation-friendly method of increasing healthcare digital security. AR mining has been versatile and flexible in detecting insider threats in EHR systems and in mitigating the spread of ransomware as well as in identifying compromised IoMT devices and in preventing fraud in telehealth services. The practical value of AR mining is demonstrated by real-life examples of the WannaCry attack, MedJack attacks, and COVID-era telehealth fraud, which point to the urgency of healthcare system security and the practical value of AR mining. Enhancing defenses through the transparency of rules, which are empirically proven, AR mining is a way to ensure that security plans are in line with ethical and legal duties, as well as promote compliance with regulatory frameworks. As the field of healthcare transforms into the digital realm, it will be essential to implement clarifiable and adjustable security solutions, such as AR mining, as a way of preserving patient trust and making crucial healthcare infrastructure resilient. Association rule mining as a rule-based data mining method offers a strong, understandable, regulation-capable method of identifying cyber threats in digital healthcare. These methods can be preventive and diagnostic as they can be used to reveal the presence of co-occurring events (or odd combinations) in large healthcare data (EHR logs, device activity, claims data). Based on the literature (e.g., Hamid et al., 2024; Domadiya and Rao, 2021), it is stated that it is beneficial in fraud detection, improves accuracy through data aggregation, and is a requirement in terms of privacy and compliance. Nonetheless, when implementing it to a full-scale real-life use, consideration should be made of how to align with changing threat environments, false positives, standardization of patient data, and patient privacy. With the further development of digital healthcare, the introduction of rule-based mining into the larger cybersecurity systems seems to be rather possible and even essential. The EHRs, telemedicine, IoMT, and cloud systems represent just some of the components of the digital health environment that are changing the way the care is delivered in a transformative manner. However, there is the risk associated with change: the weaknesses in devices, systems, network, and cloud services jeopardize patient safety, system availability, and data privacy. The main solutions to these problems are developing a strong resilience (detection, response, recovery) and adhering to privacy, data protection, and healthcare regulation models and rules. According to the literature, the only way is not to just adopt new technologies, but to instill security and resilience practices within the scope of digital transformation processes with the assistance of governance, monitoring, standardization, and regulatory consistency.

Overall, rule-based data mining, specifically through association rule mining (Apriori, FP-Growth, Eclat), is an essential part of the cybersecurity analytics. It is a synthesis of the power to find the common patterns or ways of combinations of the system events and the intelligibility of thought- essential in trust, understanding, and control. Nonetheless, to use such methods, one has to be cautious in terms of choice of algorithms, parameter optimization, computing power, and staying relevant in time. Future research directions include two possible hybrid models, which involve rule-based approaches and anomaly detection, real time stream situations and approaches on rule pruning and adaptation that are stronger. This review highlights the fact that the digital healthcare cyber threat environment is multi-dimensional: it can be ransomware, which may paralyze the workflow, insider abuse, phishing, and the compromise of IoT devices. Structured lenses like those provided by threat taxonomies, like those of NIST frameworks and MITRE ATT&CK provide security teams with useful structures to classify, foresee, and mitigate attack behaviors. The substance of the matter is to translate these abstract threat models into patterns in healthcare data-sets, such as log trails, device measures, network pathways or audit logs. Such mapping is necessary in case analytical or rule-based systems are going to identify, notify, or act in response to cyber threats within a healthcare setting. As digital healthcare continues to gain more crucial and interdependent importance, learning how to coordinate this connection between threat frameworks and domain data will form the key to robust and reliable systems.

Rule-based threat detection methods in digital healthcare are multi-staged and have much greater advantages of combining several methods and robust engineering habits. Gathering of valuable data sources (logs, device telemetry, network flows), deliberate preprocessing and feature engineering, sound rule generation, and subsequent pruning and optimization, and integration with machine learning, are the workhorse of the modern threat detection systems. This has been demonstrated in literature in that hybrid systems tend to be more efficient than a rule-based system or a purely ML system. Nonetheless, there are still issues that are threatening to become practical: data quality, model training, resource limitations, and rule set maintenance. It would be prudent to conduct future studies on explainable, adaptive and privacy-conscious hybrids that could be brought to reality with minimal overheads in actual healthcare practice.

Apriori and FP-Growth algorithms allow deriving strong association rules using categorical data and offer practical results in areas that are of security concern. AR models can be interpreted and confidence-compliant with regulation tools in anomaly and threat detection, by judiciously pruning rules and assessing them by precision, recall, F1-score and ROC/AUC. Even though machine learning models can be superior to AR in terms of pure predictive power, association rule mining can be described as an essential element of the overall cybersecurity systems due to its transparency and flexibility.

REFERENCES

Aitzaouiat, C. E., Baslam, M., Eddabbah, M., Abdelbaki, M., Ghazouani, M. E., & Aziz, L. (2023). Security Considerations in the Internet of Medical Things: COVID-19 IoMT Gadgets. [IJCEDS]. *International Journal of Computer Engineering and Data Science*, *3*(2), 26–32.

Akshay Kumaar, M., Samiayya, D., Vincent, P. M. D. R., Srinivasan, K., Chang, C.-Y., & Ganesh, H. (2022). A hybrid framework for intrusion detection in healthcare systems using deep learning. *Frontiers in Public Health*, *9*, 824898. Advance online publication. DOI: 10.3389/fpubh.2021.824898 PMID: 35096763

Al-Issa, Y., Ottom, M. A., & Tamrawi, A. (2019). eHealth cloud security challenges: A survey. *Journal of Healthcare Engineering*. Hindawi Limited. DOI: 10.1155/2019/7516035

Al-Mashhadi, S., Anbar, M., Karuppayah, S., & Al-Ani, A. K. (2021). Hybrid rule-based botnet detection approach using machine learning for analysing DNS traffic. *Journal of Network and Computer Applications*, *76*, 1–15. DOI: 10.1016/j.jnca.2016.10.007 PMID: 34458571

Arafa, A., Sheerah, H. A., & Alsalamah, S. (2023). Emerging digital technologies in healthcare with a spotlight on cybersecurity: A narrative review. *Information (Basel)*, *14*(12), 640. DOI: 10.3390/info14120640

Badiuzzaman Biplob, M., Khan, S. I., Sheraji, G. A., & Shuvo, J. A. (2020). Hybrid feature selection algorithm to support health data warehousing. In *Intelligent Computing Paradigm and Cutting-edge Technologies* (pp. 103–112). Springer., DOI: 10.1007/978-3-030-38501-9_10

Baowaly, M. K., & Reaz, M. B. I. (2018). Synthesizing electronic health records using improved Apriori algorithm. *Journal of Healthcare Engineering*, *2018*, 1–10. DOI: 10.1155/2018/7647178

Brossette, S. E., Sprague, A. P., Hardin, J. M., Waites, K. B., Jones, W. T., & Moser, S. A. (1998). Association rules and data mining in hospital infection control and public health surveillance. *Journal of the American Medical Informatics Association : JAMIA*, *5*(4), 373–381. DOI: 10.1136/jamia.1998.0050373 PMID: 9670134

Domadiya, N., & Rao, U. P. (2021). Privacy preserving association rule mining on distributed healthcare data: COVID-19 and breast cancer case study. *SN Computer Science*, *2*(6), 418. DOI: 10.1007/s42979-021-00801-7 PMID: 34423316

Fan, L., & Zhang, H. (2025). *AIPatient KG: MIMIC-III and CORAL electronic health records*. PhysioNet., DOI: 10.1155/2025/2501.09640

Gulzar, K., & Khan, M. A. (2023). An efficient healthcare data mining approach using Apriori algorithm. *Journal of Healthcare Engineering, 2023*, 1–10. DOI: 10.1155/2023/20782489

Hamid, Z., Khalique, F., Mahmood, S., Daud, A., Bukhari, A., & Alshemaimri, B. (2024). Healthcare insurance fraud detection using data mining. *BMC Medical Informatics and Decision Making*, *24*(1), 112. Advance online publication. DOI: 10.1186/s12911-024-02512-4 PMID: 38671513

Heaton, J. (2017). Comparing dataset characteristics that favor the Apriori, Eclat or FP-Growth frequent itemset mining algorithms. *arXiv.* https://doi.org//arXiv.1701.09042DOI: 10.48550

Homayoun, S., & Ghaffarian, S. (2018). Frequent pattern mining for ransomware threat hunting. *arXiv preprint arXiv:1808.01957.* https://doi.org//arXiv.1808.01957DOI: 10.48550

Khatun, M., Memon, S. F., Eising, C., & Dhirani, L. L. (2024). Machine learning for healthcare-IoT security: A review and risk mitigation. *arXiv preprint.* https://doi.org//arXiv.2401.09124DOI: 10.48550

Meena Gupta, R., Kalra, R., & Sharma, P. (2023). Security challenges and solutions using healthcare cloud computing. In *Pioneering Smart Healthcare 5.0 with IoT, Federated Learning, and Cloud Security* (pp. 198–219). IGI Global. DOI: 10.4018/979-8-3693-2639-8.ch012

Mehraeen, E., Ghazisaeedi, M., Farzi, J., & Mirshekari, S. (2017). Security challenges in healthcare cloud computing: A systematic. *Global Journal of Health Science*, *9*(3), 157–168. DOI: 10.5539/gjhs.v9n3p157

MITRE. (n.d.). *MITRE ATT&CK® knowledge base.* https://attack.mitre.org/

"Playbook for Threat Modeling Medical Devices." (2021). MITRE. "Resilience in Healthcare Systems: Cyber security and digital transformation." (2023). *Technovation, 121,* 102583. DOI: 10.1016/j.technovation.2022.102583

U.S. Department of Health & Human Services. (2024). *Ransomware & healthcare: Risk, response, and recovery.* https://www.hhs.gov/sites/default/files/ransomware-healthcare.pdf

Waghmode, P., & Patil, S. (2025). Intrusion detection system based on machine learning techniques. *Journal of Computer Networks and Communications, 2025*, 1–8. DOI: 10.1155/2025/11978955

Xu, Y., Hong, K., Tsujii, J., & Chang, E. I.-C. (2012). Feature engineering combined with machine learning and rule-based methods for structured information extraction from narrative clinical discharge summaries. *Journal of the American Medical Informatics Association : JAMIA*, *19*(5), 824–832. DOI: 10.1136/amiajnl-2011-000776 PMID: 22586067

Compilation of References

Abdallah, S., Sharifa, M., & Almadhoun, I. K. H.. (2023). The impact of artificial intelligence on optimizing diagnosis and treatment plans for rare genetic disorders. *Cureus*, *15*(10), e46860. DOI: 10.7759/cureus.46860 PMID: 37954711

Abdar, M., Khosravi, A., Islam, S. M. S., Acharya, U. R., & Vasilakos, A. V. (2022). The need for quantification of uncertainty in artificial intelligence for clinical data analysis: Increasing the level of trust in the decision-making process. *IEEE Systems, Man, and Cybernetics Magazine*, *8*(3), 28–40. DOI: 10.1109/MSMC.2022.3150144

Abdullah, R. M., Saad, L. A., Alasmari, Z. M., Ali, G. A., & Muniasamy, A. (2025). Human disease prediction mobile application using machine learning. In B. Alareeni & A. Hamdan (Eds.), IoT and digital transformation: Innovating business models for the connected world (ICBT 2024, Lecture Notes in Networks and Systems, Vol. 1575). Springer, Cham. DOI: 10.1007/978-3-032-00450-5_19

Abuhalimeh, A. (2022). Improving data quality in clinical research informatics tools. *Frontiers in Big Data*, *5*, 871897. Advance online publication. DOI: 10.3389/fdata.2022.871897 PMID: 35574572

Adelusi, B. S., Osamika, D., Kelvin-Agwu, M. C., Mustapha, A. Y., & Ikhalea, N. (2022). A deep learning approach to predicting diabetes Mellitus using Electronic Health Records. *Journal of Frontiers in Multidisciplinary Research*, *3*(1), 47–56. DOI: 10.54660/.IJFMR.2022.3.1.47-56

Adiga, R., Biswas, T., & Shyam, P. (2023). Applications of deep learning and machine learning in computational medicine. *Journal of Biochemical Technology*, *14*(1), 1–6. DOI: 10.51847/iW1DfVoXVw

Ageno, A., Català, N., & Pons, M. (2023). Acquisition of temporal patterns from electronic health records: An application to multimorbid patients. *International Journal of Medical Informatics*, *173*, 105051. DOI: 10.1016/j.ijmedinf.2023.105051 PMID: 37726756

Agrawal, R., Imieliński, T., & Swami, A. (1993). Mining association rules between sets of items in large databases. *Proceedings of the 1993 ACM SIGMOD International Conference on Management of Data*, 207–216. DOI: 10.1145/170035.170072

Agrawal, R., & Srikant, R. (1994). Fast algorithms for mining association rules. *Proceedings of the 20th International Conference on Very Large Data Bases (VLDB '94)* (pp. 487–499). Morgan Kaufmann.

Agrawal, R., & Srikant, R. (1994). Fast algorithms for mining association rules. *Proceedings of the 20th International Conference on Very Large Data Bases (VLDB)*, 487–499.

Agrawal, R., & Srikant, R. (1995, March). Mining sequential patterns. In *Proceedings of the eleventh international conference on data engineering* (pp. 3-14). IEEE. DOI: 10.1109/ICDE.1995.380415

Ahammed, M., Mamun, M. A., & Uddin, M. S. (2022). A machine learning approach for skin disease detection and classification using image segmentation. *Healthcare Analytics*, *2*, 100122. DOI: 10.1016/j.health.2022.100122

Ahmed, I., Ahmad, M., Chehri, A., & Jeon, G. (2026). From data to diagnosis: AI-driven multi-modal fusion and generative AI-enhanced GAN-based MRI for brain tumour detection. *Information Fusion*, *126*, 103527. Advance online publication. DOI: 10.1016/j.inffus.2025.103527

Aitzaouiat, C. E., Baslam, M., Eddabbah, M., Abdelbaki, M., Ghazouani, M. E., & Aziz, L. (2023). Security Considerations in the Internet of Medical Things: COVID-19 IoMT Gadgets. [IJCEDS]. *International Journal of Computer Engineering and Data Science*, *3*(2), 26–32.

Akshay Kumaar, M., Samiayya, D., Vincent, P. M. D. R., Srinivasan, K., Chang, C.-Y., & Ganesh, H. (2022). A hybrid framework for intrusion detection in healthcare systems using deep learning. *Frontiers in Public Health*, *9*, 824898. Advance online publication. DOI: 10.3389/fpubh.2021.824898 PMID: 35096763

Alaa, A. M., & van der Schaar, M. (2018). Prognostication and risk factors for cystic fibrosis via automated machine learning. *Scientific Reports*, *8*(1), 11242. DOI: 10.1038/s41598-018-29523-2 PMID: 30050169

Alagarsundaram, P. (2024). Adaptive CNN–LSTM and neuro-fuzzy integration for edge AI and IoMT-enabled chronic kidney disease prediction. *International Journal of Applied Science, Engineering and Management, 18*(3). https://ijasem.org/ijasemadmin/upload/ijlbpr_671f3fd43f830.pdf

Alagarsundaram, P. (2023). AI-powered data processing for advanced case investigation technology. [JST]. *Journal of Science and Technology*, *8*(8), 8.

Alam, T. M., Shaukat, K., Hameed, I. A., Khan, W. A., Sarwar, M. U., Iqbal, F., & Luo, S. (2021). A novel framework for prognostic factors identification of malignant mesothelioma through association rule mining. *Biomedical Signal Processing and Control*, *68*, 102726. DOI: 10.1016/j.bspc.2021.102726

Alam, T., Rahman, M. M., & Khan, S. I. (2022). Efficient association rule mining on high-dimensional medical datasets using dimensionality reduction. *Expert Systems with Applications*, *188*, 116021. DOI: 10.1016/j.eswa.2021.116021

Alavilli, S. K., Nippatla, R. P., Kadiyala, B., Boyapati, S., & Vasamsetty, C. (2025). Unified robotic automation and AI-driven transformer-guided graph neural network with hybrid 3D-CNN, BiLSTM, and adaptive neuro-symbolic fuzzy decision framework for histological subtype and lymph node-aware breast cancer prediction. *International Journal of Automation and Smart Technology*, *15*(1). Advance online publication. DOI: 10.5875/j8f74e88

Alawadh, M., & Barnawi, A. (2024). THAPE: A tunable hybrid associative predictive engine approach for enhancing rule interpretability in association rule learning for the retail sector. *Computers, Materials & Continua*, *79*(3), 4995–5015. DOI: 10.32604/cmc.2024.048762

Aldegheri, L., Cipullo, C., Rosso, N., Catamo, E., Casagranda, B., Giraudi, P., de Manzini, N., Palmisano, S., & Robino, A. (2025). Polygenic Score for Body Mass Index Is Associated with Weight Loss and Lipid Outcomes After Metabolic and Bariatric Surgery. *International Journal of Molecular Sciences*, *26*(15), 7337. Advance online publication. DOI: 10.3390/ijms26157337 PMID: 40806468

Alexopoulos, T. (2023). On global maritime oil piracy: An association rules analysis. *Preprint*. DOI: 10.21203/rs.3.rs-3289329/v1

Alghobiri, M. (2023). Exploring the attributes of influential users in social networks using association rule mining. *Preprint*. https://doi.org/DOI: 10.21203/rs.3.rs-3150435/v1

Al-Halhouli, A. A., Albagdady, A., Alawadi, J. F., & Abeeleh, M. A. (2021). Monitoring symptoms of infectious diseases: Perspectives for printed wearable sensors. *Micromachines*, *12*(6), 620. DOI: 10.3390/mi12060620 PMID: 34072174

Ali, A., Ali, H., Saeed, A., Ahmed Khan, A., Tin, T. T., Assam, M., Ghadi, Y. Y., & Mohamed, H. G. (2023). Blockchain-powered healthcare systems: Enhancing scalability and security with hybrid deep learning. *Sensors (Basel)*, *23*(18), 7740. DOI: 10.3390/s23187740 PMID: 37765797

Alici-Karaca, D., Akay, B., Yay, A., Suna, P., Nalbantoglu, O. U., Karaboga, D., Basturk, A., Balcioglu, E., & Baran, M. (2022). A new lightweight convolutional neural network for radiation-induced liver disease classification. *Biomedical Signal Processing and Control*, *73*, 103463. DOI: 10.1016/j.bspc.2021.103463

Al-Issa, Y., Ottom, M. A., & Tamrawi, A. (2019). eHealth cloud security challenges: A survey. *Journal of Healthcare Engineering*. Hindawi Limited. DOI: 10.1155/2019/7516035

Al-Mashhadi, S., Anbar, M., Karuppayah, S., & Al-Ani, A. K. (2021). Hybrid rule-based botnet detection approach using machine learning for analysing DNS traffic. *Journal of Network and Computer Applications*, *76*, 1–15. DOI: 10.1016/j.jnca.2016.10.007 PMID: 34458571

Alzubaidi, L., Zhang, J., Humaidi, A. J., Al-Dujaili, A., Duan, Y., Al-Shamma, O., … Farhan, L. (2021). *Review of deep learning: concepts, CNN architectures, challenges, applications, future directions. Journal of Big Data* (Vol. 8). Springer International Publishing. DOI: 10.1186/s40537-021-00444-8

Amin, A., Talib, R., Raza, S., & Javed, S. (2014). Extract association rules to minimize the effects of dengue by using a text mining technique. *International Journal of Computer Science and Mobile Computing*, *3*(4), 394–400.

Amorim, J. P., Abreu, P. H., Fernandez, A., Reyes, M., Santos, J., & Abreu, M. H. (2023). Interpreting deep machine learning models: An easy guide for oncologists. *IEEE Reviews in Biomedical Engineering*, *16*, 192–207. DOI: 10.1109/RBME.2021.3131358 PMID: 34847043

Anandhavalli, M., Ghose, M. K., & Gauthaman, K. (2010e). Mining frequent and associated gene expression patterns from spatial gene expression data: A proposed approach. In S. Ranka et al. (Eds.), *Contemporary computing: Third International Conference, IC3 2010* (pp. 119–130). Springer. https://doi.org/DOI: 10.1007/978-3-642-14834-7_12

Anandhavalli, M., & Ghose, M. K. (2008). Mining gene expression data for association rules using mutual information based on entropy. *International Journal of Information Technology and Knowledge Management*, *1*(2), 559–567.

Anandhavalli, M., Ghose, M. K., & Gauthaman, K. (2009). Mining spatial gene expression data using negative association rules. *International Journal of Computer Science and Information Security*, *6*(1), 117–120.

Anandhavalli, M., Ghose, M. K., & Gauthaman, K. (2010). Association rule mining in genomics. *International Journal of Computer Theory and Engineering*, *2*(2), 269–273. DOI: 10.7763/IJCTE.2010.V2.151

Anandhavalli, M., Ghose, M. K., & Gauthaman, K. (2010). Interestingness measure for mining spatial gene expression data using association rules. *Journal of Computing*, *2*(1), 110–114.

Anandhavalli, M., Ghose, M. K., & Gauthaman, K. (2010). Mining spatial gene expression data using association rules. *Malaysian International Journal of Computer Science and Security*, *3*(1), 351–357.

Anandhavalli, M., Ghose, M. K., & Gauthaman, K. (2010a). Analysis of associate genes of spatial gene expression data for association rules. *International Journal of Computer Applications in Engineering. Technology and Sciences*, 2(1), 473–477.

Anandhavalli, M., Ghose, M. K., & Gauthaman, K. (2010c). Interestingness measure for mining spatial gene expression data using association rule. *Journal of Computing*, *2*(1), 110–114. https://arxiv.org/ftp/arxiv/papers/1001/1001.3498.pdf

Anandhavalli, M., Sudhanshu, S. K., Kumar, A., & Ghose, M. K. (2009). Optimized association rule mining using genetic algorithm. *Journal of Advances in Information Mining*, *1*(1), 1–4. DOI: 10.9735/0975-3265

Angermueller, C.. (2016, July). Deep learning for computational biology. *Molecular Systems Biology*, •••, 29. PMID: 27474269

Angermueller, C.. (2017, April). Deepcpg: Accurate prediction of single-cell DNA methylation states using deep learning. *Genome Biology*.

Anuja, A., Ambikesh, J., Mayank, G., Prakhar, M., & Chandra, S. S. (2021). Brain tumor segmentation of MRI images using processed image driven U-net architecture. *Computers*, *10*(11), 1–39.

Apiletti, D., Baralis, E., Cerquitelli, T., & Chiusano, S. (2017). Frequent itemsets mining for big data: A comparative analysis. In *Big data research: Advances in theory and applications* (pp. 53–66). Springer International Publishing., DOI: 10.1016/j.bdr.2017.06.006

Arafa, A., Sheerah, H. A., & Alsalamah, S. (2023). Emerging digital technologies in healthcare with a spotlight on cybersecurity: A narrative review. *Information (Basel)*, *14*(12), 640. DOI: 10.3390/info14120640

Araujo, L., Martínez-Romo, J., Bisbal, O., Sanchez-de-Madariaga, R., Portilla, J., Portilla, I., Merino, E., García, G., Agea, I., Sánchez-Payá, J., Rodríguez, J. C., Giner, L., Reus, S., Boix, V., Torrus, D., Pérez, V., Portilla, J., Gómez, J. L., Hernández, J., & Telleria, P. (2022). Discovering HIV-related information by means of association rules and machine learning. *Scientific Reports*, *12*(1), 18208. DOI: 10.1038/s41598-022-22695-y PMID: 36307506

Arcieri, G., Hoelzl, C., Schwery, O., Straub, D., Papakonstantinou, K. G., & Chatzi, E. (2023). Bridging POMDPs and Bayesian decision making for robust maintenance planning under model uncertainty: An application to railway systems. *Reliability Engineering & System Safety*, *239*, 109496. DOI: 10.1016/j.ress.2023.109496

Arumuga, P. (2013). Association rule mining and medical application: A detailed survey. *International Journal of Computer Applications*, *80*(4), 10–19. DOI: 10.5120/13967-1698

Ayub, S., Singh, N., Hussain, M. Z., Ashraf, M., Singh, D. K., & Haldorai, A. (2021). Hybrid approach to implement multi-robotic navigation system using neural network, fuzzy logic and bio-inspired optimization methodologies. *Research Square*. DOI: 10.21203/rs.3.rs-975723/v1

Babanejaddehaki, G., An, A., & Papagelis, M. (2025). Disease outbreak detection and forecasting: A review of methods and data sources. *ACM Transactions on Computing for Healthcare*, *6*(2), 1–40. DOI: 10.1145/3708549

Badawy, M., Ramadan, N., & Hefny, H. A. (2023). Healthcare predictive analytics using machine learning and deep learning techniques: A survey. *Journal of Electrical Systems and Information Technology*, *10*(1), 40. DOI: 10.1186/s43067-023-00108-y

Badhon, B., Kabir, M., Xu, S., & Kabir, M. (2019). A survey on association rule mining based on evolutionary algorithms. *International Journal of Computers and Applications*, *43*(1), 1–11. DOI: 10.1080/1206212X.2019.1612993

Badiuzzaman Biplob, M., Khan, S. I., Sheraji, G. A., & Shuvo, J. A. (2020). Hybrid feature selection algorithm to support health data warehousing. In *Intelligent Computing Paradigm and Cutting-edge Technologies* (pp. 103–112). Springer., DOI: 10.1007/978-3-030-38501-9_10

Bakar, W. A. W. A., Man, M., Man, M., & Abdullah, Z. (2020). i-Eclat: Performance enhancement of Eclat via incremental approach in frequent itemset mining. *Telkomnika*, *18*(1), 562–570. DOI: 10.12928/telkomnika.v18i1.13497

Bansal, R., Rajput, N., & Khanna, M. (2025). Enhancing quantum support vector machine for healthcare applications using custom feature maps. *Knowledge-Based Systems*, *320*, 113669. DOI: 10.1016/j.knosys.2025.113669

Baowaly, M. K., & Reaz, M. B. I. (2018). Synthesizing electronic health records using improved Apriori algorithm. *Journal of Healthcare Engineering*, *2018*, 1–10. DOI: 10.1155/2018/7647178

Bao, X. (2025). Research on pose estimation algorithm for visual robot grasping target objects based on Unet-DGN-L2. *Applied and Computational Engineering*, *177*(1), 48–58. DOI: 10.54254/2755-2721/2025.BJ25397

Barredo Arrieta, A., Díaz-Rodríguez, N., Del Ser, J., Bennetot, A., Tabik, S., Barbado, A., Garcia, S., Gil-Lopez, S., Molina, D., Benjamins, R., Chatila, R., & Herrera, F. (2020). Explainable Artificial Intelligence (XAI): Concepts, taxonomies, opportunities and challenges toward responsible AI. *Information Fusion*, *58*, 82–115. DOI: 10.1016/j.inffus.2019.12.012

Baryakova, T. H., Pogostin, B. H., Langer, R., & McHugh, K. J. (2023). Overcoming barriers to patient adherence: The case for developing innovative drug delivery systems. *Nature Reviews. Drug Discovery*, *22*(5), 387–409. DOI: 10.1038/s41573-023-00670-0 PMID: 36973491

Bays, H. E., Agarwala, A., German, C., Satish, P., Iluyomade, A., Dudum, R., Thakkar, A., Rifai, M. A., Mehta, A., Thobani, A., Al-Saiegh, Y., Nelson, A. J., Sheth, S., & Toth, P. P. (2022). Ten things to know about ten cardiovascular disease risk factors–2022. *American Journal of Preventive Cardiology*, *10*, 100342. DOI: 10.1016/j.ajpc.2022.100342 PMID: 35517870

Beaufrère, A., Ouzir, N., Zafar, P. E., Laurent-Bellue, A., Albuquerque, M., Lubuela, G., Grégory, J., Guettier, C., Mondet, K., Pesquet, J. C., & Paradis, V. (2024). Primary liver cancer classification from routine tumor biopsy using weakly supervised deep learning. *JHEP Reports : Innovation in Hepatology*, *6*(3), 101008. Advance online publication. DOI: 10.1016/j.jhepr.2024.101008 PMID: 38379584

Bélair, J., Glass, L., an der Heiden, U., & Milton, J. (1995). Dynamical disease: Identification, temporal aspects and treatment strategies of human illness. *Chaos (Woodbury, N.Y.)*, *5*(1), 1–7. DOI: 10.1063/1.166069 PMID: 12780147

Bellazzi, R., & Zupan, B. (2008). Predictive data mining in clinical medicine: Current issues and guidelines. *International Journal of Medical Informatics*, *77*(2), 81–97. DOI: 10.1016/j.ijmedinf.2006.11.006 PMID: 17188928

Benjamens, S., Dhunnoo, P., & Meskó, B. (2020). The state of artificial intelligence-based FDA-approved medical devices and algorithms: An online database. *NPJ Digital Medicine*, *3*(1), 118. Advance online publication. DOI: 10.1038/s41746-020-00324-0 PMID: 32984550

Bhujade, V., Janwe, N. J., & Meshram, C. (2011). Discriminative Features Selection in Text Mining Using TF-IDF Scheme. *[IJCTT]. International Journal of Computer Trends and Technology*, *1*(3), 277–280.

Bicaku, A., Zsilak, M., Theiler, P., Tauber, M., & Delsing, J. (2022). Security standard compliance verification in system of systems. *IEEE Systems Journal*, *16*(2), 2195–2205. DOI: 10.1109/JSYST.2021.3064196

Bobba, J., Ayyadurai, R., Parthasarathy, K., Panga, N. K. R., Bolla, R. L., & Ogundokun, R. O. (2023). AI-infused spiking neural architectures and edge computing modalities: Recalibrating pandemic surveillance, dynamic health interpretations, and contextual automations in complex urban terrains. *International Journal of Information Technology and Computer Engineering*, *11*(2), 60–74.

Borah, A., & Nath, B. (2020). Comparative evaluation of pattern mining techniques: An empirical study. *Complex & Intelligent Systems*, *6*(4), 857–868. DOI: 10.1007/s40747-020-00226-4

Brahme, A., Kulkarni, S., & Kulkarni, M. (2022). To Devise and Implement Effective Stemming Algorithm for Text Mining and NLP for Healthcare Management. *JOURNAL OF MANAGEMENT & ENTREPRENEURSHIP*, 163

Brahme, A. (2025). Association rule mining and information retrieval using stemming and text mining techniques. *Journal of Information Systems Engineering & Management*, *10*(18s).

Briceno, O. (2022). Semi-supervised incremental learning with few examples for medical monitoring (discussing association rules as pattern representation). *BMC Medical Informatics and Decision Making*. Advance online publication. DOI: 10.1186/s12911-022-01755-3

Brossette, S. E., Sprague, A. P., Hardin, J. M., Waites, K. B., Jones, W. T., & Moser, S. A. (1998). Association rules and data mining in hospital infection control and public health surveillance. *Journal of the American Medical Informatics Association : JAMIA*, *5*(4), 373–381. DOI: 10.1136/jamia.1998.0050373 PMID: 9670134

Cao, B., Zang, X., Zhang, X., Chen, Z., Li, S., & Zhao, J. (2024). Shape control of elastic deformable linear objects for robotic cable assembly. *Advanced Intelligent Systems (Weinheim an Der Bergstrasse, Germany), 6*(7). DOI: 10.1002/aisy.202300835

Cao, J.. (2020). Temporal association rule mining: An overview considering time variable as integral component. *Wiley Interdisciplinary Reviews. Data Mining and Knowledge Discovery, 10*(4), e1367. Advance online publication. DOI: 10.1002/widm.1367

Cao, Y., Xu, L., Liu, Z., Xiao, X., Wang, M., Li, Q., Xu, H., & Yang, G. (2022). BM-RMIA: A platform for radiologists to systematically learn automated medical image analysis by three dimensional medical decision support system. *Computer Modeling in Engineering & Sciences, 131*(2), 851–863. DOI: 10.32604/cmes.2022.018424

Casanova, I. J., Campos, M., Juárez, J. M., Gomariz, A., Canovas-Segura, B., Lorente-Ros, M., & Lorente, J. A. (2024). Surprising and novel multivariate sequential patterns using odds ratio for temporal evolution in healthcare. *BMC Medical Informatics and Decision Making, 24*(1), 165. DOI: 10.1186/s12911-024-02566-4 PMID: 38872146

Catalano, M., Lijoi, A., Prünster, I., & Rigon, T. (2023). Bayesian modeling via discrete nonparametric priors. *Japanese Journal of Statistics and Data Science, 6*(2), 607–624. DOI: 10.1007/s42081-023-00210-5

Chandio, S. A., Rehman, A. U., Bano, S., Hammed, A., & Hussain, A. (2024). Enhancing trust in healthcare: The role of AI explainability and professional familiarity. *The Asian Bulletin of Big Data Management, 4*(1). Advance online publication. DOI: 10.62019/abbdm.v4i1.100

Chandrasekar, V., Sureshkumar, V., Kumar, T. S., & Shanmugapriya, S. (2020, September). Disease Prediction Based On Micro Array Classification Using Deep Learning Techniques. *Microprocessors and Microsystems, 77*, 103189. DOI: 10.1016/j.micpro.2020.103189

Chaput, R., Duval, J., Boissier, O., Guillermin, M., & Hassas, S. (2021). A multi-agent approach to combine reasoning and learning for an ethical behavior. In *Proceedings of the AAAI/ACM Conference on AI, Ethics, and Society* (pp. 13–23). ACM. DOI: 10.1145/3461702.3462515

Charan, J. K., Chandra, S., Vaissnave, V., Ragupathi, T., Satyanarayana, P., & Manjunath, T. C. (2025). Impact of Generative AI on Industries and Organizations. In Zhao, J., Kumar, V., Katina, P., & Richards, J. (Eds.), *Humans and Generative AI Tools for Collaborative Intelligence* (pp. 509–528). IGI Global Scientific Publishing., DOI: 10.4018/979-8-3693-8332-2.ch022

Chen, C., Zheng, X., Liao, S., Chen, S., Liang, M., Tang, K., Yin, M., Liu, H., & Ni, J. (2024). The diabetes mellitus multimorbidity network in hospitalized patients over 50 years of age in China: Data mining of medical records. *BMC Public Health, 24*(1), 1433. DOI: 10.1186/s12889-024-18887-y PMID: 38811975

Cheng, L., Shi, Y., Yu, X., Li, X., Wang, X., Yan, Z., & Chen, Z. (2026). MGF-Net: Multi-granularity medical pattern fusion network for patient risk prediction. *Pattern Recognition, 172*, 112302. Advance online publication. DOI: 10.1016/j.patcog.2025.112302

Chen, M., Hao, Y., Hwang, K., Wang, L., & Wang, L. (2020). Disease prediction by machine learning over big data from healthcare communities. *IEEE Access : Practical Innovations, Open Solutions, 5*, 8869–8879. DOI: 10.1109/ACCESS.2017.2694446

Chen, S., & Guo, W. (2023). Auto-encoders in deep learning—A review with new perspectives. *Mathematics, 11*(8), 1777. DOI: 10.3390/math11081777

Chen, T.-Y. (2026). An enhanced QUALIFLEX decision-making framework incorporating power-form scoring mechanisms within a circular intuitionistic fuzzy paradigm. *Advanced Engineering Informatics, 69*, 103815. Advance online publication. DOI: 10.1016/j.aei.2025.103815

Chen, Y., Ling, M., Liu, Y., Chen, X., Li, Y., & Tong, B. (2024). Enhancing MRI image retrieval using autoencoder-based deep learning: A solution for efficient clinical and teaching applications. *Journal of Radiation Research and Applied Sciences, 17*(3), 100932. DOI: 10.1016/j.jrras.2024.100932

Chernoff, M. C., Wang, M., Anderson, J. J., & Felson, D. T. (1995). Problems and suggested solutions in creating an archive of clinical trials data…. *Controlled Clinical Trials, 16*(5), 342–355. DOI: 10.1016/0197-2456(95)00049-6 PMID: 8582152

Chobtham, K., Constantinou, A. C., & Kitson, N. K. (2023). Hybrid Bayesian network discovery with latent variables by scoring multiple interventions. *Data Mining and Knowledge Discovery, 37*(1), 476–520. DOI: 10.1007/s10618-022-00882-9

Choudhary, G. I., & Fränti, P. (2023). Predicting onset of disease progression using temporal disease occurrence networks. *International Journal of Medical Informatics, 175*, 105068. DOI: 10.1016/j.ijmedinf.2023.105068 PMID: 37104895

Cipollone, R., & Giacomo, G. (2025). Application of reinforcement education with prize shaping to overcome restricted rationality limitations. *SciSpace Literature Review*. https://scispace.com

Condori, H., Cruz, J., & Machaca, W. (2021). ResNet neural network hyperparameter tuning for rigid pavement failure assessment. *Proceedings of SACI 2021*, 317–322. DOI: 10.1109/SACI51354.2021.9465547

Cui, J., Zhao, S., & Sun, X. (2022). An association rule mining algorithm for clinical decision support. In *Proceedings of the 8th International Conference on Computing and Artificial Intelligence (ICCAI '22)* (pp. 137–143). Association for Computing Machinery. DOI: 10.1145/3532213.3532234

Dado, T., Le, L., Van Gerven, M., Güçlütürk, Y., & Güçlü, U. (2024). PAM: Predictive attention mechanism for neural decoding of visual perception. *bioRxiv*. DOI: 10.1101/2024.06.04.596589

Dai, L., Xu, H., & Zhang, Y. (2025). Automated classification of clinical diagnoses in electronic health records using transformer. *PLoS One*, *20*(9), e0329963. DOI: 10.1371/journal.pone.0329963 PMID: 40934268

Dao, C.-T., Phan, N. M. T., Ding, J.-E., Wu, C., Restrepo, D., Luo, D., Zhao, F., Liao, C.-C., Peng, W.-C., Wang, C.-T., Chen, P.-F., Chen, L., Ju, X., Liu, F., & Hung, F.-M. (2026). CURENet: Combining unified representations for efficient chronic disease prediction. *Health Information Science and Systems*, *14*(1), 7. Advance online publication. DOI: 10.1007/s13755-025-00396-w PMID: 41323159

Darrab, S., Broneske, D., & Saake, G. (2024). Exploring the predictive factors of heart disease using rare association rule mining. *Scientific Reports*, *14*(1), 18178. DOI: 10.1038/s41598-024-69071-6 PMID: 39107391

Das, A., Das, P., Panda, S. S., & Sabut, S. (2019). Detection of liver cancer using modified fuzzy clustering and decision tree classifier in CT images. *Pattern Recognition and Image Analysis*, *29*(2), 201–211. DOI: 10.1134/S1054661819020056

David, J. (2007). Association rule ontology matching approach. *International Journal on Semantic Web and Information Systems*, *3*(2), 27–49. DOI: 10.4018/jswis.2007040102

Di Bonito, L. P., Campanile, L., Iacono, M., & Di Natale, F. (2025). An eXplainable Artificial Intelligence framework to predict marine scrubbers performances. *Engineering Applications of Artificial Intelligence*, *160*, 111860. Advance online publication. DOI: 10.1016/j.engappai.2025.111860

Di Martino, F., & Delmastro, F. (2023). Explainable AI for clinical and remote health applications: A survey on tabular and time series data. *Artificial Intelligence Review*, *56*(6), 5261–5315. DOI: 10.1007/s10462-022-10304-3 PMID: 36320613

Diallo, A., Camara, F., Camara, G., & Sarr, M. (2024, December). Association Rule Mining-based Analysis of Clinical Manifestations of SARS-Cov-2 (COVID-19) Coronavirus Infection in Senegal. In *Proceedings of the 2024 5th International Conference on Intelligent Medicine and Health* (pp. 54-59).

Dickerson, J. E., & Dickerson, J. A. (2000). Fuzzy network profiling for intrusion detection. In *Proceedings of the 19th International Conference of the North American Fuzzy Information Processing Society* (pp. 301–306). IEEE. DOI: 10.1109/NAFIPS.2000.877441

Dimitsaki, S., Natsiavas, P., & Jaulent, M.-C. (2024). Causal Deep learning for the detection of adverse drug reactions: Drug-induced acute kidney injury as a case study. *Studies in Health Technology and Informatics, 316*, 803–807. DOI: 10.3233/SHTI240533 PMID: 39176914

Dixit, S., Kumar, A., & Srinivasan, K. (2023). A current review of machine learning and deep learning models in oral cancer diagnosis: Recent technologies, open challenges, and future research directions. *Diagnostics (Basel), 13*(7), 1353. DOI: 10.3390/diagnostics13071353 PMID: 37046571

Domadiya, N., & Rao, U. P. (2022). ElGamal homomorphic encryption-based privacy preserving association rule mining on horizontally partitioned healthcare data. *Journal of The Institution of Engineers (India) Series B, 103*(3), 817–830. DOI: 10.1007/s40031-021-00696-1

Domadiya, N., & Rao, U. P. (2022). ElGamal homomorphic encryption–based privacy-preserving association rule mining on horizontally partitioned healthcare data. *Journal of the Institution of Engineers (India): Series B, 103*(3), 817–830.

Domadiya, N., & Rao, U. P. (2021). Privacy preserving association rule mining on distributed healthcare data: COVID-19 and Breast Cancer case study. *SN Computer Science*, 2(6), 418. DOI: 10.1007/s42979-021-00801-7 PMID: 34423316

Dong, X., Zhou, Y., Wang, L., Peng, J., Lou, Y., & Fan, Y. (2020). Liver cancer detection using hybridized fully convolutional neural network based on deep learning framework. *IEEE Access : Practical Innovations, Open Solutions, 8*, 129889–129898. DOI: 10.1109/ACCESS.2020.3006362

Ehrenstein, V., Kharrazi, H., Lehmann, H., & Taylor, C. O. (2019). *Obtaining data from electronic health records....* AHRQ.

El-Sappagh, S. H., El-Masri, S., Riad, A. E.-D., & Elmogy, M. (2013). Data mining and knowledge discovery: Applications, techniques, challenges and process models in healthcare. [IJERA]. *International Journal of Engineering Research and Applications, 3*(3), 900–906.

Elwahsh, H., Tawfeek, M. A., Abd El-Aziz, A. A., Mahmood, M. A., Alsabaan, M., & El-shafeiy, E. (2023). A new approach for cancer prediction based on deep neural learning. *Journal of King Saud University. Computer and Information Sciences, 35*(6), 101565. DOI: 10.1016/j.jksuci.2023.101565

Fan, L., & Zhang, H. (2025). *AIPatient KG: MIMIC-III and CORAL electronic health records*. PhysioNet., DOI: 10.1155/2025/2501.09640

Fayyad, U., Piatetsky-Shapiro, G., & Smyth, P. (1996). From data mining to knowledge discovery in databases. *AI Magazine, 17*(3), 37–37.

Gaitsch, H., Franklin, R. J., & Reich, D. S. (2023). Cell-free DNA-based liquid biopsies in neurology. *Brain, 146*(5), 1758–1774. DOI: 10.1093/brain/awac438 PMID: 36408894

Gauthaman, S. A., Kumar, S. S., Kamaldheen, R., Murugesan, K., Viswanathan, M. K., Devendran, H., & Muniasamy, A. (2026). Current challenges in the pharmaceutical industry and AI's role in addressing them. In Muniasamy, A., & Karunakaran, G. (Eds.), *Applications of artificial intelligence in pharmaceuticals* (pp. 1–26). IGI Global Scientific Publishing., DOI: 10.4018/979-8-3373-2043-4.ch001

Geng, L., & Hamilton, H. J. (2006). Interestingness measures for data mining: A survey. *ACM Computing Surveys, 38*(3), 9. Advance online publication. DOI: 10.1145/1132960.1132963

Geng, X., Yang, Z., Jiao, L., Zhou, Z.-J., & Ma, Z. (2025). Association rule-based classification: A comprehensive review of methodologies and applications. *Expert Systems with Applications, 280*, 127454. DOI: 10.1016/j.eswa.2025.127454

Ghahramani, A., Prokofieva, M., & de Courten, M. P. (2025). Health promotion campaigns using social media: Association rules mining and co-occurrence network analysis of Twitter hashtags. *BMC Public Health, 25*(1), 67. Advance online publication. DOI: 10.1186/s12889-024-21255-5 PMID: 39773431

Glukhikh, I., & Glukhikh, D. (2021). Case-based reasoning with an artificial neural network for decision support in situations at complex technological objects of urban infrastructure. *Applied System Innovation, 4*(4), 73. Advance online publication. DOI: 10.3390/asi4040073

Gong, P., Cheng, L., Zhang, Z., Meng, A., Li, E., Chen, J., & Zhang, L. (2023). Multi-omics integration method based on attention deep learning network for biomedical data classification. *Computer Methods and Programs in Biomedicine, 231*, 107377. DOI: 10.1016/j.cmpb.2023.107377 PMID: 36739624

Gonzalez, C. (2024). Building human-like artificial agents: A general cognitive algorithm for emulating human decision-making in dynamic environments. *Perspectives on Psychological Science, 19*(5), 860–873. DOI: 10.1177/17456916231196766 PMID: 37906108

Gulzar, K., & Khan, M. A. (2023). An efficient healthcare data mining approach using Apriori algorithm. *Journal of Healthcare Engineering, 2023*, 1–10. DOI: 10.1155/2023/20782489

Gunasekaran, H., Ramalakshmi, K., Rex Macedo Arokiaraj, A., Deepa Kanmani, S., Venkatesan, C., & Suresh Gnana Dhas, C. (2021). Analysis of DNA sequence classification using CNN and hybrid models. *Computational and Mathematical Methods in Medicine, 2021*(1), 1835056.

Gupta, M., Gallamoza, B., Cutrona, N., & Sun, J. (2022). An extensive data processing pipeline for MIMIC-IV. *Proceedings of Machine Learning Research, 193*, 311–325. https://proceedings.mlr.press/v193/gupta22a.html

Guru Basava Aradhya, S., Chithambar Gupta, V., Raman, M. S., Singh, J., Manjunath, T. C., & Sharma, M. (2025). Health Crises and Digitalization: Digital Health. In Yıldırım, D., Yıldırım, S., & Kandpal, V. (Eds.), *Sustainable Digitalization Strategies in Business and Healthcare* (pp. 171–198). IGI Global Scientific Publishing., DOI: 10.4018/979-8-3373-5087-5.ch007

Gurusamy, V., Muniasamy, A., Gauthaman, S. A., & Abdulla, H. (2026). Human–AI collaboration in healthcare: The evolving role of healthcare professionals. In Muniasamy, A. M., Chakkaravarthy, P., & Dhas, D. J. (Eds.), *Evaluation and assessment of AI-driven systems in hospitals* (pp. 341–364). IGI Global Scientific Publishing., DOI: 10.4018/979-8-3373-2787-7.ch012

Hagendorff, T., & Danks, D. (2023). Ethical and methodological challenges in building morally informed AI systems. *AI and Ethics, 3*(2), 553–566. DOI: 10.1007/s43681-022-00188-y

Hahsler, M., Hornik, K., & Reutterer, T. (2008). Implications of probabilistic data modeling for mining association rules. *Journal of Machine Learning Research, 9*, 1–37.

Hamid, Z., Khalique, F., Mahmood, S., Daud, A., Bukhari, A., & Alshemaimri, B. (2024a). Healthcare insurance fraud detection using data mining. *BMC Medical Informatics and Decision Making*, *24*(1), 112. DOI: 10.1186/s12911-024-02512-4 PMID: 38671513

Han, J., Pei, J., & Yin, Y. (2000). Mining frequent patterns without candidate generation. *Proceedings of the 2000 ACM SIGMOD International Conference on Management of Data* (pp. 1–12). DOI: 10.1145/335191.335372

Haq, E. U., Jianjun, H., Li, K., Haq, H. U., & Zhang, T. (2023). An MRI-based deep learning approach for efficient classification of brain tumors. *Journal of Ambient Intelligence and Humanized Computing*, *14*(6), 6697–6718. DOI: 10.1007/s12652-021-03535-9

Harb, H., Alobaidi, A., & El-Bakry, H. (2020). A Hadoop-Based Platform for Patient Classification and Real-Time Monitoring. *Sensors (Basel)*, *20*(7), 1931. DOI: 10.3390/s20071931 PMID: 32235657

Haryanto, H., Winarto, H., & Juliane, C. (2024). Application of data mining techniques in healthcare: Identifying inter-disease relationships through Association Rule Mining. *Journal of Wood Science*, *3*(5), 520–529. DOI: 10.58344/jws.v3i5.597

Haug, P. J., Gardner, R. M., Tate, K. E., Evans, R. S., East, T. D., Kuperman, G., Pryor, T. A., Huff, S. M., & Warner, H. R. (1994). Decision support in medicine: Examples from the HELP system. *Computers and Biomedical Research, an International Journal*, *27*(5), 396–418. DOI: 10.1006/cbmr.1994.1030 PMID: 7813202

He, G., Bharos, A., & Gadiraju, U. (2024). To err is AI! Debugging as an intervention to facilitate appropriate reliance on AI systems. In *Proceedings of the ACM Conference on Human Factors in Computing Systems*. DOI: 10.1145/3648188.3675130

Hossain, M., Devnath, A., & Karmokar, P. (2023). *Handling Missing Values and Outliers....* Diabetes Classification Accuracy.

Hossain, P. S., Kim, K., Uddin, J., Samad, M. A., & Choi, K. (2023). Enhancing Taxonomic Categorization of DNA Sequences with Deep Learning: A Multi-Label Approach. *Bioengineering (Basel, Switzerland)*, *10*(11), 1293. DOI: 10.3390/bioengineering10111293 PMID: 38002417

Hripcsak, G., & Albers, D. J. (2013). Next-generation phenotyping of electronic health records. *Journal of the American Medical Informatics Association : JAMIA*, *20*(1), 117–121. DOI: 10.1136/amiajnl-2012-001145 PMID: 22955496

Hripcsak, G., Albers, D. J., Perotte, A., & Correll, M. (2015). Health data use and privacy: Contextual integrity, transparency, and public trust. *Journal of the American Medical Informatics Association : JAMIA*, *22*(1), 36–43.

Huang, Z., Li, Y., Bucci, V., & Haran, J. P. (2025). Decoding cancer prognosis with deep learning: The ASD-cancer framework for tumor microenvironment analysis. *mSystems*, *10*(5), e0145524. DOI: 10.1128/msystems.01455-24 PMID: 40237527

Hunyadi, I. D., Constantinescu, N., & icleanu, O.-A. (2025). Efficient Discovery of Association Rules in E-Commerce: Comparing Candidate Generation and Pattern Growth Techniques. *Applied Sciences (Basel, Switzerland)*, *15*(10), 5498. DOI: 10.3390/app15105498

Hu, Y.. (2018). Fuzzy association rules for medical decision support. *Applied Soft Computing*, *69*, 397–408.

Ibrahim, N., Akhir, N. S. M., & Hassan, F. H. (2017, October). Predictive analysis effectiveness in determining the epidemic disease infected area. In AIP conference proceedings (Vol. 1891, No. 1, p. 020064). AIP Publishing LLC. DOI: 10.1063/1.5005397

Iqbal, A. M., & Jamal, S. F. (2023). *Essential hypertension. StatPearls*. StatPearls Publishing.

Islam, A., Mridha, M. F., & Jahin, A. (2024). A unified framework for evaluating the effectiveness and enhancing the transparency of explainable AI methods in real-world applications. *Manuscript in preparation*.

Jensen, P. B., Jensen, L. J., & Brunak, S. (2012). Mining electronic health records: Towards better research applications and clinical care. *Nature Reviews. Genetics*, *13*(6), 395–405. DOI: 10.1038/nrg3208 PMID: 22549152

Jeyaraman, N., Jeyaraman, M., Yadav, S., Ramasubramanian, S., & Balaji, S. (2024). Revolutionizing healthcare: The emerging role of quantum computing in enhancing medical technology and treatment. *Cureus*, *16*(8), e67486. DOI: 10.7759/cureus.67486 PMID: 39310567

Jiang, S., Cheng, Z., Yang, L., & Shen, L. (2023). An auto-tuned hybrid deep learning approach for predicting fracture evolution. *Engineering with Computers*, *39*(5), 3353–3370. DOI: 10.1007/s00366-022-01756-w

Jiang, X., Hu, Z., Wang, S., & Zhang, Y. (2023). Deep learning for medical image-based cancer diagnosis. *Cancers (Basel)*, *15*(14), 3608. DOI: 10.3390/cancers15143608 PMID: 37509272

Jiang, X., Sun, Q., Wang, C., Li, W., Chen, W., Xu, J., & Yu, L. (2025). CT-based radiomics and deep learning to predict EGFR mutation status in lung adenocarcinoma. *Frontiers in Oncology, 15*(1597548), 1597548. DOI: 10.3389/fonc.2025.1597548 PMID: 41114339

Jin, R., & Li, X. (2023). Backdoor attack and defense in federated generative adversarial network-based medical image synthesis. *Medical Image Analysis, 90*, 102965. Advance online publication. DOI: 10.1016/j.media.2023.102965 PMID: 37804585

Ji, S., Li, X., Sun, W., Dong, H., Taalas, A., Zhang, Y., Wu, H., Pitkänen, E., & Marttinen, P. (2024). A unified review of deep learning for automated medical coding. *ACM Computing Surveys, 56*(12), 306. Advance online publication. DOI: 10.1145/3664615

Jyothi, P., & Ajitha, P. (2021, December). Computerized Prediction of Hereditary Diseases Through DNA Sequence Using Support Vector Machine (SVM). In 2021 5th International Conference on Electronics, Communication and Aerospace Technology (ICECA) (pp. 953-958). IEEE.

Jyotsna, & Reddy, P. K. (2021). An experimental approach for discovering frequent patterns. *International Journal of Circuit, Computing and Networking, 2*(1), 30–33. DOI: 10.33545/27075923.2021.v2.i1a.24

Kang'ethe, S. M. (2014). Discovering medical diagnosis patterns… (Doctoral dissertation).

Karabulut, E., Degeler, V., & Groth, P. (2024). *AE SemRL: Learning semantic association rules with autoencoders*. arXiv. https://arxiv.org/abs/2403.18133

Karim, S. A., Mohamad, U. H., & Nohuddin, P. N. E. (2025). Discovery of Interpretable Patterns of Breast Cancer Diagnosis via Class Association Rule Mining (CARM) With SHAP-Based Explainable AI (XAI). *Malaysian Journal of Fundamental and Applied Sciences, 21*(3), 2008–2031. DOI: 10.11113/mjfas.v21n3.3792

Kariotis, T. C., Prictor, M., Chang, S., & Gray, K. (2022). Impact of electronic health records on information practices in mental health contexts: Scoping review. *Journal of Medical Internet Research, 24*(5), e30405. DOI: 10.2196/30405 PMID: 35507393

Kaul, D., Raju, H., & Tripathy, B. K. (2022). Deep learning in healthcare. In D. P. Acharjya, A. Mitra, & N. Zaman (Eds.), *Deep learning in data analytics* (Studies in Big Data, Vol. 91). Springer. DOI: 10.1007/978-3-030-75855-4_6

Kaur, J., & Madan, N. (2015). Association rule mining: A survey. *International Journal of Hybrid Information Technology, 8*(7), 239–242. DOI: 10.14257/ijhit.2015.8.7.22

Kavitha, S., & Kannan, A. (2016). Mining association rules in medical data for disease prediction. *International Journal of Computer Applications*, *140*(7), 15–20.

Kazimierczak, N., Kazimierczak, W., Serafin, Z., Nowicki, P., Nożewski, J., & Janiszewska-Olszowska, J. (2024). AI in orthodontics: Revolutionizing diagnostics and treatment planning—A comprehensive review. *Journal of Clinical Medicine*, *13*(2), 344. DOI: 10.3390/jcm13020344 PMID: 38256478

Ker, J., Wang, L., Rao, J., & Lim, T. (2017). Deep learning applications in medical image analysis. *IEEE Access : Practical Innovations, Open Solutions*, *6*, 9375–9389.

Khan, S., & Parkinson, S. (2018). Eliciting and utilising knowledge for security event log analysis: An association rule mining and automated planning approach. *Expert Systems with Applications*, *113*, 20–33. DOI: 10.1016/j.eswa.2018.07.006

Kheirollahi, H. (2022). A new method of well clustering and association rule mining. *Expert Systems with Applications*, *191*, 116281. DOI: 10.1016/j.eswa.2021.116281

Khotina, V. A., Vinokurov, A. Y., Bagheri Ekta, M., Sukhorukov, V. N., & Orekhov, A. N. (2023). Creation of mitochondrial disease models using mitochondrial DNA editing. *Biomedicines*, *11*(2), 532. DOI: 10.3390/biomedicines11020532 PMID: 36831068

Kim, H., Kim, J. H., Lee, S. W., Kim, S. J., Han, K. S., Lee, S., Song, J., & Lee, H. K. (2026). Safety-aware explainable deep reinforcement learning for nephrotoxic medication management in critical care. *Biomedical Signal Processing and Control*, *112*, 108577. Advance online publication. DOI: 10.1016/j.bspc.2025.108577

Kim, S. Y., Kim, D. H., Kim, M. J., Kim, K., & Kang, J. (2024). XAI-based clinical decision support systems: A systematic review. *Journal of Healthcare Engineering*, *2024*, 1–16.

Koh, H. C., & Tan, G. (2011). Data mining applications in healthcare. *Journal of Healthcare Information Management*, *19*(2), 64–72. PMID: 15869215

Koparde, S. A., Jha, R. P., Deepthi Reddy, K., Kuchipudi, J. D., Manjunath, T. C., & Sharma, M. (2026). Generative AI in Predicting and Preventing Foodborne Illnesses. In Madaan, G., Singh, A., Chahal, B., David, A., & Singh, G. (Eds.), *Generative AI in Food Systems: Predictive Demand, Smart Supply Chains, and Sustainable Service Futures* (pp. 205–232). IGI Global Scientific Publishing., DOI: 10.4018/979-8-3373-5182-7.ch010

Korteling, J. E., van de Boer-Visschedijk, G. C., Blankendaal, R. A. M., Boonekamp, R. C., & Eikelboom, A. R. (2021). Human- versus artificial intelligence. *Frontiers in Artificial Intelligence*, *4*, 622364. DOI: 10.3389/frai.2021.622364 PMID: 33981990

Kost, R.. (2012). Exploring generalized association rule mining for disease co-occurrence discovery from ICD codes. Journal / BMC. *Medical Informatics*. Advance online publication. DOI: 10.1186/1472-6947-12-50

Kouter, K., Arčan, I. Š., & Paska, A. V. (2023). Epigenetics in psychiatry: Beyond DNA methylation. *World Journal of Psychiatry*, *13*(6), 319–330. DOI: 10.5498/wjp.v13.i6.319 PMID: 37383287

Krolevets, M., Cate, V. T., Prochaska, J. H., Schulz, A., Rapp, S., Tenzer, S., Andrade-Navarro, M. A., Horvath, S., Niehrs, C., & Wild, P. S. (2023). DNA methylation and cardiovascular disease in humans: A systematic review and database of known CpG methylation sites. *Clinical Epigenetics*, *15*(1), 56. DOI: 10.1186/s13148-023-01468-y PMID: 36991458

Kulkarni, A., & Mundhe, S. (2016). A theoretical review on text mining: Tools, techniques, applications and future challenges. *International Journal of Innovative Research in Computer and Communication Engineering*, *4*(11), 19225–19230.

Kulkarni, A., & Mundhe, S. (2017). Data mining technique: An implementation of association rule mining in healthcare. *International Advanced Research Journal in Science. Engineering and Technology*, *4*(7), 62–65.

Kumar, R. M. R., & Joghee, S. (2025). A Review on Integrating Breast Cancer Clinical Data. *Current Treatment Options in Oncology*, *26*(1), 1–13. DOI: 10.1007/s11864-024-01285-2 PMID: 39752094

Lakshmipriya, B., Pottakkat, B., & Ramkumar, G. (2023). Deep learning techniques in liver tumour diagnosis using CT and MR imaging – A systematic review. *Artificial Intelligence in Medicine*, *141*, 102557. DOI: 10.1016/j.artmed.2023.102557 PMID: 37295904

Latif, J., Xiao, C., Tu, S., Rehman, S. U., Imran, A., & Bilal, A. (2020). Implementation and use of disease diagnosis systems for electronic medical records based on machine learning: A complete review. *IEEE Access : Practical Innovations, Open Solutions*, *8*, 150489–150513. DOI: 10.1109/ACCESS.2020.3016782

Lau, J. M., Iochpe, C., Thom, L. H., & Reichert, M. (2009). *Discovery and analysis of activity pattern co-occurrences....* ICEIS.

Lee, C. H., & Yoon, H. J. (2017). Medical big data: Promise and challenges. *Kidney Research and Clinical Practice*, *36*(1), 3–11. DOI: 10.23876/j.krcp.2017.36.1.3 PMID: 28392994

Lello, L.. (2019, November). Genomic Prediction of 16 Complex Disease Risks Including Heart Attack, Diabetes, Breast and Prostate Cancer. *Scientific Reports*.

Lessanibahri, S., Gastaldi, L., & González, C. (2019). A novel pruning algorithm for mining long and maximum length frequent itemsets. *Expert Systems with Applications, 142*, 113004. DOI: 10.1016/j.eswa.2019.113004

Li, H., & Sheu, P. C. Y. (2022). A scalable association rule learning and recommendation algorithm for large-scale microarray datasets. *Journal of Biomedical Informatics, 133*, 104169.

Li, J., Chiu, T. P., & Rohs, R. (2024). Predicting DNA structure using a deep learning method. *Nature Communications, 15*(1), 1243. DOI: 10.1038/s41467-024-45191-5 PMID: 38336958

Li, M., Lv, X., Liu, Y., Wang, L., & Song, J. (2022). TCM constitution analysis method based on parallel FP-Growth algorithm in Hadoop framework. *Journal of Healthcare Engineering, 2022*, 9006096. DOI: 10.1155/2022/9006096 PMID: 36081755

Li, S., Zeng, W., Ni, X., Liu, Q., Li, W., Stackpole, M. L., Zhou, Y., Gower, A., Krysan, K., Ahuja, P., Lu, D. S., Raman, S. S., Hsu, W., Aberle, D. R., Magyar, C. E., French, S. W., Han, S.-H. B., Garon, E. B., Agopian, V. G., & Zhou, X. J. (2023). Comprehensive tissue deconvolution of cell-free DNA by deep learning for disease diagnosis and monitoring. *Proceedings of the National Academy of Sciences of the United States of America, 120*(28), e2305236120. DOI: 10.1073/pnas.2305236120 PMID: 37399400

Li, T., Liu, F., Chen, X., & Ma, C. (2024). Web log mining techniques to optimize Apriori association rule algorithm in sports data information management. *Scientific Reports, 14*(1), 24099. DOI: 10.1038/s41598-024-74427-z PMID: 39406842

Liu, B., Ma, Y., & Wong, C.-K. (2000). Classification using association rules: Weaknesses and enhancements. *Data Mining for Scientific and Engineering Applications*, 591–605.

Liu, L., Wang, X., Gui, M., Ju, F., Cao, L., & Bi, B. (2025). Investigation of multimorbidity patterns…. *Scientific Reports, 15*(1), 25741. DOI: 10.1038/s41598-025-09926-8 PMID: 40670483

Liu, Y., Chen, P. H., Krause, J., & Peng, L. (2019). How to read articles that use machine learning: Users' guides to the medical literature. *Journal of the American Medical Association, 322*(18), 1806–1816. DOI: 10.1001/jama.2019.16489 PMID: 31714992

Li, W., Han, J., & Pei, J. (2001). CMAR: Accurate and efficient classification based on multiple class-association rules. *Proceedings of the 2001 IEEE International Conference on Data Mining*, 369–376.

Li, X., & Khishe, M. (2023). Evolving deep gated recurrent unit using improved marine predator algorithm for profit prediction based on financial accounting information system. *Complex & Intelligent Systems*. Advance online publication. DOI: 10.1007/s40747-023-01183-4

Lopez-Terrada, D., Alaggio, R., Da'vila, M. T., Czauderna, P., Hiyama, E., Katzenstein, H., Leuschner, I., Malogolowkin, M., Meyers, R., Ranganathan, S., Tanaka, Y., Tomlinson, G., Fabre', M., Zimmermann, A., & Finegold, M. J. (2014). Towards an international pediatric liver tumor consensus classification. *Modern Pathology*, *27*(3), 472–491. DOI: 10.1038/modpathol.2013.80 PMID: 24008558

Lyu, G. (2025). Data-driven decision making in patient management: A systematic review. *BMC Medical Informatics and Decision Making*, *25*(1), 239. DOI: 10.1186/s12911-025-03072-x PMID: 40598137

Lyu, L., Yu, H., & Yang, Q. (2023). Privacy-preserving collaboration in federated healthcare systems. *IEEE Transactions on Knowledge and Data Engineering*, *35*(2), 189–202. DOI: 10.1109/TKDE.2021.3057850

Ma, H., Huang, Q., Zhang, H., Song, H., Zhang, B., Liu, Y., & Zhang, L. (2025). Discovering sequential patterns and interrelations among multiple diseases in electronic medical records using cSPADE algorithm. *Archives of Public Health = Archives Belges de Santé Publique*, *83*(1), 100. DOI: 10.1186/s13690-025-01589-1 PMID: 40211318

Mahbod, A., Schaefer, G., Wang, C., Ecker, R., & Ellinger, I. (2019). Skin lesion classification using hybrid deep neural networks. *Proceedings of ICASSP 2019*, 1229–1233. DOI: 10.1109/ICASSP.2019.8683352

Maheshwari, V. C., Osman, N. A., Daud, H., Kurniati, A., & Yousaf, W. (2024). Detecting and Adapting to Concept Drift in Large-Scale Internet of Medical Things Data Streams: A Drift-Oriented Framework. DOI: 10.21203/rs.3.rs-3982655/v1

Makubhai, S. S., Pathak, G. R., & Chandre, P. R. (2024). The X-Factor of healthcare. In *Advances in Healthcare Information Systems and Administration* (pp. 113–140). IGI Global. DOI: 10.4018/979-8-3693-7277-7.ch004

Maletzky, A., Böck, C., Tschoellitsch, T., Roland, T., Ludwig, H., Thumfart, S., Giretzlehner, M., Hochreiter, S., & Meier, J. (2022). Lifting hospital electronic health record data treasures: Challenges and opportunities. *JMIR Medical Informatics*, *10*(10), e38557. DOI: 10.2196/38557 PMID: 36269654

Manias, G., Azqueta-Alzúaz, A., Damiani, A., Danti, M., & Maniatakos, V. (2023). An enhanced standardization and qualification mechanism for heterogeneous healthcare data. *Studies in Health Technology and Informatics*, *306*, 153–157. DOI: 10.3233/SHTI230092 PMID: 37203637

Manjunath, R., & Kwadiki, K. (2022). Automatic liver and tumour segmentation from CT images using deep learning algorithm. *Results in Control and Optimization*, *6*, 100087. DOI: 10.1016/j.rico.2021.100087

Manolitsis, I., Feretzakis, G., Tzelves, L., Kalles, D., Loupelis, E., Katsimperis, S., Kosmidis, T., Anastasiou, A., Koutsouris, D., Kofopoulou, S., Verykios, V. S., Skolarikos, A., & Varkarakis, I. (2022). Using association rules in antimicrobial resistance in stone disease patients. In *Studies in Health Technology and Informatics*. IOS Press., DOI: 10.3233/SHTI220765

Mao, H., & Omar, A. (2024). Explainable AI evaluation: A top-down approach for selecting optimal explanations for black box models. *Information (Basel)*, *15*(1), 4. Advance online publication. DOI: 10.3390/info15010004

Martínez-García, M., & Hernández-Lemus, E. (2022). Data integration challenges for machine learning in precision medicine. *Frontiers in Medicine*, *8*, 784455. DOI: 10.3389/fmed.2021.784455 PMID: 35145977

Martínez-Romero, M.. (2019). Using association rule mining and ontologies to generate real-time clinical suggestions. *Database : The Journal of Biological Databases and Curation*. Advance online publication. DOI: 10.1093/database/baz059 PMID: 31210270

Matsumura, Y., Yamashita, T., & Kitagaki, H. (2017). Mining association rules of combination medication patterns in medical prescriptions. *Journal of Biomedical Informatics*, *68*, 138–148. DOI: 10.1016/j.jbi.2017.03.004

McIntosh, T. R., Susnjak, T., Liu, T., Watters, P., Xu, D., Liu, D., Nowrozy, R., & Halgamuge, M. N. (2024). From COBIT to ISO 42001: Evaluating cybersecurity frameworks for opportunities, risks, and regulatory compliance in commercializing large language models. *Computers & Security*, *144*, 103964. Advance online publication. DOI: 10.1016/j.cose.2024.103964

Meena Gupta, R., Kalra, R., & Sharma, P. (2023). Security challenges and solutions using healthcare cloud computing. In *Pioneering Smart Healthcare 5.0 with IoT, Federated Learning, and Cloud Security* (pp. 198–219). IGI Global. DOI: 10.4018/979-8-3693-2639-8.ch012

Mehraeen, E., Ghazisaeedi, M., Farzi, J., & Mirshekari, S. (2017). Security challenges in healthcare cloud computing: A systematic. *Global Journal of Health Science*, *9*(3), 157–168. DOI: 10.5539/gjhs.v9n3p157

Mei, P., & Zhang, F. (2024). A framework for processing large-scale health data in medical higher-order correlation mining by quantum computing in smart healthcare. *Frontiers in Digital Health*, *6*, 1502745. DOI: 10.3389/fdgth.2024.1502745 PMID: 39633967

Meng, C., Trinh, L., Xu, N., Enouen, J., & Liu, Y. (2022). Interpretability and fairness evaluation of deep learning models on MIMIC-IV dataset. *Scientific Reports*, *12*(1), 7166. DOI: 10.1038/s41598-022-11012-2 PMID: 35504931

Meskó, B., & Topol, E. J. (2023). The imperative for regulatory oversight of large language models (or generative AI) in healthcare. *NPJ Digital Medicine*, *6*(1), 120. Advance online publication. DOI: 10.1038/s41746-023-00873-0 PMID: 37414860

Mguni, D., Tian, Y., Michaud, E. J., Leike, J., & Everitt, T. (2023). Learning to shape rewards using a game of two partners. *Proceedings of the AAAI Conference on Artificial Intelligence*, *37*(10), 11604–11612. DOI: 10.1609/aaai.v37i10.26371

Mienye, I. D., & Swart, T. G. (2025). Deep autoencoder neural networks: A comprehensive review and new perspectives. *Archives of Computational Methods in Engineering*, *32*(7), 3981–4000. DOI: 10.1007/s11831-025-10260-5

Miotto, R., Wang, F., Wang, S., Jiang, X., & Dudley, J. T. (2018). Deep learning for healthcare: Review, opportunities, and challenges. *Briefings in Bioinformatics*, *19*(6), 1236–1246. DOI: 10.1093/bib/bbx044 PMID: 28481991

Mishra, B. R., Selvakumar, P., Kaur, R., Kalshetti, P., Mishra, K. K., Sharma, M., & Manjunath, T. C. (2025). Innovation and Digital Transformation in the Public Sector Entities. In Santos Ferreira, A., & Lourenço dos Santos, C. (Eds.), *Enhancing Public Sector Accountability and Services Through Digital Innovation* (pp. 409–436). IGI Global Scientific Publishing., DOI: 10.4018/979-8-3693-9251-5.ch013

Miswan, N. H., Yusof, R. M., & Ahmad, M. (2021). Association Rules Mining for Hospital Readmission: A Case Study. *Mathematics*, *9*(21), 2706. DOI: 10.3390/math9212706

MITRE. (n.d.). *MITRE ATT&CK® knowledge base.* https://attack.mitre.org/

Moral, C., de Antonio, A., Imbert, R., & Ramírez, J. (2014). A survey of stemming algorithms in information retrieval. *Information Research, 19*(1), n1.

Mu, T., & Zheng, S. (2025). Modeling bounded rationality in multi-agent simulations using rationally inattentive reinforcement learning. *OpenReview*. https://openreview.net/forum?id=DY1pMrmDkm

Mubarakali, A., & AlJarullah, A. (2025). IoT and XAI-driven data aggregation framework for intelligent decision-making in smart healthcare systems. *Sustainable Computing : Informatics and Systems, 48*, 101179. Advance online publication. DOI: 10.1016/j.suscom.2025.101179

Muniasamy, A., Bhatnagar, R., & Karunakaran, G. (2021). Predicting COVID-19 spread in Saudi Arabia using artificial intelligence techniques—Proposing a shift towards a sustainable healthcare approach. In A. Hassanien, R. Bhatnagar, & A. Darwish (Eds.), Artificial intelligence for sustainable development: Theory, practice and future applications (Studies in Computational Intelligence, Vol. 912, pp. 59–78). Springer, Cham. DOI: 10.1007/978-3-030-51920-9_6

Muniasamy, A., Tabassam, S., Hussain, M. A., Sultana, H., Muniasamy, V., & Bhatnagar, R. (2020). Deep Learning for Predictive Analytics in Healthcare. In: Hassanien, A., Azar, A., Gaber, T., Bhatnagar, R., F. Tolba, M. (eds) The International Conference on Advanced Machine Learning Technologies and Applications (AMLTA2019). AMLTA 2019. Advances in Intelligent Systems and Computing, vol 921. Springer, Cham. DOI: 10.1007/978-3-030-14118-9_4

Muniasamy, A. (2025). Revolutionizing health monitoring: Integrating transformer models with multi-head attention for precise human activity recognition using wearable devices. *Technology and Health Care, 33*(1), 395–409. DOI: 10.3233/THC-241064 PMID: 39269866

Muniasamy, A. (2026). Quantum Computing in Drug Discovery: Revolutionizing Pharmaceutical Research. In Muniasamy, A., & Karunakaran, G. (Eds.), *Applications of Artificial Intelligence in Pharmaceuticals* (pp. 59–96). IGI Global Scientific Publishing., DOI: 10.4018/979-8-3373-2043-4.ch003

Muniasamy, A., & Alasmari, A. (2025). Integrating Bayesian and convolution neural network for uncertainty estimation of cataract from fundus images. *Computer Modeling in Engineering & Sciences, 143*(1), 569–592. DOI: 10.32604/cmes.2025.060484

Muniasamy, A., Alquhtani, S. A. S., Alshehri, A. H., Begum, A., & Sabahath, A. (2025). Investigating hybrid quantum-assisted classical and deep learning model for MRI brain tumor classification. *Journal of Image and Graphics, 13*(1), 123–129. DOI: 10.18178/joig.13.1.123-129

Muniasamy, A., Alquhtani, S. A. S., Bilfaqih, S. M., Balaji, P., & Karunakaran, G. (2023). Lung cancer histopathology image classification using transfer learning with convolution neural network model. *Technology and Health Care*, *32*(2), 1199–1210. DOI: 10.3233/THC-231029 PMID: 37270826

Muniasamy, A., & Asiri, F. (2025). Advanced human activity recognition on wearables with multi-scale sparse attention. *Multimedia Tools and Applications*, *84*(30), 36623–36652. DOI: 10.1007/s11042-024-20475-6

Muniasamy, A., Begum, A., Sabahath, A., Yaqub, H., & Karunakaran, G. (2024). Coronary heart disease classification using deep learning approach with feature selection for improved accuracy. *Technology and Health Care*, *32*(4), 1991–2007. DOI: 10.3233/THC-231807 PMID: 38339946

Muniasamy, A., Ghose, M. K., & Gauthaman, A. (2010). Fast association rule mining algorithm for spatial gene expression data. *Global Journal of Computer Science and Technology*, *9*(5), 11–17. https://files.eric.ed.gov/fulltext/ED508175.pdf

Muniasamy, A., & Karunakaran, G. (2026). Challenges and future directions: Emerging trends and limitations in ML and optimization for healthcare. In Muniasamy, A. (Ed.), *Integrative machine learning and optimization algorithms for disease prediction* (pp. 339–368). IGI Global Scientific Publishing., DOI: 10.4018/979-8-3373-1087-9.ch012

Muniasamy, V., Eljailani, I. M., & Anandhavalli, M. (2019). Student's performance assessment and learning skill towards Wireless Network Simulation tool - Cisco Packet Tracer. *International Journal of Emerging Technologies in Learning*, *14*(7), 196–208. DOI: 10.3991/ijet.v14i07.10351

Munusamy, S., & Jothi, K. R. (2025). Blockchain-enabled federated learning with edge analytics for secure and efficient electronic health records management. *Scientific Reports*, *15*(1), 27524. DOI: 10.1038/s41598-025-12225-x PMID: 40721766

Muralidhar, A. (2015). The Sharpe ratio revisited: What it really tells us. *Journal of Performance Measurement, 19*(3).

Murray, J., & Cohen, A. L. (2016). Infectious disease surveillance. *International encyclopedia of public health*, 222.

Muruga Priya, P.. "Microarray based Disease Prediction using Deep Learning Techniques", *7th International Conference on Computing Methodologies and Communication (ICCMC)*, 23-25 Feb. 2023.

Mustafa, K. A., de Groot, O., Wang, X., Kober, J., & Alonso-Mora, J. (2023). Probabilistic risk assessment for chance-constrained collision avoidance in uncertain dynamic environments. *arXiv.* /arXiv.2302.10846DOI: 10.1109/ICRA48891.2023.10161490

Nag, A. (2025). Balancing trustworthiness and efficiency in AI systems: A comprehensive analysis of trade-offs and strategies. *SciSpace.* https://scispace.com

Naidenova, X., Ganapolsky, V., Yakovlev, A., & Martirova, T. (2022). Application association rule mining in medical-biological investigations [Journal information not specified]. *Survey (London, England).*

Najjar, H., Pathak, D., Nuske, M., & Dengel, A. (2025). Intrinsic explainability of multimodal learning for crop yield simulation. *Computers and Electronics in Agriculture, 239,* 111003. Advance online publication. DOI: 10.1016/j.compag.2025.111003

Nalavade, K., & Meshram, B. B. (2014). Finding frequent item-sets using Apriori algorithm.... *IJCAIT, 6*(1), 84–92.

Nanda Prakash, N., Rajesh, V., Namakhwa, D. L., Pande, S. D., & Ahammada, S. H. (2023). A DenseNet CNN-based liver lesion prediction and classification for future medical diagnosis. *Scientific African, 20,* e01629. DOI: 10.1016/j.sciaf.2023.e01629

Naue, J. (2023). Getting the chronological age out of DNA: Using insights of age-dependent DNA methylation for forensic DNA applications. *Genes & Genomics, 45*(10), 1239–1261. DOI: 10.1007/s13258-023-01392-8 PMID: 37253906

Nguyen, T. V., Zhang, J., Zhou, L., & Chen, J. (2019). A data-driven optimization of large-scale dry port location using the hybrid approach of data mining and complex network theory. *Journal of Cleaner Production, 234,* 1113–1123.

Nirupama, E., Seenivasan, S., Bhardwaj, K., Karunakaran, N. B., & Basava Aradhya, S. G., & Manjunath, T. C. (2025). Transforming Digital Supply Chains With Gamification and Metaverse Integration. In G. Malik, D. Singh, & R. Bansal (Eds.), *Addressing Practical Problems Through the Metaverse and Game-Inspired Mechanics* (pp. 123-152). IGI Global Scientific Publishing. DOI: 10.4018/979-8-3693-8886-0.ch006

Nishant, R. (2023). The formal rationality of artificial intelligence-based algorithms and the problem of bias. *Journal of Information Technology.* Advance online publication. DOI: 10.1177/02683962231176842

Oesterheld, C., Demski, A., & Conitzer, V. (2023). A theory of bounded inductive rationality. *Electronic Proceedings in Theoretical Computer Science, 379,* 421–440. DOI: 10.4204/EPTCS.379.33

Ojala, T., Pietikäinen, M., & Maenpaa, T. (2002). Multiresolution grayscale and rotation invariant texture classification with local binary patterns. *IEEE Transactions on Pattern Analysis and Machine Intelligence*, *24*(7), 971–987. DOI: 10.1109/TPAMI.2002.1017623

Ojo, A., & Adeyemo, A. (2012). Framework for knowledge discovery from journal articles using text mining techniques. *African Journal of Computing and ICT*, *5*(2). www.ajocict.net

Ordonez, C. (2006). Association rule discovery with the train and test approach for heart disease prediction. *IEEE Transactions on Information Technology in Biomedicine*, *10*(2), 334–343. DOI: 10.1109/TITB.2006.864475 PMID: 16617622

Ordonez, C., Omiecinski, E., de Braal, L., Santana, C. A., Ezquerra, N., Taboada, J. A., & Cooke, D. (2001). Mining constrained association rules to predict heart disease. *Proceedings of the IEEE International Conference on Data Mining*, 433–440. DOI: 10.1109/ICDM.2001.989549

Öztürk, Ş., Ahmad, R., & Akhtar, N. (2020). Variants of Artificial Bee Colony algorithm and its applications in medical image processing. *Applied Soft Computing*, *97*, 106799.

Padma, A., Chithanuru, V., Uppamma, P., & VishnuKumar, R. (2024). Exploring Explainable AI in Healthcare. In *Advances in Healthcare Information Systems and Administration* (pp. 199–233). IGI Global. DOI: 10.4018/979-8-3693-5468-1.ch011

Papadimitroulas, P., Brocki, L., Christopher Chung, N., Marchadour, W., Vermet, F., Gaubert, L., Eleftheriadis, V., Plachouris, D., Visvikis, D., Kagadis, G. C., & Hatt, M. (2021). Artificial intelligence: Deep learning in oncological radiomics and challenges of interpretability and data harmonization. [AIFB]. *Physica Medica*, *83*, 108–121. DOI: 10.1016/j.ejmp.2021.03.009 PMID: 33765601

Patel, V. L., Shortliffe, E. H., Stefanelli, M., Szolovits, P., Berthold, M. R., Bellazzi, R., & Abu-Hanna, A. (2009). The coming of age of artificial intelligence in medicine. *Artificial Intelligence in Medicine*, *46*(1), 5–17. DOI: 10.1016/j.artmed.2008.07.017 PMID: 18790621

Patil, D., Rane, N. L., Desai, P., & Rane, J. (2024). Machine learning and deep learning: Methods, techniques, applications, challenges, and future research opportunities. In *Trustworthy Artificial Intelligence in Industry and Society*. Deep Science Publishing., DOI: 10.70593/978-81-981367-4-9_2

Penev, Y., Buchanan, T. R., Ruppert, M. M., & Johnson, K. B. (2024). Electronic health record data quality and performance assessments: A scoping review. *JMIR Medical Informatics*, *12*, 12. DOI: 10.2196/58130 PMID: 39504136

Peng, M., Sundararajan, V., Williamson, T., Minty, E. P., Smith, T. C., Doktorchik, C. T. A., & Quan, H. (2018). Exploration of association rule mining for coding consistency and completeness assessment in inpatient administrative health data. *Journal of Biomedical Informatics*, *79*, 41–47. DOI: 10.1016/j.jbi.2018.02.001 PMID: 29425732

Peng, S., Shen, F., Wen, A., & Wu, B. (2019). Detecting lifestyle risk factors for chronic kidney disease with comorbidities: Association rule mining analysis of web-based survey data. *Journal of Medical Internet Research*, *21*(4), e13508. DOI: 10.2196/14204 PMID: 31821152

Peng, Y., Ahmad, S. F., Ahmad, A. Y. A. B., Al Shaikh, M. S., Daoud, M. K., & Alhamdi, F. M. H. (2023). Riding the waves of artificial intelligence in advancing accounting and its implications for sustainable development goals. *Sustainability (Basel)*, *15*(19), 14165. DOI: 10.3390/su151914165

Perell, K., Vincent, M., Vainer, B., Petersen, B. L., Federspiel, B., Møller, A. K., Madsen, M., Hansen, N. R., Friis-Hansen, L., Nielsen, F. C., & Daugaard, G. (2015). Development and validation of a microRNA-based diagnostic assay for primary tumor site classification of liver core biopsies. *Molecular Oncology*, *9*(1), 68–77. DOI: 10.1016/j.molonc.2014.07.015 PMID: 25131495

Pouriyeh, S., Vahid, S., Sannino, G., De Pietro, G., Arabnia, H. R., & Gutierrez, J. (2017). A comprehensive investigation and comparison of machine learning techniques in the domain of heart disease. *Computer Methods and Programs in Biomedicine*, *165*, 25–39.

Prabavathy, K., & Sumathi, P. (2013). Text mining: Interpreting knowledge discovery from biomed articles. *The SIJ Transactions on Computer Science Engineering & its Applications (CSEA)*, *1*(2), 33–36.

Prados-Torres, A., Calderón-Larrañaga, A., Hancco-Saavedra, J., Poblador-Plou, B., & van den Akker, M. (2014). Multimorbidity patterns: A systematic review. *Journal of Clinical Epidemiology*, *67*(3), 254–266. DOI: 10.1016/j.jclinepi.2013.09.021 PMID: 24472295

Prasad, M. S. G., Kumar, N. N., & Shah, M. A., & B. R., S. (2022). FOEH: Frequent pattern mining performance optimization over large transactional data in extended Hadoop MapReduce. *International Journal on Computer Science and Engineering*, *10*(4), 260–264.

Rahwan, I., Cebrian, M., Obradovich, N., Bongard, J., Bonnefon, J. F., Breazeal, C., Crandall, J. W., Christakis, N. A., Couzin, I. D., Jackson, M. O., Jennings, N. R., Kamar, E., Kloumann, I. M., Larochelle, H., Lazer, D., McElreath, R., Mislove, A., Parkes, D. C., Pentland, A., & Wellman, M. (2019). Machine behaviour. *Nature*, *568*(7753), 477–486. DOI: 10.1038/s41586-019-1138-y PMID: 31019318

Rai, N. S., Jain, S., & Jain, A. (2014). Mining interesting positive and negative association rule based on improved genetic algorithm. *International Journal of Advanced Computer Science and Applications*, *5*(1).

Rai, V. K., Chakraborty, S., & Chakraborty, S. (2023). Association rule mining for prediction of COVID-19. *Decision Making: Applications in Management and Engineering*, *6*(1), 365–378. DOI: 10.31181/dmame0317102022r

Rajasekar, V., Vaishnnave, M. P., Premkumar, S., Sarveshwaran, V., & Rangaraaj, V. (2023). Lung cancer disease prediction with CT scan and histopathological images feature analysis using deep learning techniques. *Results in Engineering*, *18*, 101111. DOI: 10.1016/j.rineng.2023.101111

Rajesh, C.. (2023, November). An evolutionary Chameleon Swarm Algorithm based network for 3D medical image segmentation. *Expert Systems with Applications*, *239*, •••.

Ramalakshmi, K., & Srinivasa Raghavan, V. (2021). Soft computing-based edge-enhanced dominant peak and discrete Tchebichef extraction for image segmentation and classification using DCML-IC. *Soft Computing*, *25*(1), 2635–2646. DOI: 10.1007/s00500-020-05306-8

Ramalakshmi, K., & Srinivasa Raghavan, V. (2023). Enhanced prediction using deep neural network-based image classification. *Imaging Science Journal*, *71*(5), 472–483. DOI: 10.1080/13682199.2023.2183621

Raman, M. S., Koppa, K. B., Chithambar Gupta, V., Bhat, V. A., & Guru Basava Aradhya, S. (2025). Digital Transformation and Sustainability Artificial Intelligence and Sustainable Development. In Yıldırım, D., Yıldırım, S., & Kandpal, V. (Eds.), *Effects of Digitalization and Circular Economy on Sustainable Policy and Climate Change Prevention* (pp. 69–96). IGI Global Scientific Publishing., DOI: 10.4018/979-8-3693-9909-5.ch003

Ramon-Gonen, R., Dori, A., & Shelly, S. (2023). Towards a practical use of text mining approaches in electrodiagnostic data. *Scientific Reports*, *13*(1), 45758. DOI: 10.1038/s41598-023-45758-0 PMID: 37945618

Rana, S., Mondal, M. N. I., & Islam, M. R. (2025). Unveiling Purchase Patterns... *ECCE 2025*.

Raposo, V. L. (2025). The fifty shades of black: About black box AI and explainability in healthcare. *Medical Law Review*, *33*(1), fwaf005. Advance online publication. DOI: 10.1093/medlaw/fwaf005 PMID: 39916325

Rashid, M., Kwok, C. S., Gale, C. P., Doherty, P., Olier, I., Sperrin, M., Kontopantelis, E., Peat, G., & Mamas, M. A. (2017). Impact of co-morbid burden on mortality in patients with coronary heart disease, heart failure, and cerebrovascular accident: A systematic review and meta-analysis. *European Heart Journal. Quality of Care & Clinical Outcomes*, *3*(1), 20–36. DOI: 10.1093/ehjqcco/qcw025 PMID: 28927187

Rav, D.. (2017, January). Deep Learning for Health Informatics. *IEEE Journal of Biomedical and Health Informatics*, *21*(1), •••. PMID: 28055930

Ravikumar, A. S., Atamuratova, Z., Ashirova, A., Jurayev, K., & Hayitova, M. (2025). Comprehensive evaluation of AI-driven systems in modern hospital environments. In *Advances in Computational Intelligence and Robotics* (pp. 61–88). IGI Global Scientific Publishing. DOI: 10.4018/979-8-3373-2787-7.ch003

Ravikumar, A. S., Saparbaevich, B. R., Kumar A., S., Jumaniyozova, M., & Toshova, S. (2025). AI-enhanced clinical decision-making through a collaborative approach. In *Advances in Computational Intelligence and Robotics* (pp. 249–280). IGI Global Scientific Publishing. DOI: 10.4018/979-8-3373-3311-3.ch010

Ravikumar, R. N., Aarthi, S., Dilshodbek, A., Satheesh Kumar, A., Eshkaraev, S., & Shanmugam, K. B. (2025). Integrating blockchain, smart contracts, and AI for decentralized healthcare in the metaverse. In *Blockchain-Based Healthcare Management in the Metaverse* (pp. 261–294). IGI Global Scientific Publishing., DOI: 10.4018/979-8-3373-1225-5.ch010

Ravindran, U., & Gunavathi, C. (2023). A survey on gene expression data analysis using deep learning methods for cancer diagnosis. *Progress in Biophysics and Molecular Biology*, *177*, 1–13. DOI: 10.1016/j.pbiomolbio.2022.08.004 PMID: 35988771

Raza, A.. (2023, January). Predicting Genetic Disorder and Types of Disorder Using Chain Classifier Approach. *Genes*. PMID: 36672812

Raza, A., Tran, K. P., Koehl, L., & Li, S. (2021). Designing ECG monitoring healthcare system with federated transfer learning and explainable AI. arXiv. https://arxiv.org/abs/2105.1249

Razzak, M. I., Imran, M., & Xu, G. (2020). Big data analytics for preventive medicine. *Neural Computing & Applications, 32*(9), 4417–4451. DOI: 10.1007/s00521-019-04095-y PMID: 32205918

Rebelo de Sá, C., Azevedo, P., Soares, C., Jorge, A., & Knobbe, A. (2017). Preference rules for label ranking: Mining patterns in multi-target relations. *Information Fusion, 40*, 112–125. DOI: 10.1016/j.inffus.2017.07.001

Reham, R.. (2022, June). Boosting chameleon swarm algorithm with consumption AEO operator for global optimization and feature selection. *Knowledge-Based Systems, 246*, •••.

Ren, Q., Hu, C., Xu, M., & Song, J. (2026). Association rule mining of damage severities in autonomous vehicle rear-end crashes with supplementary built environment data. *Reliability Engineering & System Safety, 265*, 111589. Advance online publication. DOI: 10.1016/j.ress.2025.111589

Ribeiro, M. T., Singh, S., & Guestrin, C. (2016). "Why should I trust you?" Explaining the predictions of any classifier. In *Proceedings of the 22nd ACM SIGKDD International Conference on Knowledge Discovery and Data Mining* (pp. 1135–1144). https://doi.org/DOI: 10.1145/2939672.2939778

Rotaru-Zavaleanu, A. D., Lungulescu, C. V., Bunescu, M. G., Vasile, R. C., Gheorman, V., Gresita, A., & Dinescu, V. C. (2024). Occupational Carpal Tunnel Syndrome…. *Frontiers in Public Health, 12*, 1407302. DOI: 10.3389/fpubh.2024.1407302 PMID: 38841666

Russell, S. J., & Norvig, P. (2021). *Artificial intelligence: A modern approach* (4th ed.). Pearson.

Sajjaa, V. R., & Kalluri, H. K. (2021). Classification of brain tumors using fuzzy c-means and VGG16. *Turkish Journal of Computer and Mathematics Education, 12*(9), 2103–2113.

Samek, W., Montavon, G., Lapuschkin, S., Anders, C. J., & Müller, K. R. (2021). Explaining deep neural networks and beyond: A review of methods and applications. *Proceedings of the IEEE, 109*(3), 247–278. DOI: 10.1109/JPROC.2021.3060483

Sandeep Pushyamitra Pattyam. (2021). Artificial Intelligence for Healthcare Diagnostics: Techniques for Disease Prediction, Personalized Treatment, and Patient Monitoring. *Journal of Bioinformatics and Artificial Intelligence, 1*(1 SE-Articles), 309–343. Retrieved from https://biotechjournal.org/index.php/jbai/article/view/99

Sangma, J. W. (2020). Clustering-based hybrid approach for identifying associations in data. *PubMed*. https://pubmed.ncbi.nlm.nih.gov/32931587

Sarker, I. H. (2021). Machine learning: Algorithms, real-world applications and research directions. *SN Computer Science*, *2*(3), 160. DOI: 10.1007/s42979-021-00592-x PMID: 33778771

Scheffer, T. (2001). Finding association rules that trade support optimally against confidence. *PKDD*, 424–435.

Sekti, B. A. (2025a). Adversarial Machine Learning in Industrial Cybersecurity: Challenges and Solutions. In *AI-Enhanced Cybersecurity for Industrial Automation* (pp. 363–386). IGI Global Scientific Publishing. DOI: 10.4018/979-8-3373-3241-3.ch018

Sekti, B. A. (2025b). Information Security Awareness. In *User-Centric Cybersecurity Implications for Sustainable Digital Transformation* (pp. 111–145). DOI: 10.4018/979-8-3373-3171-3.ch004

Sekti, B. A. (2025c). Machine Learning vs. AI: Key Concepts. In *Implementing Enterprise Cybersecurity With AI* (pp. 1–27). DOI: 10.4018/979-8-3373-2252-0.ch001

Shackelford, S. J., Proia, A. A., Martell, B., & Craig, A. N. (2015). Toward a global cybersecurity standard of care.... *Tex. Int'l LJ*, *50*, 305.

Shakil, K.A., Anis, S., & Alam, M. (2015). Dengue disease prediction using weka data mining tool. *ArXiv, abs/1502.05167.*

Shan, Z., & Miao, W. (2023). COVID-19 patient diagnosis and treatment data mining algorithm based on association rules. *Expert Systems: International Journal of Knowledge Engineering and Neural Networks*, *40*(4), e12814. Advance online publication. DOI: 10.1111/exsy.12814 PMID: 34898798

Shichkina, Y., Petrov, M., & Roza, F. (2022). Determination of significant parameters.... *Mathematics*, *10*(7), 1133. DOI: 10.3390/math10071133

Shneiderman, B. (2020). Human-centered artificial intelligence: Reliable, safe & trustworthy. *International Journal of Human-Computer Interaction*, *36*(6), 495–504. DOI: 10.1080/10447318.2020.1741118

Shrestha, A., Zikos, D., & Fegaras, L. (2021). An annotated association mining approach for extracting and visualizing interesting clinical events. *International Journal of Medical Informatics*, *148*, 104366. DOI: 10.1016/j.ijmedinf.2020.104366 PMID: 33485216

Shu, X., & Ye, Y. (2023). Knowledge discovery: Methods from data mining and machine learning. *Social Science Research*, *110*, 102817. DOI: 10.1016/j.ssresearch.2022.102817 PMID: 36796993

Sidhu. (2025). Deep learning approaches for enhancing healthcare data security. *International Journal of Research and Review in Applied Science, Humanities, and Technology*, 242–247. DOI: 10.71143/y1dhmw84

Simmachan, T., Lerdpraserdpakorn, N., Deesrisuk, J., Sriwipat, C., Shakya, S., & Boonkrong, P. (2025). A penalized regression and machine learning approach for quality-of-life prediction in psoriasis patients. *Healthcare Analytics*, *8*, 100417. Advance online publication. DOI: 10.1016/j.health.2025.100417

Simonyan, K., & Zisserman, A. (2014). Very deep convolutional networks for large-scale image recognition. *arXiv preprint arXiv:1409.1556.*

Sindiramutty, S. R., Tee, W. J., Balakrishnan, S., Kaur, S., Thangaveloo, R., Jazri, H., Khan, N. A., Gharib, A., & Manchuri, A. R. (2024). Explainable AI in Healthcare Application. In *Advances in Computational Intelligence and Robotics* (pp. 123–176). IGI Global. DOI: 10.4018/978-1-6684-6361-1.ch005

Singh, K. N., & Mantri, J. K. (2024). An intelligent recommender system using machine learning association rules and rough set for disease prediction from incomplete symptom set. *Decision Analytics Journal, 11*, 100468. DOI: 10.1016/j.dajour.2024.100468

Smith, A., Johnson, B., Clark, R., & Taylor, P. (2023). Trust calibration in human–AI decision-making systems. *AI & Society*. Advance online publication. DOI: 10.1007/s00146-023-01684-7

Sogandi, F. (2024). Identifying diseases symptoms and general rules using supervised and unsupervised machine learning. *Scientific Reports*, *14*(1), 17956. Advance online publication. DOI: 10.1038/s41598-024-69029-8 PMID: 39095606

Soria-Comas, J., & Domingo-Ferrer, J. (2021). Differential privacy in data mining for health information systems. *Computers in Biology and Medicine*, *134*, 104441. DOI: 10.1016/j.compbiomed.2021.104441

Sowan, B., Zhang, L., Matar, N., Zraqou, J., Omar, F., & Alnatsheh, A. (2025). A novel lift adjustment methodology… *Decision Analytics Journal, 100582.*

Spooner, A., Mohammadi, G., Sachdev, P., Brodaty, H., & Sowmya, A. (2022). Temporal pattern mining for analysis of longitudinal clinical data: Identifying risk factors for Alzheimer's disease. *Preprint.* https://doi.org//arXiv.2209.04793DOI: 10.48550

Srinadh, V. (2022). Evaluation of Apriori, FP-growth and Eclat…. *International Journal of Health Sciences*, •••, 7475–7485. DOI: 10.53730/ijhs.v6nS2.6729

Sumathy, K. L., & Chidambaram, M. (2013). Text mining: Concepts, applications, tools and issues-an overview. *International Journal of Computer Applications, 80*(4). Advance online publication. DOI: 10.5120/13851-1685

Sundaresan, B., Shirafkan, F., Ripperger, K., & Rattay, K. (2023). The role of viral infections in the onset of autoimmune diseases. *Viruses, 15*(3), 782. DOI: 10.3390/v15030782 PMID: 36992490

Sutton, R. S., & Barto, A. G. (2018). *Reinforcement learning: An introduction* (2nd ed.). MIT Press.

Tandan, M., Acharya, Y., Pokharel, S., & Timilsina, M. (2021). Discovering symptom patterns of COVID-19 patients using association rule mining. *Computers in Biology and Medicine, 131*, 104249. DOI: 10.1016/j.compbiomed.2021.104249 PMID: 33561673

Tarekegn, A. N., Ullah, M., & Cheikh, F. A. (2024). Deep Learning for Multi-Label Learning: A Comprehensive Survey. *arXiv preprint arXiv:2401.16549.*

Thabtah, F. (2007). A review of associative classification mining. *The Knowledge Engineering Review*, *22*(1), 37–65. DOI: 10.1017/S0269888907001026

Thaler, R. H., & Sunstein, C. R. (2008). *Nudge: Improving decisions about health, wealth, and happiness*. Yale University Press.

Thaljaoui, A., & El-Bouzidi, A. (2022). Integrated Bayesian and association-rules methods for autonomous decision making to support COVID-19 management. *Medical & Biological Engineering & Computing*. Advance online publication. DOI: 10.1007/s11517-022-02677-y PMID: 36205834

Thanikachalam, R., Muniasamy, A., Alasmari, A., & Thavasimuthu, R. (2025). EffNet-CNN: A semantic model for image mining and content-based image retrieval. *Computer Modeling in Engineering & Sciences, 143*(2), 1971–2000. DOI: 10.32604/cmes.2025.063063

Ting, H. W., Chien, T. Y., & Liao, C. C. (2022). Diseases that occur prior to spontaneous intracerebral hemorrhage: Identification of predisposing and risk factors using lag sequential analysis. *Journal of Healthcare Engineering*, *2022*, 9733712. DOI: 10.1155/2022/9733712 PMID: 35368939

Tversky, A., & Kahneman, D. (1974). Judgment under uncertainty: Heuristics and biases. *Science*, *185*(4157), 1124–1131. DOI: 10.1126/science.185.4157.1124 PMID: 17835457

Tyagi, S., Macesic, N., Peleg, A., & Ramakrishnaiah, Y. (2023). EHR-QC: A streamlined pipeline for automated electronic health records standardisation and preprocessing to predict clinical outcomes. *International Journal of Medical Informatics, 174*, 105058.

U.S. Department of Health & Human Services. (2024). *Ransomware & healthcare: Risk, response, and recovery.* https://www.hhs.gov/sites/default/files/ransomware-healthcare.pdf

Upadhyaya, A., Mishra, M., & Saxena, A. (2024). User preferences for AI-based healthcare apps: An association mining analysis. *SN Computer Science, 5*(5), 273. Advance online publication. DOI: 10.1007/s42979-024-02739-y

Vallée, A. (2025). Digital twins for personalized medicine require epidemiological data and mathematical modeling: Viewpoint. *Journal of Medical Internet Research, 27*, e72411. DOI: 10.2196/72411 PMID: 40762974

Varghese, A., Varghese, J., Biju, J., Thomas, R., & Thomas, M. (2024). Explainable AI in Healthcare Applications. [IRJAEM]. *International Research Journal on Advanced Engineering and Management*, 2(12), 3671–3679. DOI: 10.47392/IRJAEM.2024.0545

Vineela, M., ... (2022). "Prediction of Genetic Diseases Based On DNA", Journal of Engineering Sciences Vol 13 Issue 07, JULY/2022 ISSN:0377-9254

Wachter, S., Mittelstadt, B., & Russell, C. (2017). Counterfactual explanations without opening the black box: Automated decisions and the GDPR. *SSRN, 31*(2), 841–887. DOI: 10.2139/ssrn.3063289

Waghmode, P., & Patil, S. (2025). Intrusion detection system based on machine learning techniques. *Journal of Computer Networks and Communications, 2025*, 1–8. DOI: 10.1155/2025/11978955

Wang, W., Ferrari, D., Haddon-Hill, G., & Curcin, V. (2023). Electronic health records as source of research data… *Machine Learning for Brain Disorders*, 331–354.

Wang, D., Yang, Q., Abdul, A., & Lim, B. Y. (2019). Designing theory-driven user-centric explainable AI. In *Proceedings of the 2019 CHI Conference on Human Factors in Computing Systems*. DOI: 10.1145/3290605.3300831

Wang, J., Li, Y., Zhang, Y., & Zhang, J. (2021). Scalable association rule mining for precision medicine. *Journal of Biomedical Informatics, 118*, 103778. DOI: 10.1016/j.jbi.2021.103778

Wang, M., Tan, Y., Shi, Y., Wang, X., Liao, Z., & Wei, P. (2020). Diabetes and sarcopenic obesity…. *Frontiers in Endocrinology*, *11*, 568. DOI: 10.3389/fendo.2020.00568 PMID: 32982969

Wang, X., & Jin, Z. (2025). Multi-region infectious disease prediction modeling based on spatio-temporal graph neural network and the dynamic model. *PLoS Computational Biology*, *21*(1), e1012738. DOI: 10.1371/journal.pcbi.1012738 PMID: 39787070

Wang, Y., Kung, L., & Byrd, T. A. (2018). Big data analytics: Understanding its capabilities and potential benefits for healthcare organizations. *Technological Forecasting and Social Change*, *126*, 3–13. DOI: 10.1016/j.techfore.2015.12.019

Wang, Y., Song, Z., & Zhang, L. (2024). Detection of safety signs using computer vision based on deep learning. *Applied Sciences (Basel, Switzerland)*, *14*(6), 2556. DOI: 10.3390/app14062556

Warale, P. N., Limbore, N. V., Anute, N., Ahluwalia, G. K., & Raut, A. (2025). AI-Enhanced Customer Engagement and Experience: Chatbots, Virtual Assistants, and AI-Powered Customer Interactions. In Hussain, Z., Khan, A., Uzir, M., Sharipudin, M., & Shaheen, A. (Eds.), *Impacts of AI-Generated Content on Brand Reputation* (pp. 335–362). IGI Global Scientific Publishing., DOI: 10.4018/979-8-3373-4327-3.ch014

Wei, X. (2025). The application of data mining in dynamic monitoring of mental health trends among college students. *International Journal of Healthcare Information Systems and Informatics*, *20*(1), 1–18. DOI: 10.4018/IJHISI.391363

Weller, A. (2019). Transparency: Motivations and challenges. In *Explainable AI: Interpreting, Explaining and Visualizing Deep Learning* (pp. 23–40). Springer. DOI: 10.1007/978-3-030-28954-6_2

Wright, A., et al. (2013). Validation of an Association Rule Mining-Based Method to Identify Medication–Problem Associations in Clinical Data. Journal / AMIA / medical informatics paper. DOI: 10.1186/1472-6947-13-129

Wu, J., Meng, H., Zhou, L., Wang, M., Jin, S., Ji, H., Liu, B., Jin, P., & Du, C. (2024). Habitat radiomics and deep learning fusion nomogram to predict EGFR mutation status in stage I non-small cell lung cancer: A multicenter study. *Scientific Reports*, *14*(1), 15877. DOI: 10.1038/s41598-024-66751-1 PMID: 38982267

Wu, W.-T., Li, Y.-J., Feng, A.-Z., Li, L., Huang, T., Xu, A.-D., & Lyu, J. (2021). Data mining in clinical big data: The frequently used databases, steps, and methodological models. *Military Medical Research*, *8*(1), 44. DOI: 10.1186/s40779-021-00338-z PMID: 34380547

Wu, Z., Guo, C., Chen, J., Ding, S., & Zheng, Y. (2025). Integrating temporal association rules into intelligent prediction system for metabolic dysfunction-associated fatty liver disease. *Decision Support Systems*, *195*, 114467. DOI: 10.1016/j.dss.2025.114467

Xiang, D., & Cai, W. (2021). Privacy protection and secondary use of health data: Strategies and methods. *BioMed Research International*, *2021*(1), 6967166. DOI: 10.1155/2021/6967166 PMID: 34660798

Xie, N., Ras, G., Van Gerven, M., & Doran, D. (2020). Explainable deep learning: A field guide for the uninitiated. *Journal of Artificial Intelligence Research*, *73*, 329–397. DOI: 10.1613/jair.1.12280

Xu, C., Chen, X., Zhu, G., Yi, H., Chen, S., Yu, Y., Jiang, E., Zheng, Y., Zhang, F., Wang, J., & Feng, S. (2023). Utility of plasma cell-free DNA next-generation sequencing for diagnosis of infectious diseases in patients with hematological disorders. *The Journal of Infection*, *86*(1), 14–23. DOI: 10.1016/j.jinf.2022.11.020 PMID: 36462587

Xu, W., Zhao, Q., Zhan, Y., Wang, B., & Hu, Y. (2022). Privacy-preserving association rule mining based on electronic medical system. *Wireless Networks*, *28*(1), 303–317. DOI: 10.1007/s11276-021-02846-1

Xu, Y., Hong, K., Tsujii, J., & Chang, E. I.-C. (2012). Feature engineering combined with machine learning and rule-based methods for structured information extraction from narrative clinical discharge summaries. *Journal of the American Medical Informatics Association : JAMIA*, *19*(5), 824–832. DOI: 10.1136/amiajnl-2011-000776 PMID: 22586067

Yadav, S., Singh, D. M. K., & Kumar, P. (2023). Data mining applications for enhancing healthcare services: A comprehensive review. *International Journal of Engineering Technology and Management Sciences*, *7*(5), 325–333. DOI: 10.46647/ijetms.2023.v07i05.038

Yamamoto, H., Kayanuma, G., Nagashima, T., Toda, C., Nagayasu, K., & Kaneko, S. (2023). Early detection of adverse drug reaction signals…. *Drug Safety*, *46*(4), 371–389. DOI: 10.1007/s40264-023-01278-4 PMID: 36828947

Yamamoto, S., Kanca, O., Wangler, M. F., & Bellen, H. J. (2024). Integrating non-mammalian model organisms in the diagnosis of rare genetic diseases in humans. *Nature Reviews. Genetics*, *25*(1), 46–60. DOI: 10.1038/s41576-023-00633-6 PMID: 37491400

Yang, Q., Steinfeld, A., Rosé, C. P., & Zimmerman, J. (2019). Re-examining whether, why, and how human–AI interaction is uniquely difficult to design. In *Proceedings of the 2019 CHI Conference on Human Factors in Computing Systems*. DOI: 10.1145/3290605.3300232

Ye, J., Wang, S., Yang, X., & Tang, X. (2021, December). Gene prediction of aging related diseases based on DNN and Mashup. *BMC Bioinformatics*, *22*(1), 17. DOI: 10.1186/s12859-021-04518-5 PMID: 34920719

Yin, F., Zhao, H., Lu, S., Shen, J., Li, M., Mao, X., Li, F., Shi, J., Li, J., Dong, B., Xue, W., Zuo, X., Yang, X., & Fan, C. (2023). DNA-framework-based multidimensional molecular classifiers for cancer diagnosis. *Nature Nanotechnology*, *18*(6), 677–686. DOI: 10.1038/s41565-023-01348-9 PMID: 36973399

Yuan, T., Wu, L., Li, S., Zheng, J., Li, N., Xiao, X., Zhang, H., Fei, T., Xie, L., Zuo, Z., Li, D., Huang, P., Feng, H., Cao, Y., Yan, N., Wei, X., Shi, L., Sun, Y., Wei, W., & Zuo, E. (2024). Deep learning models incorporating endogenous factors beyond DNA sequences improve the prediction accuracy of base editing outcomes. *Cell Discovery*, *10*(1), 20. DOI: 10.1038/s41421-023-00624-1 PMID: 38378648

Zaki, M. J. (2000). Scalable algorithms for association mining. *IEEE Transactions on Knowledge and Data Engineering*, *12*(3), 372–390. DOI: 10.1109/69.846291

Zeng, C., Jian, Y., Zhuo, C., Li, A., Zeng, C., & Zhao, Y. (2024). Evaluation of DNA–protein complex structures using the deep learning method. *Physical Chemistry Chemical Physics*, *26*(1), 130–143. DOI: 10.1039/D3CP04980A PMID: 38063012

Zhang, H., & Qie, Y. (2023). Applying deep learning to medical imaging: A review. *Applied Sciences (Basel, Switzerland)*, *13*(18), 10521. DOI: 10.3390/app131810521

Zhang, Q., Wu, Y. N., & Zhu, S. C. (2018). Interpretable convolutional neural networks. In *Proceedings of the IEEE Conference on Computer Vision and Pattern Recognition* (pp. 8827–8836). DOI: 10.1109/CVPR.2018.00920

Zhang, X., Dong, X., Saripan, M. I., Du, D., Wu, Y., Wang, Z., Cao, Z., Wen, D., Liu, Y., & Marhaban, M. H. (2023). Deep learning PET/CT-based radiomics integrates clinical data: A feasibility study to distinguish between tuberculosis nodules and lung cancer. *Thoracic Cancer*, *14*(19), 1802–1811. DOI: 10.1111/1759-7714.14924 PMID: 37183577

Zhang, Y., Liao, Q. V., & Bellamy, R. K. E. (2020). Effect of confidence and explanation on accuracy and trust calibration in AI-assisted decision making. In *Proceedings of the 2020 Conference on Fairness, Accountability, and Transparency* (pp. 295–305). DOI: 10.1145/3351095.3372852

Zhang, Y., Wang, F., Hu, J., & Wu, X. (2022). Discovering multimorbidity patterns from electronic health records using association rule mining. *BMC Medical Informatics and Decision Making*, *22*(1), 95. DOI: 10.1186/s12911-022-01800-1 PMID: 35392890

Zhao, L., Liu, S., An, Y., Cai, W., Li, B., Wang, S. H., Liang, P., Yu, J., & Zhao, J. (2023). A unified end-to-end classification model for focal liver lesions. *Biomedical Signal Processing and Control*, *86*, 105260. DOI: 10.1016/j.bspc.2023.105260

Zhao, Y. (2024). A metaheuristic perspective on extracting numeric association rules. *Archives of Computational Methods in Engineering*. Advance online publication. DOI: 10.1007/s11831-024-10254-1

Zhou, W. (2025). Research on deep learning algorithms and applications in robotic arm control. *Applied and Computational Engineering*, *181*(1), 147–153. DOI: 10.54254/2755-2721/2025.GL26702

Zhou, Y., Du, J., Liu, Y., Qiu, Y., & Wang, T. (2021). CD Loss: A class-center based distribution loss for discriminative feature learning in medical image classification. *Lecture Notes in Computer Science*, *12889*, 630–640. Advance online publication. DOI: 10.1007/978-3-030-87358-5_51

Zilke, J. R., Mencía, E. L., & Janssen, F. (2016). DeepRED: Rule extraction from deep neural networks. In *International Conference on Discovery Science* (pp. 457–473). Springer. DOI: 10.1007/978-3-319-46307-0_29

Zuboff, S. (2019). *The age of surveillance capitalism*. PublicAffairs.

About the Contributors

Anandhavalli Muniasamy is an Associate Professor in the Department of Informatics and Computer Systems, College of Computer Science at King Khalid University (KKU), Saudi Arabia. She holds a Ph.D. in Computer Science & Engineering from SMIT, Sikkim Manipal University, India. Her research expertise spans data mining, data analytics, artificial intelligence (AI), soft computing, and data science, with a particular focus on machine learning and deep learning applications in healthcare data analysis. She has an impressive academic and research portfolio, having published over 40 research articles in prestigious international journals, conferences, and book chapters. She has actively participated in more than 35 national and international conferences, presenting her work on cutting-edge computational techniques and contributing to edited book publications. A recognized innovator, she holds four patents, demonstrating her expertise in advanced computational methodologies. As a Principal Investigator (PI) and Co-Principal Investigator (Co-PI), she has led five university-funded research projects and served as PI for a funded project supported by the All India Council for Technical Education (AICTE). Beyond her research, she has been a dedicated manuscript reviewer for leading international journals for over a decade and a Ph.D. thesis examiner for multiple universities. She is frequently invited to deliver guest lectures and serves as an editorial board member for various renowned journals and conferences. She is an active member of professional organizations such as IEEE, the International Association of Engineers (IAENG), the Computer Society of India (CSI), and the International Association of Computer Science and Information Technology (IACSIT). Her current research focuses on leveraging AI-driven techniques in healthcare analytics, particularly machine learning and deep learning, to address complex challenges in medical data analysis and drive innovative solutions in her field.

***

Rana Alshehri is a graduate of Information Systems from King Khalid University, Saudi Arabia. Her interests include data analysis, data mining, and machine learning.

Fotima Axmedova is a distinguished faculty member in the Department of Clinical Sciences at Ma'mun University, Urgench, Uzbekistan. She holds a Ph.D. in Clinical Sciences, with her research focusing on medical diagnostics, therapeutic methodologies, and clinical data analytics. Her academic interests include advancing evidence-based medical education, exploring innovative healthcare interventions, and improving patient-centered care through interdisciplinary research. Throughout her career, Mrs. Axmedova has actively contributed to national and international research collaborations, publishing scholarly papers in reputed journals and presenting at professional conferences. She is deeply committed to mentoring students and fostering scientific inquiry within clinical education. Her work reflects a strong dedication to enhancing healthcare outcomes through academic excellence and applied medical research.

Syeda Meraj Bilfaqih is a Lecturer in the Department of Computer Science at King Khalid University (KKU), Saudi Arabia. with a Master of Computer Applications from Osmania University, India, and is currently pursuing a Ph.D. at SR University, Warangal. Beyond her academic contributions, she has been actively involved in curriculum development, student mentorship, and research collaborations. She is passionate about fostering innovation and integrating emerging technologies into education and industry applications. As an active member of the research community, she regularly participates in professional workshops, conferences, and journal reviews. Her current research focuses on leveraging AI-driven techniques for advanced data analysis, particularly in the domains of machine learning and cybersecurity, aiming to develop intelligent systems that enhance decision-making and efficiency in various applications.

Ashwini Brahme MCA, Ph.D. (Computer Management), MBA (HR, Marketing) having as 20 years academic experience, working as Associate Professor at Yashaswi's International Institute of Management Science (IIMS), Chinchwad, Pune recognized as Ph.D. Guide in the subject of Computer Management and currently guiding 5 Ph.D. research scholars . She has published more than 35 research papers in National and International Journals and Conferences, 2 copyrights, 1 patent and 1 Book. She is an active member of the curriculum designing of MCA course in SPPU, skill development courses.

Rajashree K. C is a Biomedical Engineer with a Master's in Business Administration from Saveetha University, specializing in Hospital Management and Marketing, and holds a Ph.D. in Healthcare Management. An energetic and enthusiastic professor, she excels in academics and as a multitasker, organizing seminars, workshops, cultural programs, and other extra-curricular activities. She serves as the Coordinator of NSS Unit of Saveetha School of Management, leading them to achieve multiple accolades including the Best Club award. A prominent researcher with publications in Web of Science, Scopus, and UGC-listed journals, she actively enhances her expertise through conferences, workshops, MOOCs, and certifications, including Quality Coordination in Hospitals. Awarded the "Young Academician Award" and "Young Teacher Award," she is passionate about innovation, student skill development, and inspiring young minds through exemplary teaching and mentorship.

Shiney Chib is a distinguished academic leader and administrator currently serving as the Dean – Academics at Datta Meghe Institute of Management Studies, Nagpur, Maharashtra. In this pivotal role, she is responsible for providing strategic academic leadership, ensuring excellence in curriculum design, teaching–learning processes, and academic governance. With extensive experience in higher education, Dr. Chib plays a key role in strengthening academic frameworks, implementing outcome-based education, and aligning institutional practices with regulatory and accreditation requirements. She actively contributes to academic planning, faculty development initiatives, and continuous quality improvement within the institution. As Dean – Academics, Dr. Shiney Chib oversees academic policy formulation, program delivery, assessment systems, and student-centric learning approaches. She is deeply committed to fostering an environment that promotes innovation, research orientation, ethical values, and professional competence among students and faculty members. Dr. Chib is recognized for her academic insight, administrative acumen, and dedication to educational excellence. Her leadership has been instrumental in enhancing academic standards, interdisciplinary learning, and institutional effectiveness at Datta Meghe Institute of Management Studies.

Shruthi A.G. is an MBBS graduate from MAHSA University with a strong interest in the integration of artificial intelligence (AI) in the medical field. She has actively contributed to impactful research, authoring five book chapters focused on data visualization and healthcare innovation. Shruthi is dedicated to leveraging emerging technologies such as AI to improve healthcare delivery and patient outcomes. She has also attended multiple surgical and Obstetrics & Gynaecology workshops in Malaysia, strengthening her clinical skills and hands-on experience. Additionally, she completed her internship at Apollo Hospital, Madurai, gaining broad exposure to patient care across various specialties.

Osama Hassan is a Computer Science graduate and holds a Master's degree in Information Systems with a focus on Data Science from King Khalid University. He specializes in cybersecurity, data analytics, and artificial intelligence, with hands-on experience working as a detection engineer in a full Security Operations Center SOC environment, where he monitored threats and handled real-world security incidents. His research interests include deep learning and optimizing neural networks for imbalanced skin disease image classification, reflecting his strong foundation in AI and applied machine learning. In addition to his technical background, he has practical experience in business operations and real estate, giving him a well-rounded perspective that bridges technology and commercial strategy.

Pratik Kalbande is a final-year MBA student at the Datta Meghe Institute of Management Studies, Nagpur, Maharashtra. He is currently pursuing his Master of Business Administration with a strong focus on developing managerial, analytical, and leadership skills. As a management student, Pratik actively engages in academic learning, case studies, presentations, and institutional activities that enhance his understanding of business concepts and real-world applications. He demonstrates a keen interest in professional growth, teamwork, and practical exposure to organizational environments. Pratik Kalbande aspires to build a successful career in management by applying his academic knowledge, ethical values, and problem-solving abilities in dynamic business settings. He is motivated to continuously learn and adapt in order to meet the evolving challenges of the corporate and entrepreneurial landscape.

Babaqul Khudayqulov is a distinguished academic affiliated with the Department of Basic Medical Sciences at Termez University of Economics and Service, Termez, Uzbekistan. His educational and research pursuits focus on foundational and applied aspects of medical sciences, contributing to the advancement of healthcare education and biomedical understanding in Uzbekistan. Dr. Khudayqulov has been actively involved in teaching and mentoring students, fostering interdisciplinary learning that bridges medical theory with practical healthcare applications. His scholarly interests encompass human physiology, public health, and the integration of clinical science, reflecting a commitment to improving educational standards and community well-being through evidence-based medical education and research.

Venkata Sivakumar Musam graduated in Information Technology from JNTU in the year 2006. I have started my career as a QA analyst in 2008 from nisum technologies and learned the QA concepts and applied those in the work. I have learned more about web applications and their functionality and architecture to perform the QA role.

Nagendra Kumar Musham has Bachelor's Degree in Electrical and Electronic Engineer from Acharya Nagarjuna University (2005). Currently working as Senior Software Developer at Celer Systems Inc.

P. Praveen Kumar holds an MCom, MBA, and PhD in Finance from Pondicherry University. He secured the University 1st Rank in his Under Graduation. His teaching interests include Financial Accounting, Financial Management, Mergers & Acquisitions, Security Analysis & Portfolio Management, and other finance-related courses. His research interests extend to interdisciplinary areas.

P. Selvakumar is currently an Associate Professor in the Department of Science and Humanities at Nehru Institute of Technology, Coimbatore, Tamil Nadu, India. Prior to joining Nehru Institute of Technology, he held positions as an Assistant Professor in the Department of Science and Humanities various engineering colleges in Coimbatore, Tamil Nadu, India, spanning from 2011 to 2023. Dr.P. Selvakumar's academic and research interests lie primarily in the field of phytochemistry. He has made significant contributions to his field, with an impressive record that includes 30 journal publications, 12 patents, and 20 conference papers. Additionally, he has organized 5 seminars and conferences, further demonstrating his commitment to academic and scientific exchange. Throughout his career, Dr. P.Selvakumar has been recognized for his dedication and excellence in teaching, having been honored with several awards, including the Best Teacher Awards. He holds a prominent position in the academic community, contributing actively to research.

Ravikumar R. Natarajan is an experienced academician with over 12+ years of teaching and research expertise across institutions in India, the UAE, and the Maldives. He currently serves as an Assistant Professor at Marwadi University, Rajkot, specializing in Machine Learning, Recommender Systems, and AI-driven applications in healthcare and security. He holds a Ph.D. in Machine Learning and Recommender Systems from Amity University, Jaipur, a Master of Engineering in CSE from VMRF University, Salem, and a Bachelor of Engineering in CSE from Anna University. He also has a MiniMBA from the Swiss eLearning Institute. Dr. Ravikumar has authored more than 8+ multiple SCIE/Scopus-indexed journal articles, 25+ IEEE/Springer conference papers, and co-authored a book on Artificial Intelligence. He has also published 9 patents and contributed 70+ book chapters in emerging domains such as Federated Learning, Blockchain, and Digital Twins for IGI Global, Wiley and Springer publisher. He actively mentors students through initiatives like the Research Activities Club (RAC) and Student Research Internship Training (SRIT), promoting innovation and research culture

Srujal Rajani is a dedicated student at the STEM College, Royal Melbourne Institute of Technology (RMIT), Melbourne, Australia. She is pursuing her studies in the field of science, technology, engineering, and mathematics, with a keen interest in innovation and applied research. Srujal is passionate about leveraging emerging technologies to address real-world challenges and contribute to sustainable development. At RMIT, she actively engages in academic and research activities that foster creativity, critical thinking, and interdisciplinary collaboration, reflecting her commitment to academic excellence and professional growth within the global STEM community.

Aarthi S is a dedicated Assistant Professor in Computer Science with over six years of teaching experience. She is currently pursuing her Ph.D. at Marwadi University, Gujarat, and holds an M.Phil. and MCA from Bharathiar University, Tamil Nadu. Throughout her academic career, Aarthi has specialized in programming languages such as C++, Java, and C, and contributed to research in recommender systems and AI-related data privacy. She has published journal articles, contributed to book chapters, and actively participated in technical workshops. Known for her student mentorship and engagement in academic events, Aarthi remains committed to fostering innovation and excellence in computer science education.

Kavitha Bharathi Shanmugam is working as Associate Professor in Computer Technology, Kongu Engineering College, and Perundurai. She has industrial experience and 20 years of experience in Teaching. She completed her UG degree in Computer Science, MCA from Vellalar College for Women, M.phil degree from Bharathiar University, Coimbatore and Ph.D from Anna University, Chennai.Her area of interest in Mobile Grid Computing and Internet of Things. She has published more than 30 papers in National and International Journals, Presented more than 15 papers in national and International conferences, Completed two Projects for academics and organized various funded programs, Seminars and Workshops, Published 2 books. Guided more than 100 UG, PG projects in various emerging trends in technology such as Internet of Things, Mobile Application Development, Augmented and Virtual Reality.

Prithi Samuel is currently working as an Assistant Professor in the Department of Computational Intelligence at SRM Institute of Science and Technology, Kattankulathur Campus, Chennai. She has completed her Ph.D. in Information and Communication Engineering from Anna University, Chennai. She has got over 16 years of teaching experience in reputed engineering colleges in Coimbatore and Chennai. She is a pioneer researcher in the areas of Automata Theory, Deep learning, Machine Learning, Computational Intelligence Techniques, and Natural Language Processing. She has published papers in leading International Journals and International Conferences and published books and book chapters in Wiley, IEEE Press, Taylor and Francis, Springer and Elsevier.

Binastya Anggara Sekti has been a lecturer at the Faculty of Computer Science, Esa Unggul University, Jakarta, since 2016. He is actively involved in the Artificial Intelligence and Information Security Study Group. He holds a Bachelor's degree in Informatics Engineering from the Bandung Institute of Technology and a Master's degree in Information Systems Management from Trisakti University, Jakarta. Prior to entering academia, he accumulated over 25 years of professional experience as an IT practitioner in various companies across Jakarta. His work focused on developing data centers for internet service providers and delivering IT solutions for the manufacturing and oil & gas sectors. His research interests include artificial intelligence, cybersecurity, and the development of IT infrastructure.

Mohsin Shaikh is a professor of management with over 24 years of experience in teaching, research and administration. He is a Phd research guide and has guided 10 students for their PhD. He has published papers in national and international journals and has presented papers in national and international conferences. He has authored 5 books. His area of interest is HRM, Entrepreneurship and strategy

Sujatha S. is currently working as an Assistant Professor in the Department of Computer Science and Engineering at Chaitanya Bharathi Institute of Technology in Proddatur. She completed her M.Tech in CSE from JNTUA in Ananthapuram. Her research includes one patent and a book chapter published with a well-known academic publisher. She has also participated in national and international conferences. With over six years of teaching experience, she has held academic positions at various colleges and universities. She has taught subjects such as Cloud Computing, Computer Networks, Internet of Things (IoT), Database Management Systems (DBMS), Computer Science, and Machine Learning to both undergraduate and postgraduate students. Her area of interests is Neural Networks in Deep Learning, Artificial Intelligence and Machine Learning, particularly in intelligent systems and data-driven modeling.

Geetha Priya Thiagarajan is a Digital Transformation Manager at HCLTech with over 18 years of experience in project and operations management. A PMP® certified professional and Lean Six Sigma Green Belt, she has led large-scale automation, P2P, supply chain, and finance transformation initiatives across global clients. Her expertise spans digital transformation, vendor management, procurement, banking, and ERP modules including IM, WM, and SD. Recognized with multiple performance awards, she has successfully managed onsite and offshore transitions and consistently delivered cost-efficient, high-impact business outcomes.

K. V. S. V. Trinadh Reddy is an Associate Professor in the Department of Electronics and Communication Engineering at Cambridge Institute of Technology, K. R. Puram, Bengaluru. He is a highly dedicated and committed academician with over 22 years of rich teaching experience, spanning both online and offline modes of instruction. He has taught core engineering subjects such as Analog Electronics, Control Systems, Signals & Systems, and Network Analysis, and has mentored more than 80,000 students preparing for GATE and Engineering Services examinations. His teaching outreach has been delivered through reputed platforms and institutions including MADE EASY and Unacademy, earning him wide recognition among students nationwide. With extensive academic and professional experience in engineering education, research, and student development, Dr. Reddy has made significant contributions in the areas of Digital Image Processing and emerging technologies such as Internet of Things (IoT) and Artificial Intelligence & Machine Learning. Driven by a strong passion for student growth, innovation, and academic excellence, he continuously adopts advanced teaching–learning methodologies, actively engages in mentoring and guidance, and contributes meaningfully to institutional development initiatives.

Humara Yaqub has done Master of Computer Applications (MCA) degree from the University of Kashmir and has more than 13 years of rich teaching experience in higher education. Throughout my academic career, I have been actively involved in teaching, research, and curriculum development, contributing significantly to student learning and academic excellence. I have published over 10 research papers in reputed national and international journals and have also authored two book chapters published in Scopus-indexed volumes, reflecting the quality and impact of my research work. In addition to my formal qualifications, I have completed 12 online certification courses from well-known and globally recognized platforms such as Coursera and Huawei, demonstrating my commitment to continuous professional development and staying updated with emerging technologies. My primary research interests include Artificial Intelligence, Machine Learning, Computer Networks, and Database Systems.

Index

A

B

C

D

E

F

G

H

I

K

L

M

P

R

S

T

www.ingramcontent.com/pod-product-compliance
Lightning Source LLC
LaVergne TN
LVHW080911300926
849162LV00003B/646